SMALL ANIMAL DENTAL EQUIPMENT, MATERIALS AND TECHNIQUES

A Primer

SMALL ANIMAL DENTAL EQUIPMENT, MATERIALS AND TECHNIQUES

A Primer

Jan Bellows

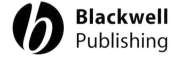

Blackwell Publishing

Jan Bellows, DVM, is a veterinarian with more than 25 years of experience in small animal medicine and surgery. He is a board certified veterinary dentist as well as a boarded companion animal specialist. Dr. Bellows sees dental referrals at Hometown Animal Hospital and Dental Clinic in Weston, Florida.

©2004 Blackwell Publishing

Blackwell Publishing Professional
2121 State Avenue, Ames, Iowa 50014, USA

Orders:	1-800-862-6657
Office:	1-515-292-0140
Fax:	1-515-292-3348
Web site:	www.blackwellprofessional.com

Blackwell Publishing Ltd
9600 Garsington Road, Oxford OX4 2DQ, UK
Tel.: +44 (0)1865 776868

Blackwell Publishing Asia
550 Swanston Street, Carlton, Victoria 3053, Australia
Tel.: +61 (0)3 8359 1011

Authorization to photocopy items for internal or personal use, or the internal or personal use of specific clients, is granted by Blackwell Publishing, provided that the base fee is paid directly to the Copyright Clearance Center, 222 Rosewood Drive, Danvers, MA 01923. For those organizations that have been granted a photocopy license by CCC, a separate system of payments has been arranged. The fee code for users of the Transactional Reporting Service is ISBN-13: 978-0-8138-1898-6/2004.

First edition, 2004

This publication contains information relating to general principles for the delivery of dental treatment, and should not be construed as specific instructions for individual animals. The author and publisher are not responsible (as a matter of product liability, negligence, or otherwise) for any injury resulting from any material contained herein. Every attempt has been made to ensure that product numbers are correct; however, the author cautions the reader to check correctness with the distributor before order placement.

Library of Congress Cataloging-in-Publication Data

Bellows, Jan.
  Small animal dental equipment, materials, and techniques / Jan Bellows.— 1st ed.
    p. cm.
  ISBN-13: 978-0-8138-1898-6
  ISBN-10: 0-8138-1898-2 (alk. paper)
  1. Veterinary dentistry. I. Title.
  SF867.B456 2004
  636.089'76—dc22
                                    2003023655

The last digit is the print number: 9 8 7 6 5 4

This book is dedicated to Allison, my wife; our children Wendi, David, and Lauren; our pets present and past—Pepper, Daisy, Chelsea, Lacey, Bailey, Casey, Molly, and Dylan; and to my colleagues, patients, and clients, from whom I have learned so much.

Contents

Foreword

In the past twenty years, our profession has experienced the transformation of dentistry from the delivery of rudimentary dental services to a highly sophisticated art and science. As both the veterinarian and the public have recognized this trend, the demand for comprehensive dental care has grown in an almost exponential manner. This increased interest in dental techniques has led to the availability of many seminars and textbooks on the subject.

One of the difficulties discovered by practitioners who want to incorporate a more comprehensive dental department into their practice has been how to get started. Due in large part to the growth rate of the discipline, there has been a tendency for continuing educational sources to concentrate on the important pathophysiology of dental diseases rather than the "nuts and bolts" of how to obtain the proper equipment and materials to treat these problems.

Anyone who is contemplating increasing his or her ability to deliver dental treatment to patients will find the information in this text invaluable. The author has gone back to basics to fill in that gap between limited and advanced dental services.

Small Animal Dental Equipment, Materials, and Techniques takes the mystery away from unfamiliar dental terms and techniques. The reader will learn how to establish an efficient dental operatory and perform many of the day-to-day techniques required to truly raise his or her level of dental services.

It is indeed a great honor to have been asked to write the Foreword for a book that deals with a subject so dear to my heart. I congratulate Dr. Bellows for his persistence and hard work in producing this textbook.

Thomas W. Mulligan, D.V.M.
Diplomate, American Veterinary Dental College

Preface

Small Animal Dental Equipment, Materials, and Techniques was born out of a need to inform and share information with veterinarians, technicians, and human dentists. As in other areas of veterinary medicine and surgery, there are scores of methods, materials, and types of equipment used to perform dental care. The book's goal is to clearly explain how to choose dental equipment and materials and how to perform basic and intermediate dental procedures based on examination findings. Some advanced procedures are included for completeness, and are noted as such.

Veterinary educators stress that practitioners "do no harm." The veterinarian must appreciate and fully understand the science behind the procedures outlined in this book *before* performing them on clinical cases. Dentistry is not a step-by-step cookbook endeavor. Often there are procedural complications or cases that occur with other than "textbook" presentations. For those who attempt dental procedures without proper equipment, materials, and knowledge, there is the potential to make a patient worse from the experience. The reader is advised to practice these procedures on cadaver specimens and dental models. Proficiency can be obtained by working with human or veterinary dentists and attending veterinary dental hands-on wet labs—coupled with reading, reading, and more reading. Results should be evaluated by someone knowledgeable

before attempting clinical cases. The reader is advised to contact the American Veterinary Dental College or the American Veterinary Dental Society for a list of continuing education opportunities.

My goal was not to write a text that listed *all* equipment, materials, and techniques available for patient care. I have included those materials, equipment, and techniques that I and many of my colleagues have found valuable in the practice of veterinary dentistry. Where useful, I have included a summary of the manufacturer's instructions. The reader is advised to consult with the complete directions before product use.

It is important for veterinarians to find their own sources of material and service and develop a relationship with those suppliers. Burns Veterinary Supply, Cislak Manufacturing Inc., and Henry Schein Company are leaders in supporting veterinary dentistry. Without their help, veterinary dentistry would not have advanced to where it is today. I have made every attempt to list their current product numbers where applicable.

Small Animal Dental Equipment, Materials, and Techniques provides readers with a good starting or continuation source for the dental education journey to improve the level of dental care available to animals everywhere.

Acknowledgments

As with other veterinary disciplines, there are many materials, brands of equipment, and techniques perfected for therapy. Input after review of the manuscript was supplied by veterinarians Larry Baker, Brett Beckman, Tiffany Brown, Barron Hall, Michael Morgan, John Rehak, Leonel Rocha, and Keith Stein; veterinary dentists Dan Carmichael, Ben Colmery, Gary Goldstein, Fraser Hale, Steven Holmstrom, Ira Luskin, Ken Lyon, Sandra Manfra, Brook Nemic, Frank Verstraete, and Charles Williams; human dentists Marcos Diaz, Larry Grayhills, and Amy Golden; veterinary surgeons Ken Bartels and Barbara Gores; and veterinary radiologist Ron Burk.

Industry support—both in allowing me to evaluate equipment and materials and in reviewing the manuscript—was graciously provided by Adrienne Silkowitz (Burns Veterinary Supply), Ken Zoll (Cislak Manufacturing Inc.), Linda Pappalardo and Janet Pianese (Henry Schein Company), Charles Rahner (Summit Hill), Charles Brungart and Cara Helfrich (CBi Manufacturing), Andrea Battaglia (VetSpecs), Vern Dollar (iM3), Carl Bennett and Daniel Fields (AccuVet), Steven Senia (LightSpeed Endodontics), Donald Rabinovitch, Alan Haber, and Herb Clay (AFP Imaging), and Richard Noss (Ellman International). Their input and insight improved each draft, making the final edition user friendly and a reflection of current veterinary dental practice. I acknowledge and thank every one of the reviewers.

I also thank all of those veterinarians and technicians that have shared their dental knowledge with the rest of us through textbooks, journal articles, and seminars. Where applicable, I have used much of their information in this text.

Finally, it was a sincere pleasure to work with the wonderful people at Blackwell Publishing in creating this text. Special thank-yous go out to Cheryl Garton, who baby-sat this five-year project; Nancy Albright, who corrected hundreds (thousands) of syntax errors; Tad Ringo, who guided the project to completion; and, most important, Dave Rosenbaum, who believed that small animals all over the world would benefit from this work.

SMALL ANIMAL DENTAL EQUIPMENT, MATERIALS AND TECHNIQUES

A Primer

1
The Dental Operatory

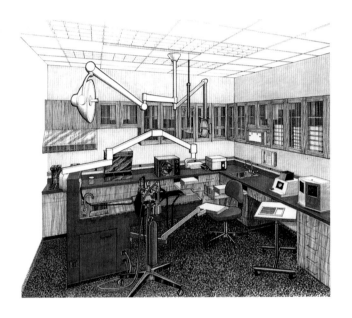

FIGURE 1.1. Veterinary dental suite, Warren Freedenfeld & Associates.

Creating the ideal place to practice dentistry is a worthwhile challenge (Figures 1.1, 1.2). By the time most practitioners realize they want to make dentistry an integral part of their practice, their facility has been built without sufficient dental planning. Fortunately, most dental equipment and materials are compact and can be adapted to fit into nearly all practice environments.

By necessity, dentistry entails special equipment. The challenge is to provide a safe and efficient area for the use and storage of dental materials, instruments, radiography unit, processor, suction, illumination, general anesthesia, and monitoring equipment.

If the practitioner has the luxury of planning the dental operatory, a 12-foot by 15-foot area is ideal; an 8-foot by 10-foot area should be the minimum operative area. If possible, space for at least two tables and a den-

tal x-ray unit should be provided.

Dental procedures require instruments and materials. If the veterinarian works alone, much time is spent acquiring these essentials. Four-handed dentistry, practiced commonly in human dentistry, employs a dental assistant who envisages what the dentist needs, then hands over the instruments and materials. In veterinary dental practice, four-handed dentistry increases the efficiency of dental procedures performed and decreases the time of anesthesia. To permit four-handed dentistry, sufficient space must be provided for one or two veterinary dental technicians to work on both sides of the animal with uninterrupted access to the head.

The dental operatory should not be located in the same room as general surgery. Bacteria-laden aerosols released during ultrasonic scaling will contaminate the room and patients. Most practices perform dental procedures in the treatment area (Figures 1.3, 1.4)

ERGONOMICS

When planning a dental operatory, attention to the mechanics of delivering dental care is important. Activities that cause excessive reaching, bending, and twisting should be limited:

- Instruments and equipment should be arranged where they can be easily grasped to avoid overreaching.
- Supplies and frequently used equipment should be placed as close as possible to the working area and working height to decrease stretching and bending.
- Enough space should be allowed to turn the whole body, using a swivel stool with back support.

The Operatory Table/Tub

The operatory table/tub should be 5–7 feet long, 2 1/2

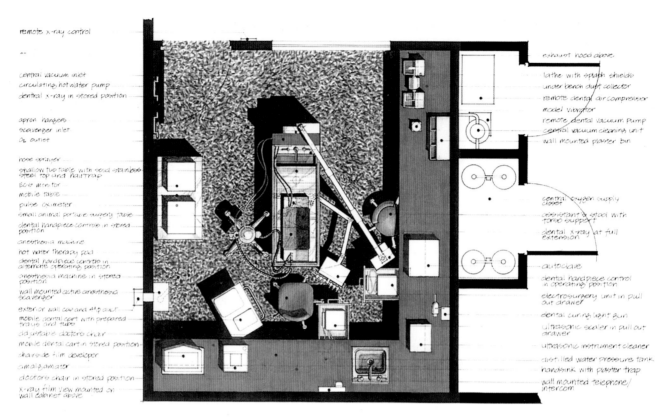

remote x-ray control

--

central vacuum inlet
circulating hot water pump
dental x-ray in stored position

apron hangers
scavenger inlet
O₂ outlet

nose sprayer
shallow tub table with solid stainless
steel top and hairtrap
ECG monitor
mobile table
pulse oximeter
small animal portable surgery table
dental handpiece controls in stored
position
anesthesia machine
hot water therapy pad
dental handpiece controls in
alternate operating position
anesthesia machine in stored
position
wall mounted active anesthesia
scavenger
exterior wall cowl and flip out
mobile dental cart with prepared
trays and tubs
adjustable doctor's chair
mobile dental cart in stored position
chairside film developer
amalgamator
doctor's chair in stored position
x-ray film view mounted on
wall cabinet above

exhaust hood above
lathe with splash shields
under bench dust collector
remote dental air compressor
model vibrator
remote dental vacuum pump
central vacuum cleaning unit
wall mounted plaster bin

central oxygen supply
closet
assistant's stool with
torso support
dental x-ray at full
extension

autoclave
dental handpiece control
in operating position
electrosurgery unit in pull
out drawer
dental curing light gun
ultrasonic scaler in pull out
drawer
ultrasonic instrument cleaner
distilled water pressure tank
handsink with plaster trap
wall mounted telephone/
intercom

FIGURE 1.2. Veterinary dental suite, Warren Freedenfeld & Associates.

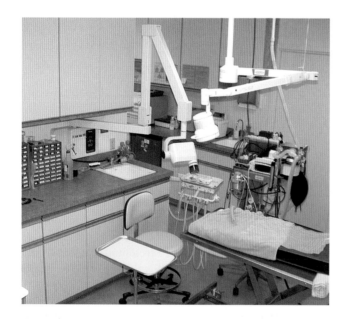

FIGURE 1.3. Dental operatory (courtesy Dr. Steven Holmstrom Animal Dental Clinic).

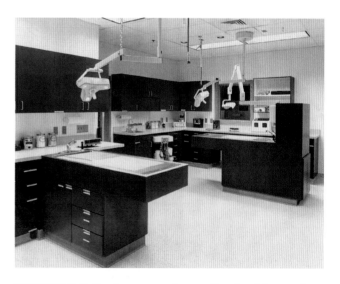

FIGURE 1.4. Rocky mountain small animal hospital dental suite, Warren Freedenfeld & Associates.

feet wide, 36 (head) and 38 (tail) inches high. If possible, two dental stations should be planned side by side to allow treatment on one table while a technician cleans teeth and performs diagnostics on the other table. Two peninsular stations allow the sharing of the dental radiograph unit, view box, chairside developer, scaler/polisher, light cure unit, and dental materials. When two tables are used, one can be shorter, because many companion animal patients are small dogs or cats (Figure 1.5):

• The working end of the table should be placed opposite from the faucet.
• Room beneath the table should be provided for the practitioner or technician's knees and access on three sides.
• A stainless steel grate can be used for animal support. To prevent instruments from falling into the sink, part of the grate can be covered with a clear drilled Plexiglas cover.
• Corian can be used as a tabletop surface, with a drain incorporated near the animal's mouth.
• A layout area should be located within three feet of the patient's head to minimize the reach for dental instruments and materials without the need to leave the stool.

Adjustable Stools on Rollers

Adjustable stools on rollers with or without backs can be placed at the patient end of the table to allow the operator to comfortably perform procedures in a seated position while maintaining good posture (Burns 952-0680, Schein 100-5307).

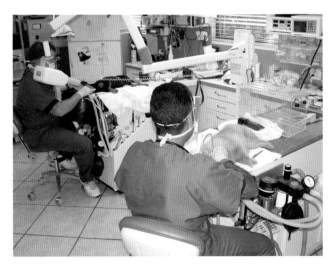

FIGURE 1.5. Dental operatory with minimal floor-based equipment Hometown Animal Hospital and Dental Clinic, Weston, Florida.

Built-in Desk

A built-in desk for note-taking should be provided as well as sufficient space for instrument and material storage within easy reach from a seated position. Effort should be made to decrease floor-based equipment (dental delivery systems, anesthesia, dental radiograph, intravenous poles).

Compressor and Suction Equipment Room

A separate room for stand-alone compressor and suction equipment should be planned if the delivery system does not have self-contained units. When possible, the stand-alone compressor and suction unit should be located away from the dental suite because of the noise and heat they generate. Some dental delivery systems are powered by nitrogen, which requires space for large H-tanks for sustained use.

UTILITIES

Utilities for dental delivery include electricity, water, and drainage. Multiple electrical grounded 110-volt receptacles are recommended to power the delivery system, light curing unit, ultrasonic scaler, light source, radiograph viewer, headlamp, monitoring equipment, and heating pad. Three four-plug grounded outlets are usually sufficient for each operatory area. Monitoring equipment may require a dedicated circuit to prevent interference from the ultrasonic scaler.

Water is used in the high-speed delivery system to prevent heat damage to surrounding tissue generated by drilling and to remove debris. If local water contains an abundance of minerals, a filter is recommended to decrease sediment collected, thereby increasing the efficiency and the life of dental handpieces. Distilled water can be used in stand-alone units where water is poured into a holding tank. Distilled water from a distiller can also be plumbed directly into the delivery system (Figure 1.6).

In time, a bacterial biofilm forms along the internal surfaces of the water lines. In human dentistry, this biofilm has been blamed for introducing pathogenic bacteria into the oral cavity. A bacterial microfilter and a chlorhexidine flushing system can be installed to decrease the biofilm (Figure 1.7).

CABINETRY

Storage of equipment and materials requires careful organization. Jumbling hand instruments, power equip-

of the operator can keep frequently used instruments and materials. A secondary location can stockpile resupply items.

Storage drawers can be arranged by dental procedure. The periodontal drawer can contain sterilized packs of hand instruments and supplies to perform gingival examinations and surgery. Other drawers are arranged in similar fashion, with radiographic, endodontic, oral surgical, restorative, and orthodontic compartments. Oversized drawers can be used for larger pieces of equipment and supplies (Figures 1.8–1.13).

Cassettes are available to store sterile instruments needed for each procedure. Advantages of using the cassette system are having all the instruments needed in one area for each procedure, and the ability to sterilize the cassette before use (Hu-Friedy).

Waste containers, including hazardous materials containers, can be built into the cabinetry (Figure 1.14).

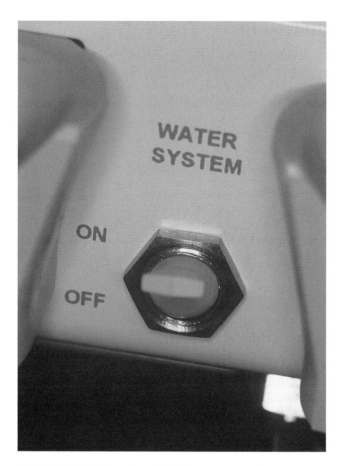

FIGURE 1.6. Most dental delivery systems have water on-off switches (iM3 pictured).

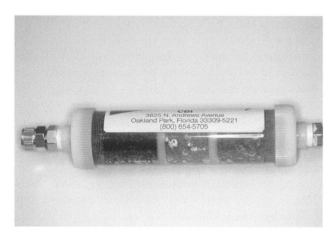

FIGURE 1.7. Water filter (CBi).

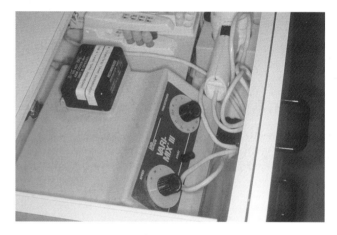

FIGURE 1.8. Cabinetry picture with dedicated discipline drawers.

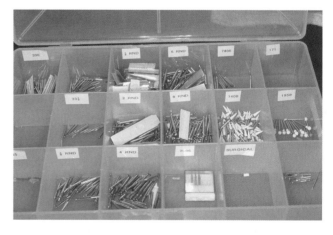

FIGURE 1.9. High/low-speed bur storage drawer.

ment, and dental materials in a group drawer results in confusion, wasted time, and poorly sterilized instruments.

At least two locations should be used for storage. For primary storage, a cabinet or drawers within easy reach

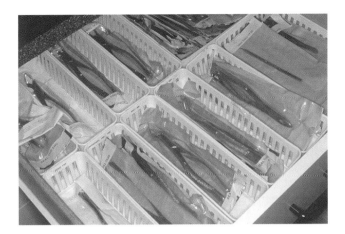

FIGURE 1.10. Sterile instrument storage.

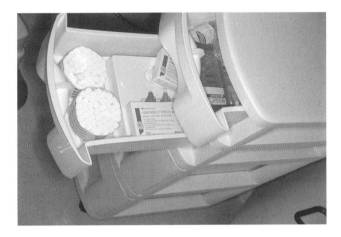

FIGURE 1.11. Plastic cabinet for dental material storage.

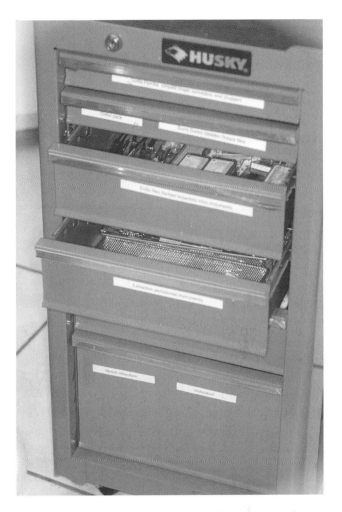

FIGURE 1.13. Tool storage unit used to organize dental materials and instruments.

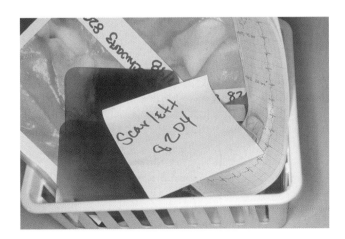

FIGURE 1.12. Bin for case pictures and case radiograph short-term storage.

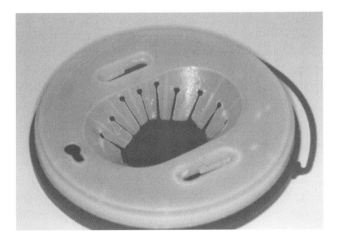

FIGURE 1.14. Hazardous material container built into cabinetry.

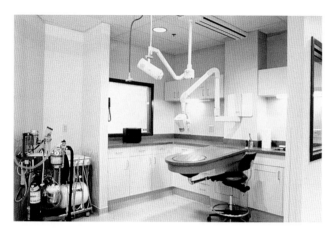

FIGURE 1.15. Illuminated operatory area.

LIGHTING

Proper lighting and magnification are fundamental to the efficient delivery of small animal dentistry. Generally, the more light the better. Spotlights combined with headlamps and fiber-optic handpieces provide optimal illumination and magnification:

- When possible, the operatory should be designed with windows to allow outside lighting.
- An overhead color-balanced dental lamp helps illuminate the oral cavity. The light should be positioned 25–30 inches (approximately an arm's length) from the oral cavity. When properly placed, the light illuminates the area to be treated without projecting shadows of the operator's hands on the oral cavity (Figure 1.15).
- Fiber optics on the high-speed handpiece additionally illuminates the working area of the handpiece (Burns 952-3893, Schein 100-1922) (Figure 1.16).
- Head-mounted spotlights accompanied with 2–4X magnifying dental telescopes also light the field of operation. As the strength of magnification increases, the width of field decreases. Clinicians who choose to wear low-powered magnification will see the entire mouth, in contrast to the preferred higher-power loupes that allow users a detailed close-up of two or three teeth. Although the power of the loupes is a well-known feature, the quality of the optics must also be considered when making a selection. Loupes manufactured with high-quality precision lenses offer users a better view because the optical resolution is much higher. Resolution enables users to see very small structures clearly (Figures 1.17–1.19).

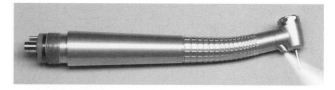

FIGURE 1.16. Fiber-optic light souce on high-speed drill (CBi).

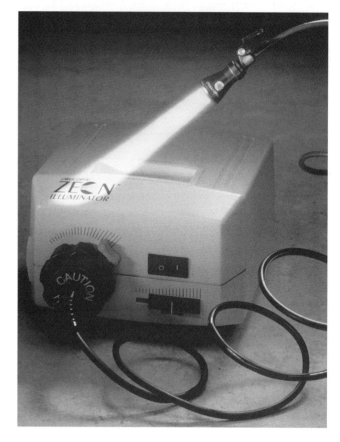

FIGURE 1.17. Zeon Illuminator System (Orascoptic).

- The two basic types of loupes are flip-up models and through-the-lens designs. Flip-ups are binoculars mounted on a pair of glasses or gargoyles. One's individual vision prescription can be installed in the lens. Through-the-lens configurations are made with the oculars mounted directly into a carrier lens in a pair of glasses. Because the magnification on a through-the-lens loupe sits closer to the eye, the field is wider than with a flip-up model (Figure 1.20).
- Veterinary technicians can also use illuminated dental telescopes to evaluate effectiveness of their teeth cleaning. Consider resolution, working angle, working distance, width, depth of field, weight, and mag-

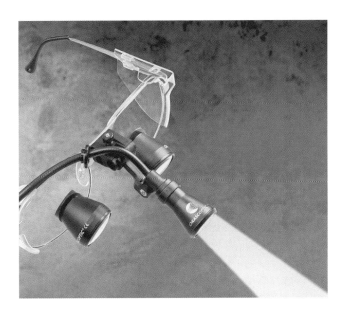

FIGURE 1.18. Through the lens telescopes (Orascoptic) with illumination.

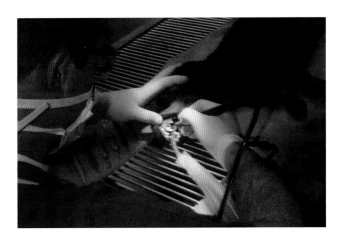

FIGURE 1.19. Illuminated patient area.

nifying power when purchasing dental telescopes (Orascoptic, Schein 566-1764, Surgitel, Designs for Vision) (Figure 1.21).

Dental Delivery Systems

Dental delivery systems help the veterinarian perform proficient veterinary dentistry. The delivery system controls water; provides pressurized air to the power drill and sonic scaler; and may offer suction, handpiece flush, and fiber-optic light options. "Silent" refrigerator compressors can be contained in the delivery unit, or larger compressors can be located remotely to minimize

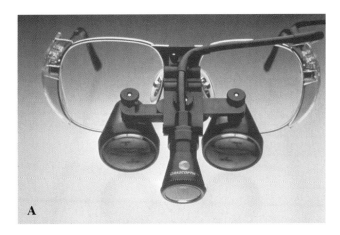

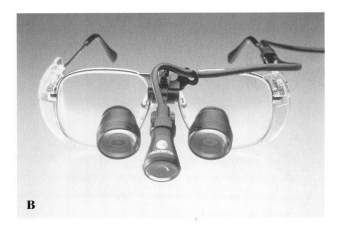

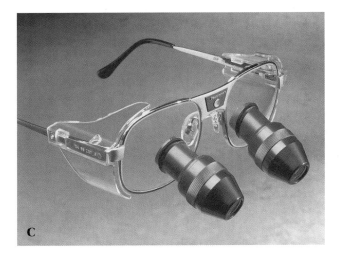

FIGURE 1.20. Flip-up telescopes with illumination (A) and through the lens telescopes with illumination (B); prismatic telescopes (C). (Orascoptic)

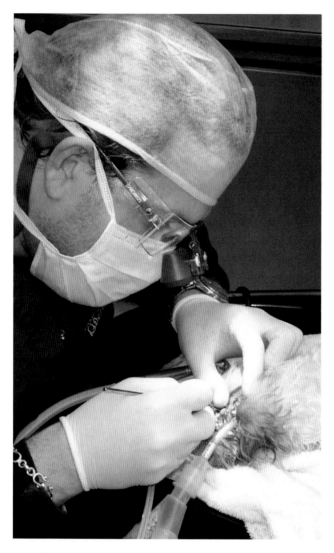

FIGURE 1.21. Hygienist gargoyle-mounted flip-up telescopes (Orascoptic).

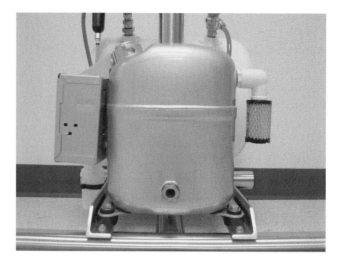

FIGURE 1.22. Silent compressor connected to the delivery system cart (iM3).

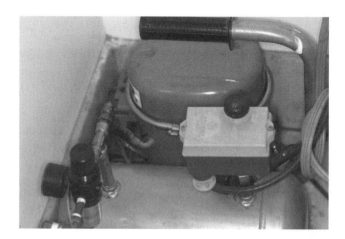

FIGURE 1.23. Remotely located stand-alone compressor.

noise. Some units are powered with nitrogen gas. Wherever the compressor is placed, easy access is essential to facilitate maintenance and repair. Compressors with adequate size to power two dental operatories occupy a minimum 3-foot by 3-foot floor space (Figures 1.22, 1.23).

Delivery units can:

- Be placed on top of the layout area (Figure 1.24).
- Reside as a stand-alone unit next to the treatment table (Schein 362-8161, Ultima 500, iM3 model GS) (Figure 1.25).
- Attach to the front or side of the treatment table.

- Be incorporated as part of the treatment table by the manufacturer (Schein 362-9483, Ultima 2000) (Figure 1.26).

Suction may be part of the delivery unit or located remotely and piped into the operatory.

Radiography

Radiography is mandatory to properly evaluate most dental cases. Human dental patients help their doctors diagnose lesions based on expressed feelings of pain, temperature, and pressure. Even with this help, radiographs are needed to evaluate the presence and extent

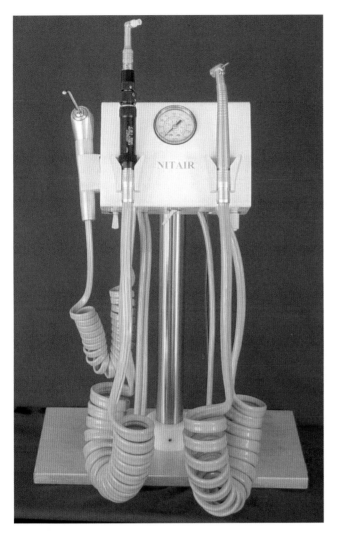

FIGURE 1.24. Table-top dental delivery unit (CBI).

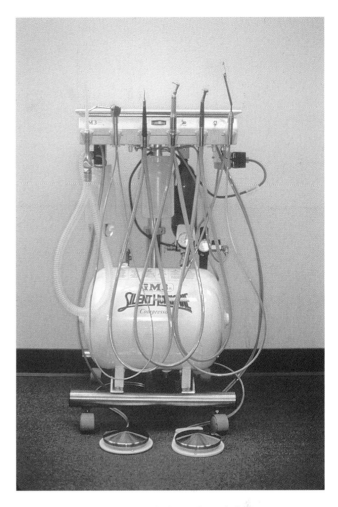

FIGURE 1.25. iM3 stand-alone dental delivery system.

of dental lesions. Radiography is the most useful diagnostic aid available to the veterinarian practicing dentistry.

Dental radiographs may be exposed with the standard radiography unit. The location and fixed nature of these units requires animal patients to be moved from the dental table to the radiograph area. With endodontic and some oral surgical procedures, patient relocation would have to be performed multiple times, which adds time and inconvenience. A dedicated dental radiograph unit is an indispensable piece of equipment in the dental operatory (Figure 1.27).

The dental radiography unit can be purchased with a retractable arm extending up to 6 feet. The unit can be positioned to reach multiple treatment tables. Floor-mounted models on rollers can be used, but due to their

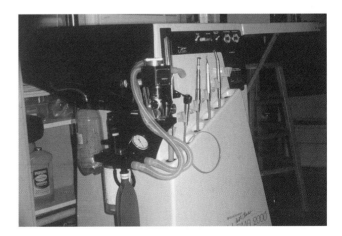

FIGURE 1.26. Ultima 2000 dental delivery system incorporated into treatment table.

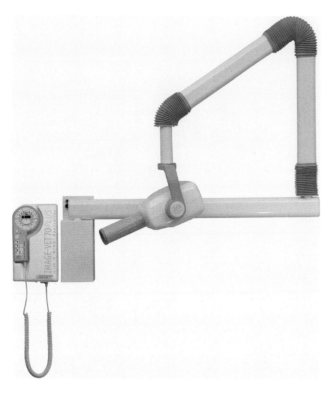

FIGURE 1.27. Dental radiography unit (Vet 70-plus-AFP imaging).

ANESTHESIA

By necessity, dentistry is performed while the animal is anesthetized. Anesthesia allows the practitioner and technician to carry out procedures on immobilized patients without pain. A properly fitted cuffed endotracheal tube must be used for patient safety. The cuff:

- Prevents the contaminated oral environment and water from entering the respiratory system.
- Aids in patient oxygenation and anesthetic delivery.
- Decreases operator-inhaled anesthetic gases.

Incorporating the anesthetic delivery system in the operatory console or mounted on the wall increases efficiency and decreases floor clutter. Canister or active suction anesthetic scavenger systems are required (see Figure 1.26).

Patient Monitoring Devices

Patient monitoring devices are essential for the maintenance of anesthesia. Some dental procedures require hours of anesthesia. Electrocardiograph monitoring, pulse oximetry, respiratory and apnea monitoring, temperature, end tidal CO_2, and blood pressure observation add to the safety of anesthesia for dental patients.

Thermal Support

Small animal dentistry requires anesthesia, which over time decreases the normal body temperature. For thermal support the clinician should provide heated water pads, blankets warmed in a dryer, and/or preheated intravenous fluid bags. Care must be taken to avoid thermal injury to skin with certain heating devices.

inherent size and bulk, create additional floor clutter. Wall-, cabinet-, tub-, or ceiling-mounted units are preferred. Most dental radiography units operate on 110 volts and require separate 30 amp circuits. Digital dental radiography is also practical to use in the veterinary setting. Space must be allowed for a laptop or computer central processing unit and screen when planning for digital dental radiography.

2
Equipping the Dental Practice

Acquiring the proper equipment to perform dentistry is one of the wisest investments a practitioner can make. There is no other branch of small animal practice wherein a relatively minimal financial investment can provide such benefit to the patient, client, and practice.

Choosing how much equipment, materials, and education to obtain is an individual decision. If dentistry is only a small part of the practice, the veterinarian may want to acquire only basic equipment and materials. If advanced dentistry is the goal, additional training, instruments, and materials are needed.

The following sections specify equipment and material examples used by the author.

BASIC ORAL EXAMINATION, ORAL HYGIENE, AND NONSURGICAL EXTRACTION

The following are recommended for basic and intermediate dental care:

- Plaque-disclosing solution (Burns 951-1218, Schein 100-2491)
- Mouth props or gags, which can be placed between the maxillary and mandibular canines or cheek teeth to keep the mouth open during dental procedures (placing props between canines is generally not recommended due to potential iatrogenic damage to the teeth and/or temporomandibular articulation (Burns 606-4183, Schein 568-8953) (Figure 2.1)
- Charts for dental examination findings (Burns 342-0691, Schein 100-8927) (Figure 2.2)
- Dental explorer (Burns 271-9105, Schein 100-4807) (Figure 2.3)

- Periodontal probe (Burns 951-8619, Schein 600-7964) (Figure 2.4)
- Oral mirror (Burns 699-1884, Schein 100-5067) (Figure 2.5)
- Intraoral radiograph film—sizes 0, 2, 3, 4—for use with standard (or dental) radiograph machine (0: Burns 833-0709, Schein 111-2822; 2: Burns 833-0717, Schein 111-2876; 3: Burns 833-0692, Schein 111-3257; 4: Burns 833-0702, Schein 111-1262)
- Chairside darkroom (Burns 951-1423, Schein 189-7385) (Figure 2.6)
- Rapid developer and fixer chemicals (Burns 952-1160, Schein 189-4910) (Figure 2.7)
- Dental hand scaler (Figure 2.8)
- Periodontal curettes—universal (McCalls 13/14 Burns 950-9535, Cislak P10 universal, P19 feline); periodontal curettes—area-specific (Schein 100-6523) (Figure 2.9); sharpening stone kit (Figure 2.10)
- Luxator kit (for the practitioner with intermediate or advanced dental surgical skills) (Burns 271-9070-85, Schein 888-3220) (Figure 2.11)
- Winged-tipped elevators (Burns 606-3204, Cislak, Schein 102-7336) (Figure 2.12)
- Extraction forceps (Burns 271-9045; Schein 100-2617, 100-5673) (Figure 2.13)
- Operator safety equipment (goggles, mask, gloves) (Figure 2.14)
- Ultrasonic scaler with at least two tips: beavertail and precision thin (Burns 263-9603, Schein 192-5824, iM3 0-0802) (Figure 2.15)
- Polishing equipment (Figure 2.16): disposable polishing angle (Figure 2.17), polishing paste
- Doxirobe gel (Figure 2.18)
- Home care products and promotional materials (Figure 2.19)
- Polaroid instant intraoral camera SLR 5 (Schein 987-2593) (Figure 2.20)

- Dental models
- Text books:
  - *Veterinary Dentistry*, Harvey and Emily; Mosby, 1993.
  - *The Practice of Veterinary Dentistry: A Team Effort*, Bellows, Iowa State University Press, 1999.
  - *Veterinary Dentistry: A Profit Center*, Eisner, AAHA Press, 1999.

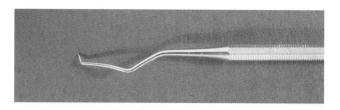

FIGURE 2.3. Dental explorer.

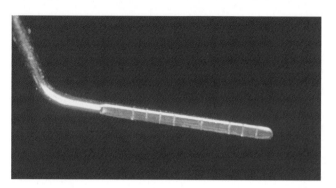

FIGURE 2.4. Goldman-Fox periodontal probe showing milllimeter markings.

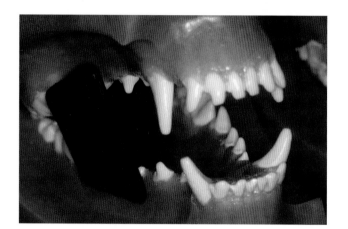

FIGURE 2.1. Mouth prop.

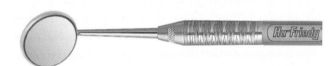

FIGURE 2.5. Oral mirror.

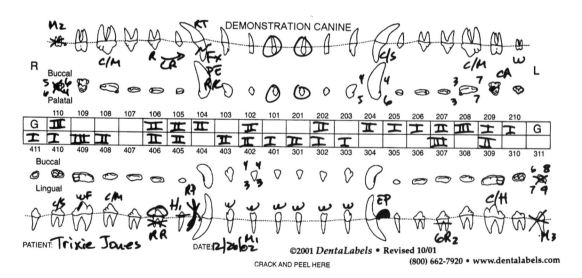

FIGURE 2.2. Dental chart (DentaLabel).

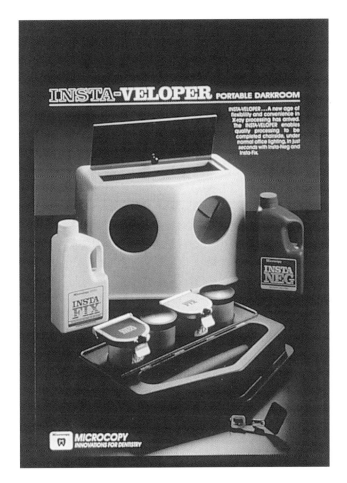

FIGURE 2.6. Chairside darkroom.

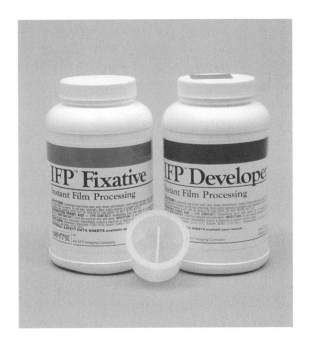

FIGURE 2.7. Rapid developer and fixer chemicals (AFP imaging).

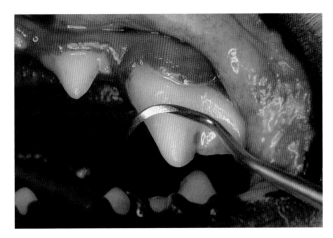

FIGURE 2.8. Hand dental scaler.

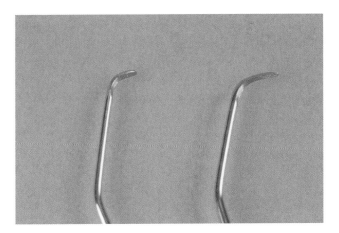

FIGURE 2.9. Periodontal curettes.

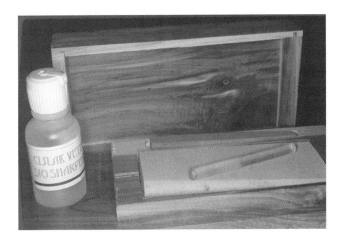

FIGURE 2.10. Sharpening stone and lubricant.

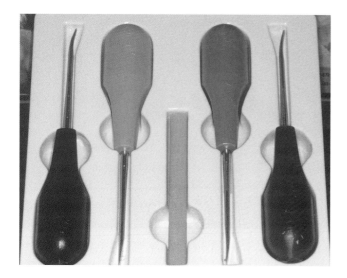

FIGURE 2.11. Dental luxator kit.

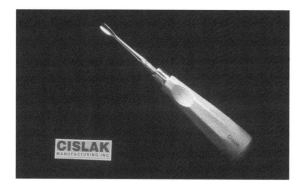

FIGURE 2.12. Winged- elevator (Cislak).

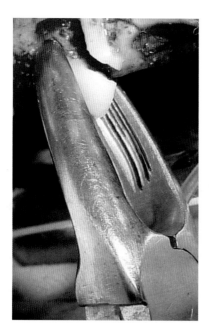

FIGURE 2.13. Extraction forceps.

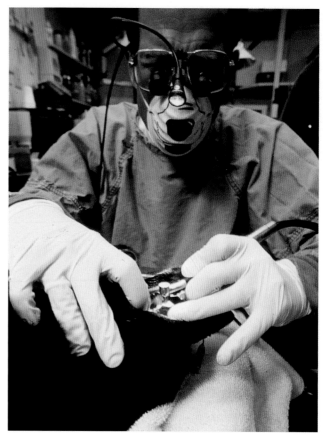

FIGURE 2.14. Appropriate respiratory and eye protection.

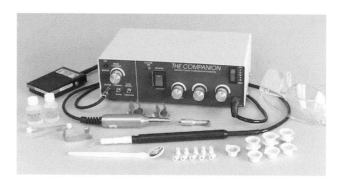

FIGURE 2.15. Ultrasonic scaler/polisher combination (CBi).

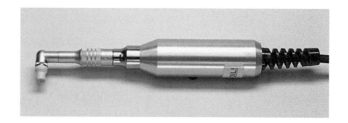

FIGURE 2.16. Slow-speed handpiece micromotor.

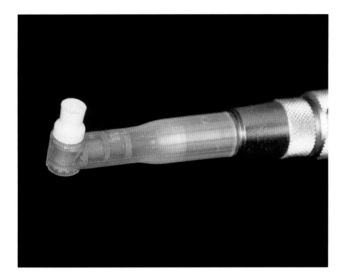

FIGURE 2.17. Disposable polishing angle.

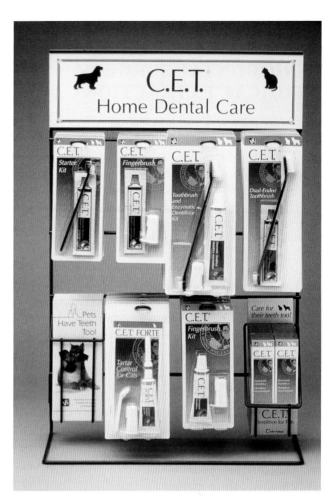

FIGURE 2.19. Home care products.

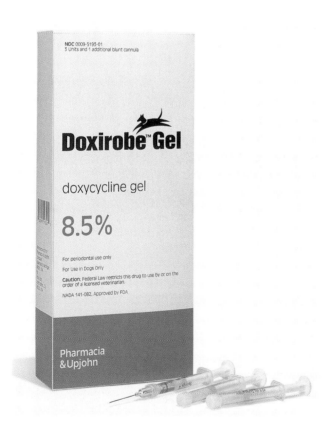

FIGURE 2.18. Doxirobe for local antibiotic insertion into properly prepared periodontal pockets.

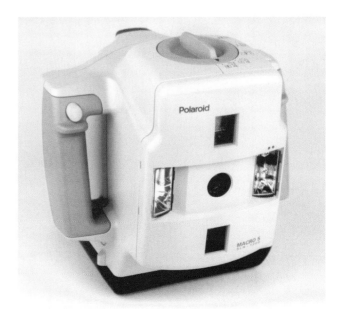

FIGURE 2.20. Polaroid intraoral instant camera.

INCREASED DIAGNOSTIC CAPABILITY, MINOR PERIODONTAL SURGERY, SURGICAL EXTRACTIONS

The following are recommended for more advanced dental care:

- Sterile instrument holders (Figure 2.21)
- Illuminated dental magnification telescopes
- Periosteal elevators—Molt (Burns 271-9008, Schein 600-1016); Freer (Schein 600-9526)) (Figure 2.22)
- Root tip pick (Burns 951-1560, Schein 100-6967, Cislak RT1 straight canine, EX 7 feline) (Figure 2.23)
- High-speed/low-speed delivery system (iM3: Burns Starter Pro 2000, 269-0413, Pro 2000 Challenger 269-0515, Pro 2000 Ultra 269-0517, NITAIR CBi; Schein: Ultima 500, 362-1875, Ultima 500 IIS, 362-3530 Ultima 500 IISF, 362-4967 Ultima 2000) (Figure 2.24)
- High-speed handpiece (Burns 953-3891, Schein 100-2231) (Figure 2.25)
- Low-speed handpiece (CBi) (Figure 2.26) contra-angle attachment (Burns 952-3750, Schein 100-8643) (Figure 2.27)

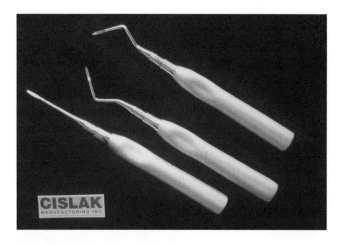

FIGURE 2.23. Root tip pick.

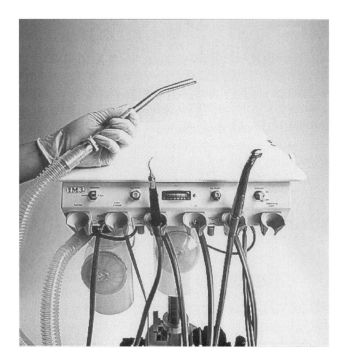

FIGURE 2.24. Self-contained dental delivery system (iM3).

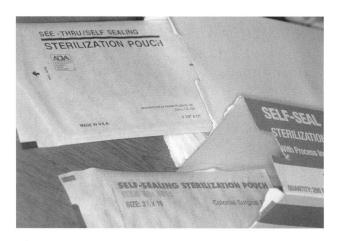

FIGURE 2.21. Sterile instrument holders.

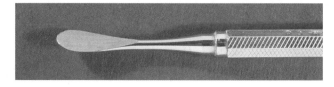

FIGURE 2.22. Molt periosteal elevator.

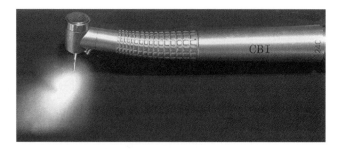

FIGURE 2.25. High-speed handpiece.

- Assortment of burs: round, inverted, pear, fissure (Burns 269-0561, Schein starter bur pack 896-0188)) (Figure 2.28)
- Dental radiograph unit (photo courtesy Dr. Steven Holmstrum) (Burns 699-6709, Schein 263-4478) (Figure 2.29)
- Education books and tools:
  - *Veterinary Dental Techniques*, Holmstrom et al., Saunders, 2004.
  - *Veterinary Dentistry: Principles and Practice*, Wiggs and Loprise, Lippincott, 1997.
  - *An Atlas of Veterinary Dental Radiology*, DeForge and Colmery, Iowa State University Press, 2000.
  - *Atlas of Canine & Feline Dental Radiography*; Mulligan, Aller, and Williams; Veterinary Learning Systems; 1998.
  - *An Introduction to Veterinary Dentistry*, Johnston. An interactive multimedia CD-ROM dental education course comprised of six chapters, including video clips; www.vetschools.ac.uk.

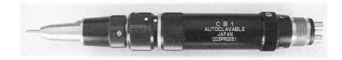

FIGURE 2.26. Low-speed handpiece.

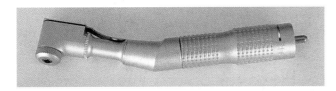

FIGURE 2.27. Contra-angle attachment.

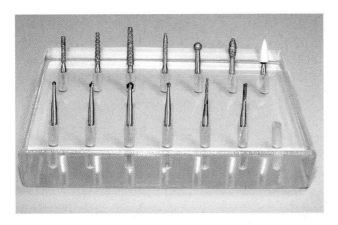

FIGURE 2.28. Bur assortment from L to R bottom row round, inverted cone, tapered fissure, cross-cut fissure; back row, diamonds and white stone.

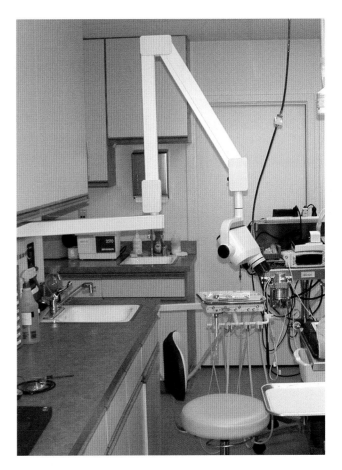

FIGURE 2.29. Dental radiograph unit.

ENDODONTICS, RESTORATION, ORTHODONTICS, AND SURGERY

The following are recommended for endodontic, restorative, and orthodontic care:

- *Endodontic materials*
  - Gates-Glidden burs (Burns 951-1370, Schein 100.6481) (Figure 2.30)
  - K-files 21–30 mm long, width sizes 8 to 140 (Burns 951-2617, 19, 65, 67, 69, 951-2765, 67, 89; Schein 100-9709, 100-4863, 100-1215, 100-5087) (Figure 2.31)
  - Hedstrom files: 30 mm, 47 mm, and 60 mm long; width sizes 10–120 (Burns 264-9458; Schein 100-7643, 100-8303) (Figure 2.32)
  - Barbed broaches: 37 mm and 47 mm long; various widths (Burns 264-9480, Schein 100-6351) (Figure 2.33)
  - Lentulo spiral paste fillers (Schein 100-3791) (Figure 2.34)

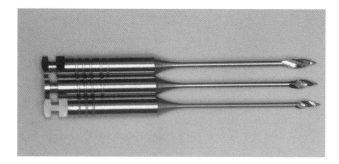

FIGURE 2.30. Gates-Glidden burs.

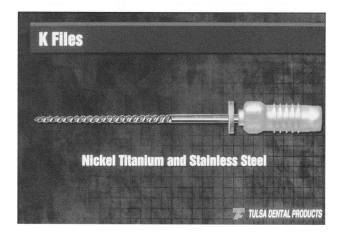

FIGURE 2.31. Kerr endodontic files.

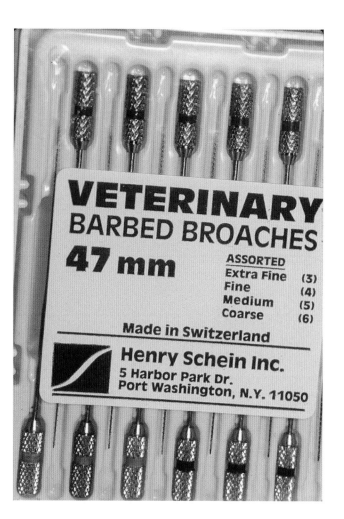

FIGURE 2.33. Barbed broaches.

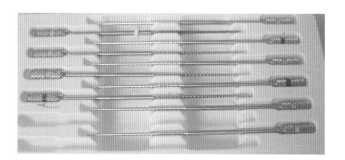

FIGURE 2.32. Hedstrom endodontic files.

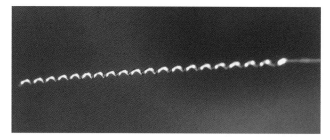

FIGURE 2.34. Lentulo spiral paste fillers.

- 23 guage and 27 gauge blunted endodontic needles (Burns 887-2305, Schein 194-2120) (Figure 2.35)
- Sodium hypochlorite solution (Burns 952-0052, Schein 100-7562) (Figure 2.36) (alternatively, 0.12% Chlorhexidine or hydrogen peroxide can be used as a root canal irrigant)

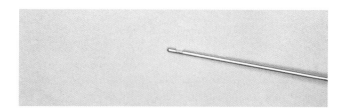

FIGURE 2.35. Endodontic slotted needles.

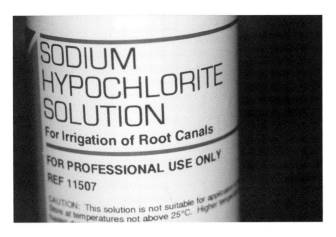

FIGURE 2.36. Root canal irrigant.

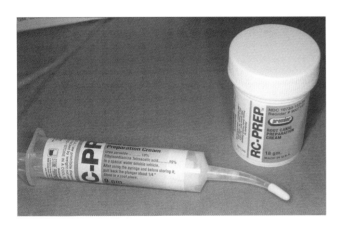

FIGURE 2.37. RC-Prep chelating material.

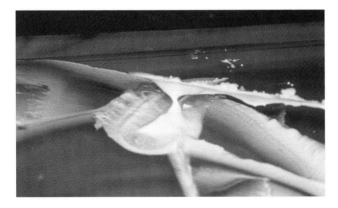

FIGURE 2.38. Mixing slab for preparing endodontic sealer.

- Root canal conditioner, file lubricant (R.C. Prep, Burns 378-4499) (Figure 2.37)
- Mixing slab (Burns 951-4160, Schein 100-4432) and spatula (Burns 950-8856, Schein 100-9387) (Figure 2.38)

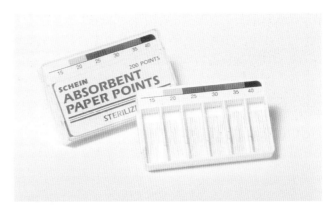

FIGURE 2.39. Assorted paper points.

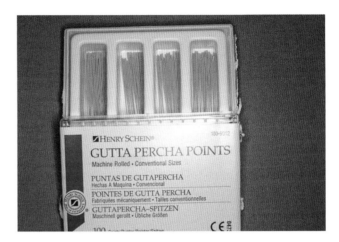

FIGURE 2.40. Assorted gutta percha points.

- Paper points: 30, 47, 60 mm long; various widths (Burns 271-7240, 41, 42, 43; Schein 100-6590) (Figure 2.39)
- Gutta percha in multiple lengths and widths (Burns 271-7215-19; Schein 100-8393, 100-8226) (Figure 2.40)
- Spreaders: small, medium, and large, the author recommends the Holmstrom plugger/spreader combination set (Cislak Holm 20,35,50,65,90; Burns 951-8916, 951-8917; Schein 100-0936, 100-2806, 100-3172) (Figure 2.41)
- Pluggers: small, medium, and large (Burns 951-8910, 14, 16; Schein 100-8337, 100-6578, 100-0971) (Figure 2.42)
- Zinc oxide-eugenol (Burns 952-3250, 951-2081; Schein 100-4540, 100-3688) (Figure 2.43)
- Non-eugenol endodontic canal sealer (Sealapex-Kerr)
- Calcium hydroxide powder and paste (paste: Burns 813-1200, Schein 100-0036; powder: Burns 950-2423, Schein 295-1036) (Figure 2.44)

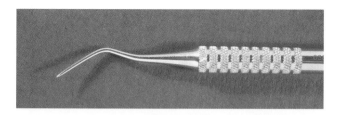

FIGURE 2.41. Endodontic spreader.

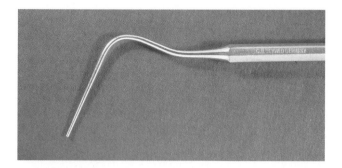

FIGURE 2.42. Endodontic plugger.

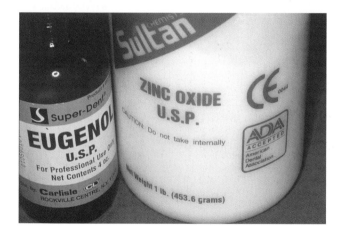

FIGURE 2.43. Zinc oxide/eugenol.

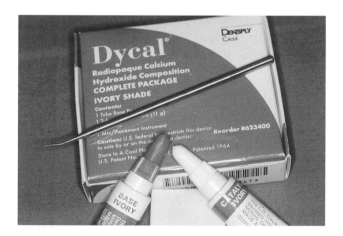

FIGURE 2.44. Calcium hydroxide paste.

- College tipped pliers (Figure 2.45)
- 10:1 reduction gear contrangle (Burns 951-4604) (Figure 2.46)

- *Restorative materials*
  - Etching gel (Burns 951-9192, Schein 100-4649) (Figure 2.47)
  - Bonding resin and brush (Burns 955-7616, Schein 100-1071)
  - Composite restorative (Burns 867-7246, Schein 777-2288) (Figure 2.48)

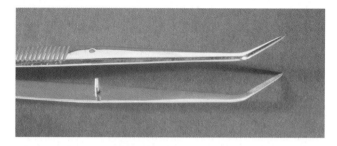

FIGURE 2.45. College tipped pliers.

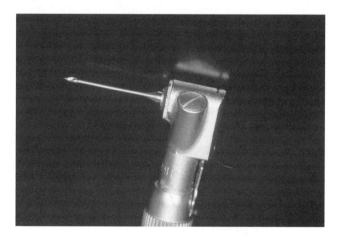

FIGURE 2.46. 10:1 contra angle reduction gear.

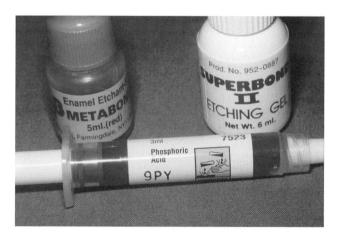

FIGURE 2.47. Etching gel/liquid.

- Light cured glass ionomer restorative (Vitrebond 3M)
- Plastic matrix strips (Burns 951-6162, Schein 100-8525)
- Curing light (Burns 955-7400, Schein 100-5151) (Figure 2.49)
- Diamond burs for crown preparation
- Finishing burs (Burns 868-0690, Schein 195-4022) (Figure 2.50)
- Polishing kit (Burns 888-3400, Schein 195-2264) (Figure 2.51)
- Polyvinylsiloxane impression material (Express 3M, Burns 867-1000, Schein 777-8798) (Figure 2.52)
- Impression trays (prefabricated or self-manufactured) (Figure 2.53)
- Cavit G (Burns 878-0360)

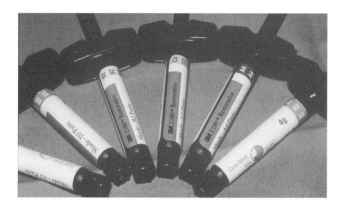

FIGURE 2.48. Light cured composite restorative.

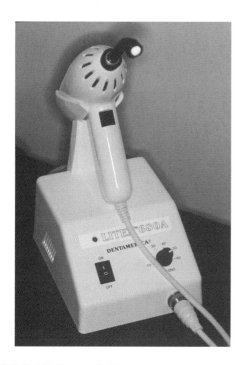

FIGURE 2.49. Curing light.

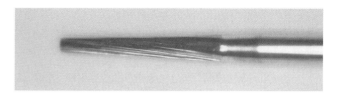

FIGURE 2.50. Finishing bur.

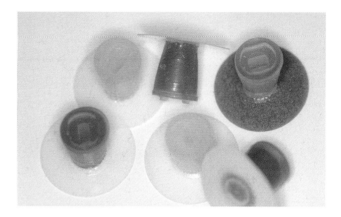

FIGURE 2.51. Polishing discs.

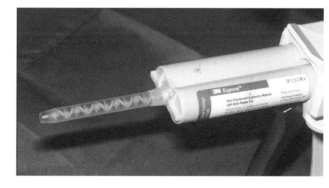

FIGURE 2.52. Impression material loaded on mixing syringe.

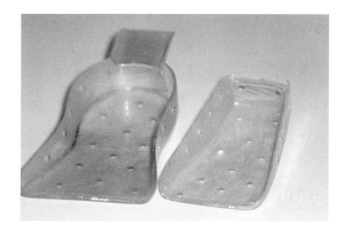

FIGURE 2.53. Impression trays.

- *Orthodontic equipment and materials*
  - Alginate (Burns 950-0460, Schein 100-5292) (Figure 2.54)
  - Boxing wax (Burns 952-2420; Schein 922-8232 thick, 922-6243 thin) (Figure 2.55)

- Wax carver (Burns 958-1084, Schein 600-0344) (Figure 2.56)
- Plaster (Burns 985-1690, Schein 569-3164 Denstone)
- Flexible mixing bowls (Burns 951-3151, Schein 547-4106) (Figure 2.57)
- Buffalo spatula (Burns 810-1230, Schein 365-7743)
- Dental vibrator (Burns 810-1568, Schein 365-3554) (Figure 2.58)
- Orthodontic buttons (Burns 075-0101, Schein 106-6684) (Figure 2.59)
- Bracket cement (Burns 878-0600, Schein 106-3732) (Figure 2.60)

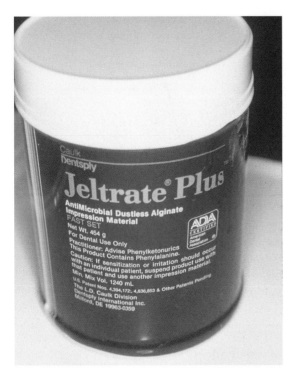

FIGURE 2.54. Alginate for dental impressions.

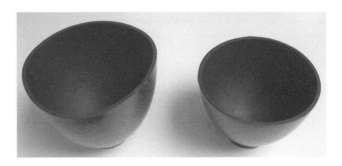

FIGURE 2.57. Flexible mixing bowls.

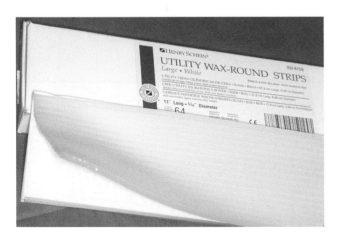

FIGURE 2.55. Wax strips.

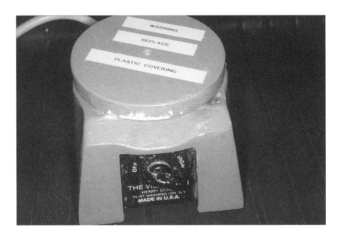

FIGURE 2.58. Dental vibrator.

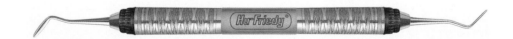

FIGURE 2.56. Wax carver.

- Elastics—Masel chain (Burns 005-1050, Schein 106-0335) (Figure 2.61)
- Acrylic repair—Jet Acrylic Repair (Burns 859-1001, Protemp Garant, Burns 878-0534, Schein 101-2894) (Figure 2.62)

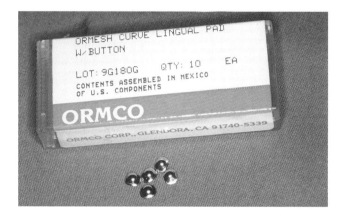

FIGURE 2.59. Orthodontic buttons (Ormco).

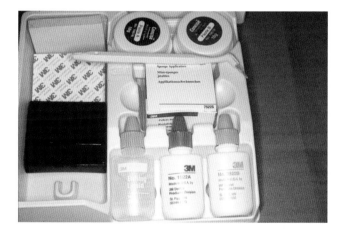

FIGURE 2.60. Orthodontic cement kit (Concise).

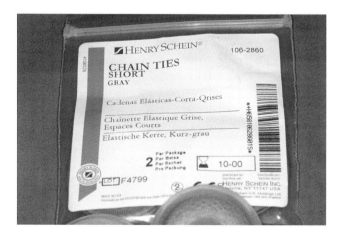

FIGURE 2.61. Masel chain—orthodontic elastics.

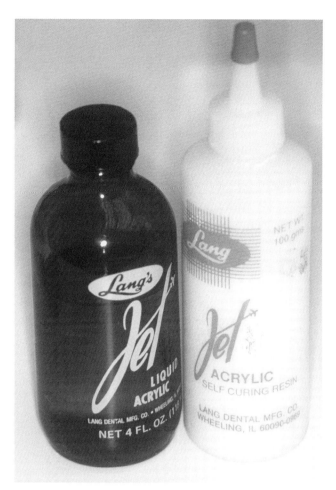

FIGURE 2.62. Jet repair acrylic.

HAND INSTRUMENTS FOR PERIODONTAL CARE

Periodontal probes and explorers are *diagnostic* hand instruments. Scalers and curettes are *working* hand instruments. Hand instruments are named after a person or the institution responsible for development.

Anatomy of the Hand Instrument

Each hand instrument has the following:

- A *handle* for grasping, which may be solid or hollow.
- A *shank* that connects the handle to the working end, allowing adaptation of the working end to the tooth surface.
- The *working end*, containing the face, cutting edge, back, and toe. Hand instruments have either one (single-ended, SE) or two (double-ended, DE) working ends (Figures 2.63, 2.64).

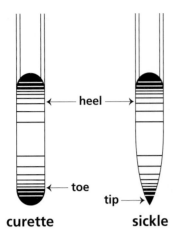

FIGURE 2.63. Curette and sickle.

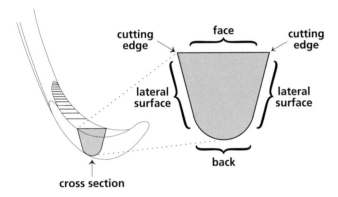

FIGURE 2.64. Cross-section of the working end of a universal curette.

Hand Positioning

Hand instruments are generally held in a modified pen grasp, which provides maximum control of the instrument and a wide range of movement. The instrument is held between the tips of the thumb and index finger, near the junction between handle and shank. The handle rests against the the thumb and knuckles.

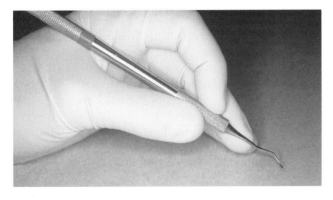

FIGURE 2.65. Modified pen grasp.

The middle finger is used to guide the instrument. The index and middle fingers are bent. The little finger (pinkie) has little function in this grasp, and should be held close to the ring finger in a relaxed, comfortable manner (Figure 2.65).

Diagnostic Hand Instruments

THE PERIODONTAL PROBE The periodontal probe is used to measure the depth of the gingival sulcus or periodontal pocket in millimeters to help evaluate the extent of support loss (Figure 2.66).

Probes vary by design and markings:

- Cross-sectional design: rectangular (flat), oval, or round
- Millimeter markings: the calibrated working end is marked at varying intervals to facilitate reading of depth measurements

COMMONLY USED PERIODONTAL PROBES The *Marquis probe* contains color-coded alternating black/yellow and silver 3 mm bands, at 3, 6, 9, and 12 mm, with a thin working end. Accurately evaluating the millimeter readings between the 3 mm markings is more difficult than with those with single millimeter markings (Figure 2.67).

The *Williams probe* is marked at 1, 2, and 3 millimeters, and then at 5, 7, 8, 9, and 10 millimeters. The spaces between 3 and 5 millimeters are important to note, because most pockets deeper than five millimeters will need surgical care (flap procedure or extraction). The Williams probe is most widely used but may be too thick to be inserted into some patient's pockets (Figure 2.68).

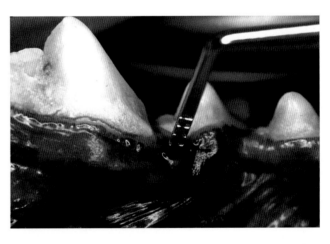

FIGURE 2.66. Periodontal probe used to evaluate sulcus/pocket depth.

The *Michigan-O probe* is marked at 3, 6, and 8 millimeters. Many veterinarians prefer this probe because it has a thin working end; however, the relatively large distance between markings makes the Michigan-O probe poorly suited for feline gingiva. The Michigan-O probe can be obtained with Williams markings, which is preferred by the author (Figures 2.69, 2.70).

The *UNC 15 probe* measures support loss up to 15 mm. It has markings at each millimeter and a black band between 4–5 mm, 9–10 mm, and 14–15 mm (Figure 2.71).

The *Goldman-Fox probe* is thin and flat. Care must be taken not to lacerate the sulcular gingiva when probing (Figure 2.72).

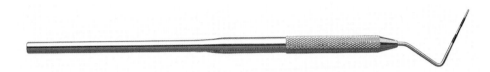

FIGURE 2.67. Marquis probe.

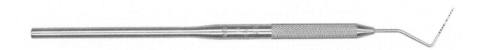

FIGURE 2.68. Williams probe.

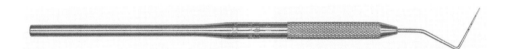

FIGURE 2.69. Michigan–O probe.

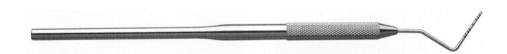

FIGURE 2.70. Michigan–O probe with Williams markings.

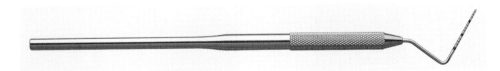

FIGURE 2.71. UNC 15 probe.

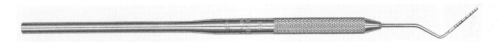

FIGURE 2.72. Goldman-Fox probe.

PROBING Inserting the periodontal probe into the gingival crevice and recording millimeter findings is called *probing*. With gentle pressure, the probe will stop where the gingiva attaches to the tooth, or at the hub of the probe if inserted into an oronasal fistula. Every professional oral hygiene procedure conducted under general anesthesia should include probing and charting. Dogs normally have less than 2 mm probing depths and cats less than 1 mm. Greater depths may indicate periodontal disease and require treatment.

Two methods of probing are *spot* and *circumferential*:

* Spot probing is the insertion and withdrawal of the probe at a single area per tooth. Because single areas do not represent the entire tooth, inaccurate readings may be obtained.
* Circumferential probing is the placing of the probe in the sulcus or pocket in at least six places (three facial, labial, or buccal, three lingual or palatal) around the tooth, recording millimeter readings. This method eliminates inaccurate readings when subgingival calculus is present, or in cases where isolated areas of vertical bone loss are present.

PROBING DEPTH The *clinical depth* or *probing depth* is the distance between the base of the pocket and the gingival margin. The probe is inserted in line with the vertical axis of the tooth and "walked" circumferentially to record at least four measurements per tooth. In addition to pathology present, the probing depth is influenced by factors such as the size of the probe, the force with which it is introduced, and the direction of penetration (Figures 2.73, 2.74).

Attachment loss (AL) or *clinical attachment level* is determined by measuring the distance from the cementoenamel junction to the pocket base (Figure 2.75). The clinical attachment loss offers greater diagnostic significance compared to the probing depth.

Clinically, the gingival margin presents:

* In its normal location, 1–2mm coronal to the CEJ where the level of attachment and the pocket depth are equal.

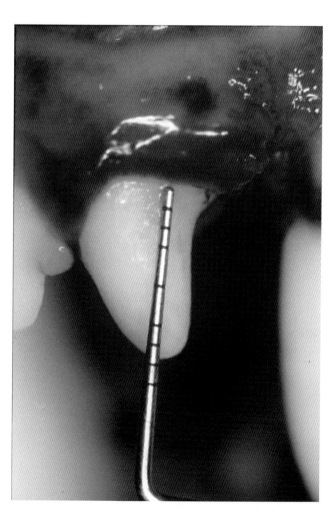

FIGURE 2.73. Before probe insertion.

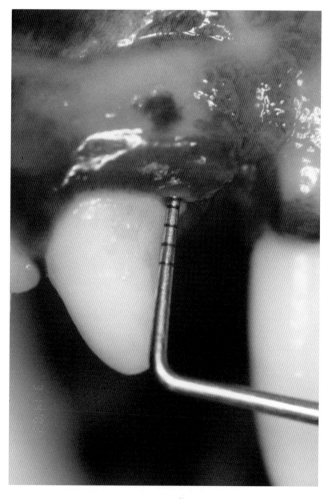

FIGURE 2.74. 7 mm probing depth.

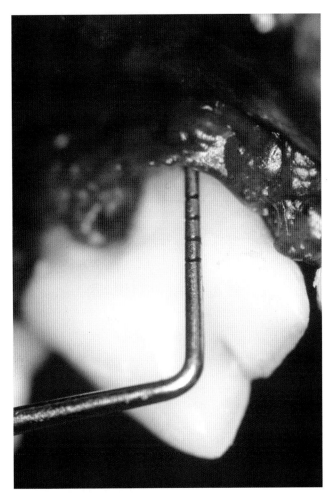

FIGURE 2.75. 9mm attachment level (loss).

- Coronal to the CEJ in cases of gingival hyperplasia. In cases of gingival hyperplasia the base remains the same, but an apparent pseudopocket forms due to excessive gingiva.
- Apical to the CEJ in cases of gingival recession. The clinical attachment level measurement is determined by adding the probing depth to the gingival recession measurement (distance between the cementoenamel junction to the gingival margin). When the gingival margin is located apical to the cementoenamel junction, the loss of attachment will be greater than the pocket depth.

Following are some examples of the clinical significance of probing depth and attachment loss:

- A Labrador retriever whose maxillary canine has a 9 mm pocket depth and an 8 mm attachment loss from Stage 4 periodontal disease may require an apical reposition flap to decrease the pocket depth and save the tooth (number 1 in (Figure 2.76).
- A boxer with a 7 mm pocket depth and a 5 mm hyperplastic gingiva (distance from the CEJ to the gingival margin) secondary to gingival hyperplasia should undergo a gingivectomy to eliminate the pseudopocket (number 2 in Figure 2.76).
- A poodle with a 2 mm pocket depth and an 8 mm attachment loss around the maxillary canine from gingival recession has a normal probing depth but significant attachment loss. Extraction may be the treatment of choice (number 3 in Figure 2.76).

DENTAL EXPLORER The *dental explorer* has a sharp point used to examine the root surface for calculus, resorptive lesions, necrotic cementum, and the crown for areas of pulpal exposure. The explorer is not

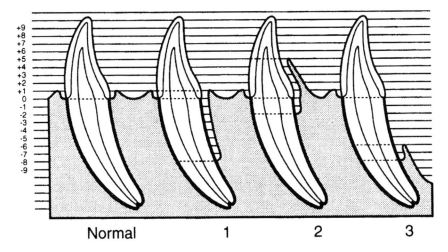

FIGURE 2.76. Normal and abnormal pocket depth and attachment levels for dogs.

used to remove calculus. The explorer's tip is the working end of the explorer.

The following describe interpretations of explorer findings:

- Normal, where there is a smooth path when the explorer is inserted and withdrawn from the sulcus or pocket
- Ledge of subgingival calculus present, where the explorer moves over the tooth surface, encounters a ledge, moves laterally over it, and returns to the tooth surface
- Fine deposits of subgingival calculus, where there is a gritty sensation as the explorer passes over fine calculus
- Carious lesion, where the explorer is pressed into a lesion and will stick or catch on withdrawal

Explorer examples include the following:

- The *number 23 shepherd's hook* is commonly paired with a probe. The hook may be too large to safely probe subgingivally in toy breeds and felines (Figure 2.77).
- The *number 17 Orban explorer* has a fine 2 mm tip that extends right angled from the shank (Figure 2.78).

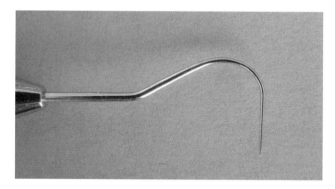

FIGURE 2.77. Number 23 shepherd's hook (CBi).

- The *ODU (Old Dominion University) number 11/12* is patterned after the Gracey 11/12 curette. Its thin tip is especially useful for examining feline odontoclastic resorptive lesions (Figure 2.79).

Working Hand Instruments

The *hand sickle scaler* is designed to remove supragingival dental deposits (plaque and calculus). A scaler's blade is triangular in cross section, with two cutting edges that converge to form a triangular point useful for working in tight interproximal spaces. The scaler is placed with blade apical to the deposit and the cutting edge contacting the tooth surface. A short, coronal pull stroke directed in line with the long axis of the tooth is used to remove supragingival debris. Examples of scalers include Cislak P-11, Towner–U15/ Jacquette-30, Goldman- 6/7.

Curettes are designed to assist in the removal of subgingival plaque and calculus. Curettes are similar to scalers, but have a smooth rounded heel opposite the cutting surface. A rounded back makes curettes less traumatic to soft tissues. Curettes are used to remove subgingival plaque and calculus, for root planing, and curettage (soft tissue removal in periodontal pockets).

Removal of calculus is beneficial because it acts as a retention site for plaque and toxins harmful to the tooth's support. Loose, free flowing plaque in the periodontal pocket causes more disease than adherent plaque. At one time it was thought that the goal of subgingival care was to create a smooth surfaced root by removing plaque and calculus-laden cementum. Every professional hygiene/teeth-cleaning visit used to be completed by hand scaling the accessible root surface smooth.

Currently, cementum removal as part of the oral hygiene visit is discouraged. Cementum contains cell-activating proteins that encourage reattachment. Dentin does not contain these proteins. The design and safety of thin, long, ultrasonic periodontal tips decrease the need to aggressively root plane teeth affected by periodontal disease. Subgingival ultrasonic treatment causes cavitation and disruption of the subgingival ecosys-

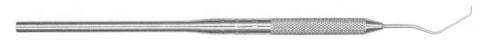

FIGURE 2.78. Number 17 Orban explorer.

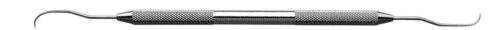

FIGURE 2.79. ODU 11/12.

tem and biofilm. It may not be necessary to follow ultrasonic scaling with hand instrumentation.

CURETTE TYPES

- *Universal curettes* have a blade with two parallel (90° to the ground) cutting edges and a rounded toe. Universal curettes can be adapted to tooth surfaces of all regions in the mouth. Both blades may be used on the front and back of a tooth without changing instruments. The working end should be parallel to the long axis of the tooth. Popular universal curettes include Columbia (Figure 2.80A), McCall (Figure 2.80B), Barnhart (Figure 2.80C), and Langer styles (Figure 2.80D).
- *Area-specific curettes* are designed to adapt to a certain area or tooth surface. Area-specific curettes are offset at 70° with only one cutting edge. The lower lateral cutting edge is used next to the tooth surface. The most common area-specific curettes are the Gracey series of seven double-ended instruments (Figure 2.81). Graceys can be used to remove deep subgingival calculus, root planing, and for curettage of the periodontal pocket. The author prefers the Gracey 1/2, 5/6, and 13/14. After-Five series curettes are designed with a thin terminal shank that is 3 mm longer than standard Gracey curettes, allowing improved access to deep periodontal pockets and root surfaces.

Use the following steps when handling a curette:

1. Hold the curette's terminal shank with a modified pen grasp, parallel to the tooth surface to engage the blade's cutting edge.
2. Insert the instrument into the pocket with the blade face parallel to the root surface below the deposit. When deep calculus lies at the bottom of a pocket, positioning the curette may damage the periodontal attachment. Ultrasonic or sonic scaling removes calculus from top to bottom, decreasing iatrogenic attachment injury.
3. Pull the instrument coronally with the engaged material toward the cementoenamel junction.
4. Repeat this process in circumferentially overlapping strokes until the root surface is smooth. Care must be taken not to remove excessive cementum (Figure 2.82).

Instrument Sharpening

Proper care of hand instruments not only prolongs the useful life, but is essential to maintain proper function. Immediately after each use, all dental instruments must be thoroughly cleaned with disinfectant, dried, and sterilized. Before sterilization, hand instruments that contain cutting surfaces (i.e., scalers and curettes) should also be lightly sharpened to maintain the cutting edges.

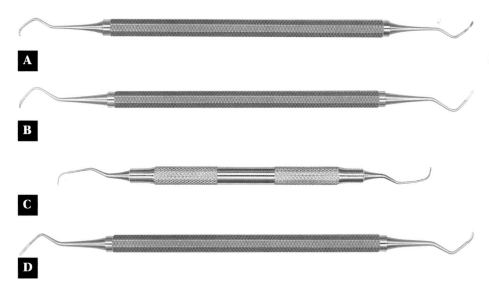

FIGURE 2.80. Universal curettes: (A) Columbia curette; (B) McCall curette; (C) Barnhart curette; (D) Langer curette.

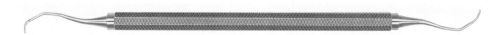

FIGURE 2.81. Gracey curette.

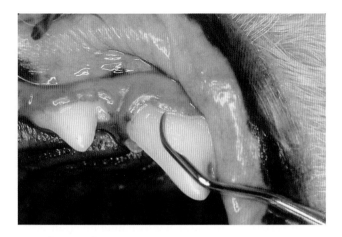

FIGURE 2.82. Using a curette.

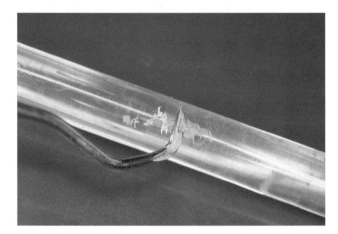

FIGURE 2.83. Plastic test stick.

A dull instrument will push calculus into the dental surface.

Methods used to determine whether an instrument requires sharpening or recontouring (reshaping) include visual inspection, comparison, and use of test sticks.

Close visual examination of an instrument can help determine the need for sharpening. The instrument is held under a bright light and examined with a magnifying glass. Dull cutting edges reflect light; sharp edges do not reflect light.

A master set of unused instruments should be available for inspection. Visual comparison of a used instrument with a new one can be used to determine sharpness and retention of the original contour.

Hard plastic test sticks can be used to determine whether an instrument requires sharpening. The instrument blade is drawn across the test stick. The sharp edge of the instrument should "grab" the stick and peel

a sliver of plastic (Figure 2.83). Dull instruments will slide across the surface.

MATERIALS FOR SHARPENING INSTRUMENTS

A variety of materials are available for proper instrument sharpening. These include sharpening stones, lubricant, gloves, alcohol soaked gauze, plastic test stick, and a magnifying glass. Mechanical sharpeners are also available (Figures 2.84, 2.85).

Types of sharpening stones include the following:

- The natural fine grit *Arkansas* stone, lubricated with oil before use (Figure 2.86)
- The synthetic fine or medium grit *India* stone, lubricated with oil before use (Figure 2.87)
- The synthetic fine or medium grit *ceramic* stone, lubricated with water before use (Figure 2.88)

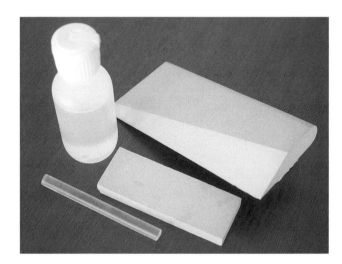

FIGURE 2.84. Sharpening equipment (CBi).

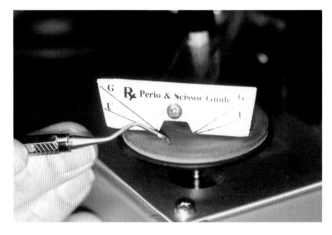

FIGURE 2.85. Mechanical instrument sharpener. (Rx Honing Machine Corporation, Mishawaka, IN)

FIGURE 2.86. Arkansas sharpening stone.

FIGURE 2.87. India sharpening stone.

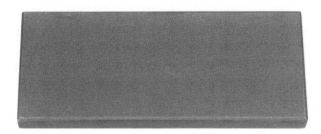

FIGURE 2.88. Ceramic stone.

Stone shapes and uses include the following:

• The *conical* Arkansas or ceramic stone can be used to remove fine metal edges from the instrument. Conical stones can also be used for lightly sharpening scalers and rounding the toe of curettes after each use.
• Arkansas or ceramic *cylindrical* stones are similar in function to the conical stone.
• Arkansas, India, or ceramic *flat* stones used for most instrument sharpening and recontouring.

Sharpening stones should be scrubbed to remove metal particles after each use, and then rinsed and autoclaved. Alternate the areas of the stone used for sharpening to prevent grooves from forming on the stone surface.

SHARPENING TECHNIQUES   The work area for sharpening should be well lit. A sturdy table that is high enough to support the operator's elbows and allow the

operator to handle the instrument at eye level will facilitate the process.

Regardless of the method used, care must be taken to avoid removing too much metal, which can damage the structural integrity of the instrument and/or alter its shape.

Follow these steps for the *moving* stone curette sharpening method:

1. Place a drop of oil on the flat stone and distribute over the face (Figure 2.89).
2. Hold the instrument's terminal shank with the point perpendicular toward the floor. The face will automatically be parallel to the floor.
3. To determine the correct edge (lower) to sharpen in an area-specific curette, hold the curette with the toe pointed toward yourself and the terminal shank perpendicular to the floor.
4. Place the stone against the instrument so that the angle between the face of the instrument and the stone is approximately 110°.
5. Move the stone up and down while maintaining the 110° angle.
6. End sharpening on a downward stroke.
7. Sharpen the opposite blade side (if it is a universal curette).
8. Wipe the tip with alcohol-soaked gauze.
9. Test the instrument with a plastic stick and/or by visual examination.

Follow these steps for the *stationary* stone curette sharpening method (Figure 2.90):

1. Place a drop of oil on the stone and distribute over the face of the stone.
2. Place the stone flat on the table.
3. Position the instrument at a 110° angle to the stone.

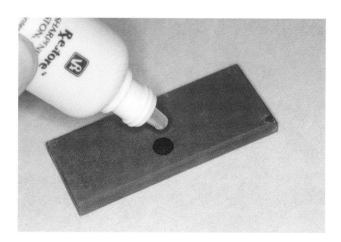

FIGURE 2.89. Oil applied to the stone.

4. Move the instrument back and forth across the stone.
5. Sharpen the other side of the blade (if universal).
6. Wipe the tip with alcohol-soaked gauze.
7. Test the instrument with a plastic test stick and/or with visual examination.

Follow these steps for the conical stone use (Figure 2.91):

1. Place a drop of oil on the conical stone.
2. Hold the instrument with the tip pointing toward the ceiling.
3. Hold the conical stone with the face of the instrument toward the stone.
4. Roll the stone between the thumb and fingers so that it comes into contact with the face of the instrument.
5. Repeat the process for 10–15 strokes against the instrument.

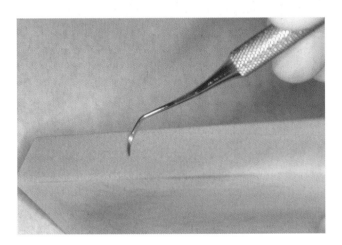

FIGURE 2.90. Stationary stone technique.

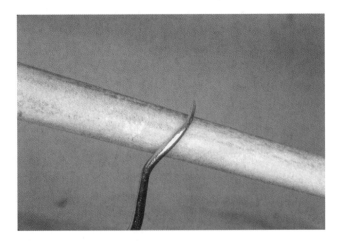

FIGURE 2.91. Sharpening with conical stone.

6. Wipe the tip with alcohol-soaked gauze.
7. Test the instrument with a plastic stick and/or by visual examination.

Power Scaling

Professional calculus and plaque removal (scaling) can be performed using hand instruments or scalers powered by electricity or gas while the animal is anesthetized. Powered scalers increase the speed and efficiency of teeth cleaning. There are three types of power-driven scalers: sonic, ultrasonic, and rotary. Because of the potential for iatrogenic damage to the gingiva and pulp, techniques for rotary scaling are not discussed in this text.

The *sonic scaler* is attached to the high-speed outlet of an air- or gas-driven delivery system. Sonic scalers are available through CBi, Star Dental, MTI, and KaVo America (Figure 2.92). In the author's opinion, sonic scalers are not appropriate for use in general veterinary dentistry because:

- Sonic scaler tips vibrate at low frequencies ranging between 3000–9000 CPS (cycles per second) and are best used to remove plaque and fresh calculus. Most veterinary patients are presented with chronic calculus accumulation.
- Sonic scalers have a wide amplitude (0.5 mm) compared to ultrasonic (0.01–0.05 mm). This wider amplitude may result in greater cementum removal when the scaler is used subgingivally compared to the ultrasonic scaler equipped with a periodontal tip for subgingival use.
- The sonic scaler unit requires continuous air pressure of 30–40 psi. A relatively large compressor (>1 hp) is needed for power. If the delivery system is nitrogen- or carbon dioxide–driven, use of sonic scalers can consume large volumes of gas, which might not be financially feasible.
- Daily lubrication is necessary for maintenance.

Ultrasonic scalers are classified as magnetostrictive or piezoelectric. Magnetostrictive units use ferromag-

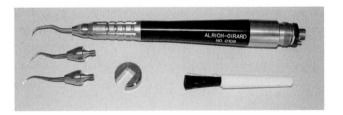

FIGURE 2.92. Sonic scaler.

netic stacks or ferrite rods to cause tip vibration. Ferromagnetic stacks are strips of laminated nickel attached with solder. When the operator wants to remove plaque and calculus from above the gingiva (supragingival), the standard P-10 or beavertail insert is selected. When subgingival use is planed, magnetostrictive thin and long subgingival After-Five (Hu-Friedy) or SLI Slimline (Dentsply Cavitron) inserts can be used

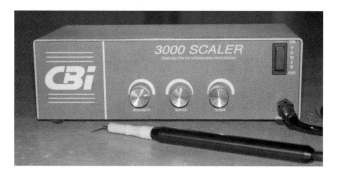

FIGURE 2.93. Magnetostrictive ultrasonic scaler.

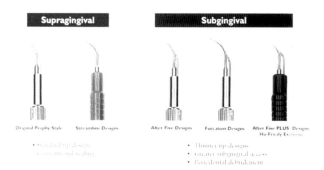

FIGURE 2.94. Subgingival and supragingival tips.

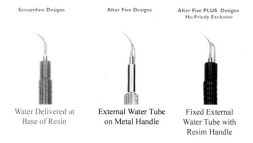

FIGURE 2.95. Water delivery variations to the tip.

safely. Thin titanium ferrite rod inserts also can be used subgingivally (Figures 2.93–2.98).

When an alternating electrical current is supplied to a wire coil in the magnetostrictive handpiece, a magnetic field is created around the stack or rod transducer, causing the tip to constrict and relax. This vibration energizes the water as it passes over the tip, producing a scouring effect to remove plaque, calculus, and stains. Bubbles are created and implode, affecting bacterial cell walls in the gingival crevice. The water mist also cools the tip and irrigates debris.

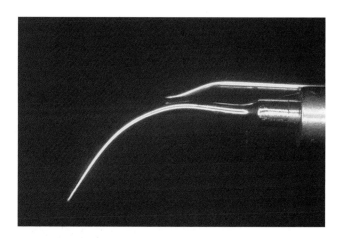

FIGURE 2.96. Periodontal ultrasonic tip.

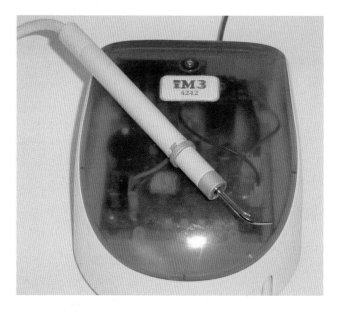

FIGURE 2.97. Ferrite rod ultrasonic scaler—iM3 Model 42-12.

When choosing an ultrasonic scaler, tip motion, frequency, and potential iatrogenic injury must be considered. Magnetostrictive tip motion is either a figure-eight pattern (ferromagnetic stack) or an elliptical pattern (ferrite rod). Magnetostrictive advocates claim elliptical tip motion is most effective because it generates pathogen-destroying cavitation bubbles 360° around the tip. In contrast, the piezo design creates bubbles only at the two ends of the back-and-forth cycle. The sonic scaler does not produce cavitation bubbles.

Frequency is the number of times the scaler tip vibrates each second. A variety of frequencies are available within the three types of ultrasonic technologies. The higher frequencies (above 40,000 Hz) may provide greater efficiency.

Ultrasonic scaling units are available in manual-tuning or auto-tuning models. Some researchers feel that better cavitation is achieved at low power settings if the scaler is slightly mistuned. Because auto-tuned scalers perfectly tune to the insert's frequency, to mistune, a manual-tuned scaler is needed. (Suppliers of manual-tuned scalers include Parkell, Ultrasonic Services, Ltd., CBi).

Ultrasonic scalers are also available with manual tuning to adjust where the spray exits the tip (Figures 2.99, 2.100, 2.101).

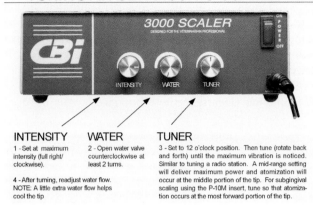

TUNING AN ULTRASONIC SCALER

INTENSITY
1 - Set at maximum intensity (full right/clockwise).

4 - After turning, readjust water flow. NOTE: A little extra water flow helps cool the tip

WATER
2 - Open water valve counterclockwise at least 2 turns.

TUNER
3 - Set to 12 o'clock position. Then tune (rotate back and forth) until the maximum vibration is noticed. Similar to tuning a radio station. A mid-range setting will deliver maximum power and atomization will occur at the middle portion of the tip. For subgingival scaling using the P-10M insert, tune so that atomization occurs at the most forward portion of the tip.

FIGURE 2.99. CBi tuneable magnetostrictive.

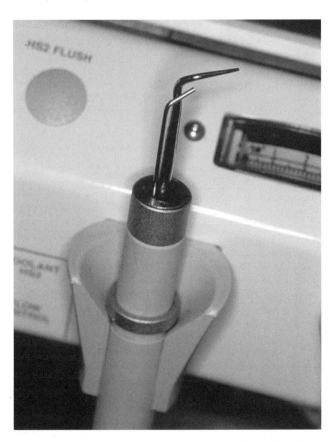

FIGURE 2.98. Ferrite rod handpiece in the iM3 high-speed delivery system.

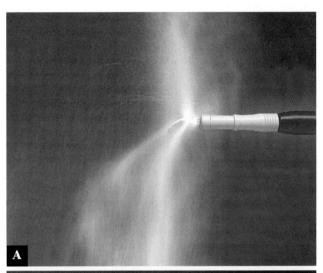

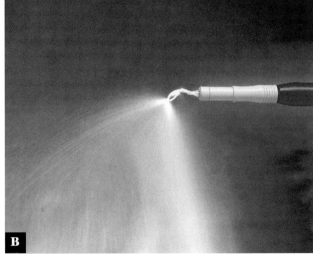

FIGURE 2.100. CBi scaler tuned for supra- (A) and subgingival (B) scaling.

TIP MOTION The most powerful surfaces of the stack scaler tip are the underside and the top; the lateral sides are the least active. To prevent trauma to the tooth surface, only the lateral sides should be used for periodontal debridement. The ferrite rod tip is equally active on all sides.

The power control on an ultrasonic scaler is used to adjust the distance that the tip travels in a specific pattern. The full range listed in Table 2.1 reflects the smallest-to-largest range of motion (lowest power setting to highest power setting) for each of the three types of ultrasonic technologies.

A piezoelectric unit is activated by dimensional changes in crystals housed within the handpiece as electricity is passed over the surface of the crystals. The resultant vibration produces tip movement (Figure 2.102).

The activity of piezoelectric scalers is limited to the last 3 mm of the tip. Magnetostrictive metal stack tips are active at the last 4 mm of tip; the magnetostrictive ferrite rod scaler is active a full 12 mm of the tip.

CHANGING TIPS Tip wear is critical to efficiency of scaling instruments and can be evaluated using a chart, which compares a tip in use with an original. A loss of 1 mm of the tip equals a 25% loss of efficiency. A 2 mm loss of the tip equals a 50% loss in efficiency and should be replaced (Figures 2.103, 2.104).

Both of the magnetostrictive types of ultrasonic tips are changed with a pull out/push in action. Both use O-rings in the handpiece or on the instrument to provide a tight fit and a seal to prevent water leakage (Figure 2.105).

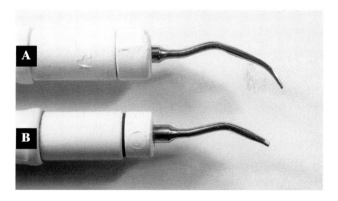

FIGURE 2.103. Normal tip (A) compared to fractured ultrasonic tip (B).

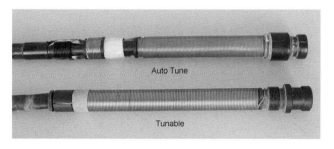

FIGURE 2.101. Auto tune and tunable magnet wands for ultrasonic insert.

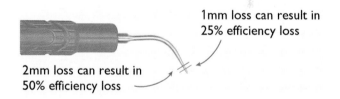

1mm loss can result in 25% efficiency loss

2mm loss can result in 50% efficiency loss

FIGURE 2.104. Chart of tip wear.

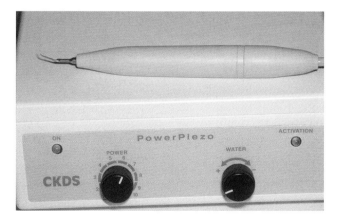

FIGURE 2.102. Piezoelectric ultrasonic scaler.

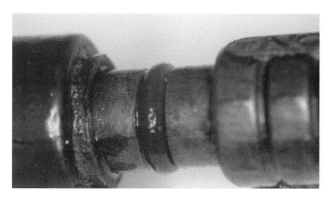

FIGURE 2.105. O-ring seal.

Table 2.1. Range of motion for types of ultrasonic technologies.

Characteristic	Magnetostrictive Metal Stack	Magnetostrictive Ferrite Rod	Piezoelectric
Tip motion pattern Range (full)	Elliptoid—figure 8 1.6 mm–2.2 mm	Elliptical—circular 0.02 mm–0.04 mm	Linear—back and forth 0.4 mm–1.2 mm
Tip activity Working area of tip	4 mm All surfaces	12 mm All surfaces	3 mm Only two sides
Frequency	18,000, 25,000, or 30,000 Hz	42,000 Hz	25,000–45,000 Hz
Caution	The metal stack generates heat and should not be used subgingivally unless equipped with special thin periodontal tips.	Rods are very fragile and prone to breakage.	Does not generate much heat, but it is more damaging to cementum when used for subgingival debridement.
Changing tips	Pull out/push in tip held by an O-ring. If a metal strip/stack unit is used, the unit must be turned on and the handpiece filled before insertion of the insert.	Pull out/push in tip held by an O-ring. The handpiece should be drained before insertion of the insert. Forcing the insert into a handpiece that contains water may cause the tip to fracture.	Tips screw on/off. Requires wrench.
Suppliers	Cavitron (Dentsply), Parkell, Coltene, Vetroson (Summit Hill), Cbi.	EMS, Amadent, Amdent, iM3 Model 42-12.	Piezon Master 400 (EMS) Young PS (Young Dental Manufacturing), Megasonic 2000 (Dentalaire)

Piezoelectric scalers require a wrench to unscrew one tip and to replace it with another (Figures 2.106–2.109).

Magnetostrictive inserts and piezoelectric tips should be cleaned and sterilized after each use. To clean, rinse thoroughly or immerse in an ultrasonic instrument-cleaning unit for twenty minutes. After removal, rinse the inserts with tap water and dry before packaging and sterilizing in a steam autoclave or gas sterilizer (Figure 2.110).

Virtually all brands of magnetostrictive inserts of the same frequencies are interchangeable. Most 30 kHz units will operate only with 30 kHz inserts (a 25 kHz insert will not fit into the handle) (Figure 2.111). Most piezoelectric scalers use tips designed specifically for each brand of scaler, which creates a problem if the manufacturer goes out of business. (Suppliers of 25 kHz scalers: Parkell, Dentsply, CBi, Summit Hill; supplier of 30 kHz scalers: Dentsply; supplier of 25/30 kHz scalers: Parkell, Whaledent.)

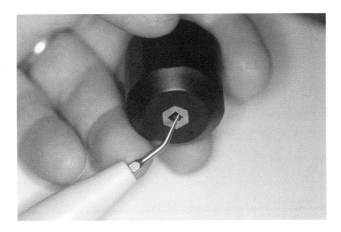

FIGURE 2.106. Tip-changing tool.

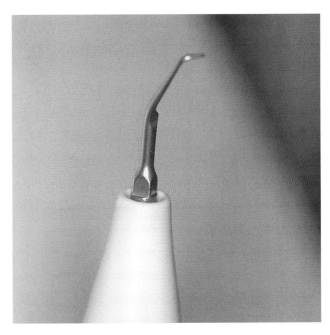

FIGURE 2.109. Piezoelectric tip in place.

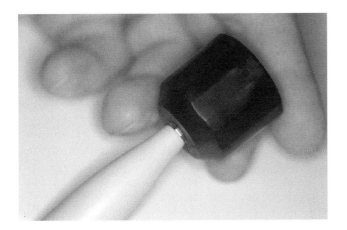

FIGURE 2.107. Tip-changing tool inserted.

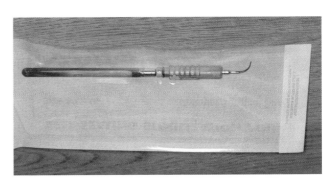

FIGURE 2.110. Sterile envelope used to store scaler insert before use.

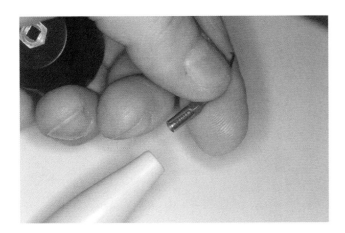

FIGURE 2.108. Tip removed.

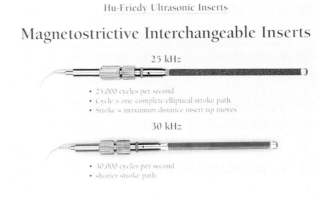

FIGURE 2.111. Two frequencies of magnetostrictive inserts.

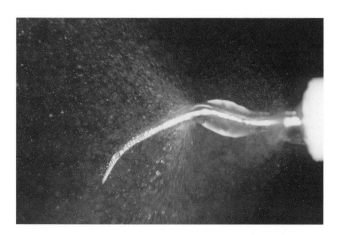

FIGURE 2.112. Adjusted water spray for supragingival scaling.

Follow these steps for the sonic/ultrasonic scaling technique:

1. Hold the handpiece lightly in a modified pen grasp.
2. Use eye, ear, and respiratory protection.
3. Hold the fulcrum or finger rest at a distance farther from the tooth than with hand instruments, because the tips do not have cutting edges.
4. Adjust water spray to deliver a steady drip with a small mist halo (Figure 2.112).
5. Apply light pressure to the tip working in a coronal-to-apical direction. The sound waves should do most of the work. Note: Efficiency decreases with increased pressure.
6. Pass the side of the working end over calculus and plaque in short, light vertical strokes. Heavy lateral pressure should be avoided.
7. Keep the lateral surface working end in constant motion. Leaving it in one place too long increases the amount of tooth material removed. Never hold the tip perpendicular to the surface of the tooth. This will either etch or groove the tooth surface.
8. Specially designed subgingival periodontal tips may be used subgingivally. To avoid iatrogenic injury, decrease the power with subgingival use.
9. After ultrasonic teeth cleaning is completed, use air from the air/water syringe to gently blow/lift off the gingival margin away from the tooth and examine for missed calculus.

DENTAL DELIVERY UNITS

Electrically Driven

Electric dental micromotors power handpieces attached to burs, disks, and polishing cups. These units accept straight, contra-angle, and prophy angle attachments.

Unfortunately, electrically driven delivery units have several drawbacks. The micromotor powered dental unit is limited in what it can do because there is no water for cooling. If used, an assistant must spray water on the field to cool the bur to prevent iatrogenic thermal damage. Additionally, micromotors operate below 30,000 RPM with high torque, causing excessive vibrations that make accurate work difficult (Figure 2.113).

Air-Driven

Compressed air or gas can be used to power handpieces for polishing, tooth sectioning, endodontics, restoration, and oral surgery. The advantages over motorized systems lie in the capability of precise cutting at higher speed, less torque, and water-cooling to prevent thermal damage to the pulp and surrounding bone.

Compressed air delivery systems consist of:

- The *compressor*, which provides pressurized air for the air-water syringe and handpieces:
  - Compressor size is important. The capacity of the compressor is related to the number of operatories and handpieces used at the same time in the practice. The compressor must be large enough to maintain pressure of 30–40 psi at a flow rate of 3 cubic feet per minute. When the compressor is too small, it will run almost continuously during use and may overheat. If a sonic scaler or more than one station is used, a minimum of a 1 hp compressor is recommended (Figure 2.114).
  - Compressors are either air- or oil-cooled. Air-cooling reduces the amount of contaminants (oil) in the line but is noisier and usually more expensive than oil-cooling. Modified refrigerator oil-cooled compressors ("silent" compressors) are commonly used in smaller self-contained delivery

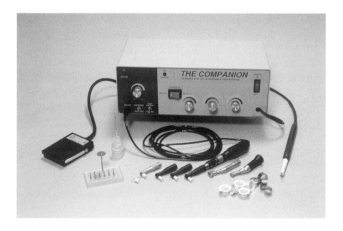

FIGURE 2.113. Electrically driven micromotor (CBi).

systems (iM3 K6500 Silent Hurricane, Schein 100-8236 Silent Surge). Unfortunately, when using an oil-cooled compressor, small particles of oil become mixed with the compressed air, which might contaminate tooth surfaces, interfering with material setting properly. Oil-free filters are available to prevent contamination (iM3, Inc. M8350).

- Compressors for dental delivery systems are either attached to the unit (self-contained) or located remotely in a nearby cabinet, closet, attic, or outside the clinic. The advantage of remote compressors include the following:

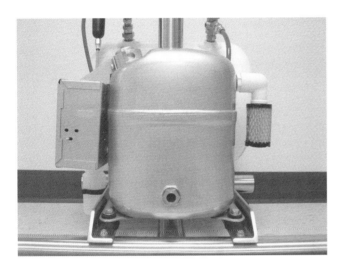

FIGURE 2.114. Compressor (iM3).

- Less noise occurs in the operatory.
- Multiple stations may be attached to one compressor.
- Less storage is required in the immediate operatory area.

- The *storage* or *air tank* holds air generated by the compressor. This stored air is used to power the dental handpieces and air/water syringe. Air tanks come in many sizes. The larger the tank size, the less "work" the compressor needs to do. Pressure inside the air storage tank varies by manufacturer between 80–120 psi. When maintenance pressure is reached, the compressor turns off. When the tank pressure drops below 60 psi, the compressor turns on to refill the tank with compressed air (Figure 2.115).
- The *water container* or *plumbing hookup* irrigates and cools the rotary instruments (Figure 2.116).
- The *assembly delivery system (control panel)* contains the air/water supply syringe, tubing for the handpieces, pressure gauge(s), switches for turning water on and off, needle valve to adjust water flow, and a switch to change from the high- to low-speed

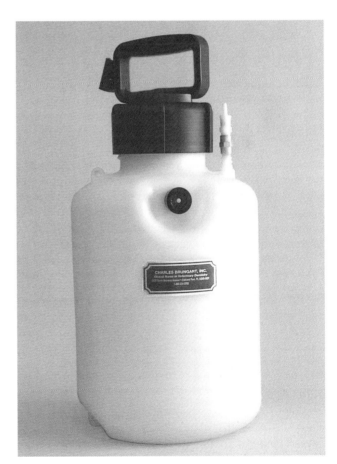

FIGURE 2.116. Water tank.

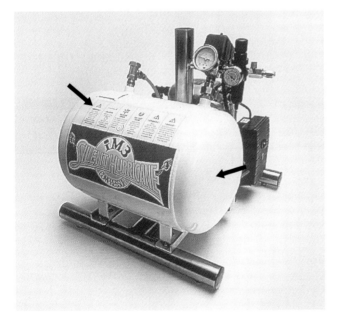

FIGURE 2.115. Storage tank (iM3).

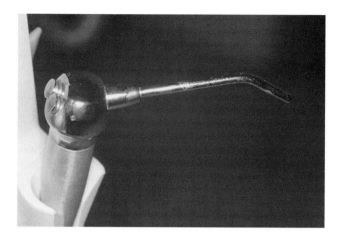

FIGURE 2.117. Three-way air/water syringe.

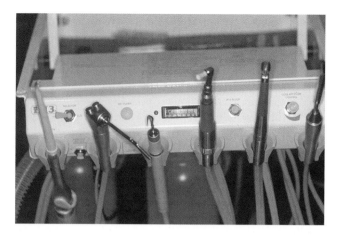

FIGURE 2.118. Control panel (iM3).

handpiece. A *three-way air/water syringe* is part of the delivery system. The syringe produces a stream of air, water, or a spray, for rinsing debris from the teeth and drying as needed during dental procedures (Figure 2.117). The control panel may be part of a cart or mounted on the dental table (Figure 2.118).

- The *foot pedal* starts and stops the system, and—in some units—controls handpiece speed.

Nitrogen-Powered

Some delivery systems use nitrogen to power handpieces. Nitrogen gas can provide clean oil-free power, which may extend the handpiece life. Because power is directly delivered from gas cylinders, compressors and air storage tanks are not necessary. There is no electrical requirement and no compressor noise. Additionally, nitrogen-driven delivery systems require less maintenance than air-driven units. The typical cost of nitrogen is less than $.50 U.S. per procedure. Nitrogen is not recommended to power air-driven sonic scalers because of the large volume of gas needed (Figure 2.119).

Filters

In-line filters that remove mineral and oil impurities from water are recommended in all types of high-speed delivery systems. Many newer units have their own water hookup for distilled water to decrease contaminants.

DENTAL HANDPIECES *Dental handpieces* are precision-built mechanical devices designed for use with rotary instruments, such as burs, stones, wheels, and discs. Handpieces can be classified according to the RPM or speed at which they operate. Handpieces that run under 100,000 RPM are classified as slow speeds.

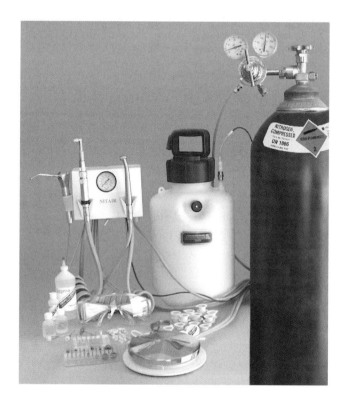

FIGURE 2.119. Nitrogen-powered delivery system: water tank, delivery unit, foot pedal.

Models running at 20,000–100,000 RPM are classified as slow-speed type II mid speed. Low speed is a subcategory of slow speed. The handpieces commonly used in veterinary medicine run less than 20,000 RPM and are classified as slow-speed type III low speeds.

The *(s)low-speed (straight) handpiece* commonly used in veterinary dentistry:

- Rotates at 5,000–20,000 RPM

- Contains forward and reverse controls
- Operates with high torque
- Generally does not use water (although some are water-equipped)
- Is used for polishing, finishing restorations, hemisection of teeth into single-rooted segments for extraction, cutting bone, and for work on dental models (Burns 952-3655, iM3 L6980, Schein 100-0701, CBi Micromite)
- Is available as one- or multiple-section units

The one-part straight handpiece accepts cutting and polishing instruments designated as *HP*. An HP designation means that the cutting or polishing instrument has a long, straight shaft that inserts directly into the straight handpiece and is tightened by rotating the collar clockwise. A prophy head, right-angled handpiece, or contra-angle may also attach to the single section unit (Figure 2.120).

The multiple-section slow-speed handpiece is composed of a low E (European type) speed motor (Figure 2.121) and a straight nose cone with a reduction gear (Figure 2.122) to drive the prophy head, right-angled handpiece, or contra-angle. Many units have a method of quickly connecting and disconnecting the motor and attachments.

The *contra-angle* attaches to the slow-speed straight handpiece to form an extension with an angle greater than 90° at the working end. Angulation provides better access to posterior teeth. The contra-angle's main use is powering burs for finishing restorations, Gates Glidden drills for pulp chamber enlargement within the crown portion of the tooth, and filling root canals using Lentulo paste fillers. (Figure 2.123) (contra-angle: Burns 951-4615, iM3 L6880).

The head of the contra-angle attachment contains either a latch or a friction type chuck, into which a den-

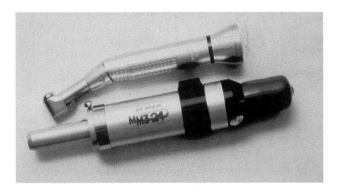

FIGURE 2.121. Slow-speed handpiece motor and nose cone.

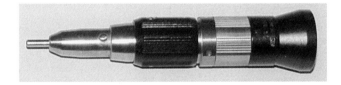

FIGURE 2.122. Slow-speed straight nose cone.

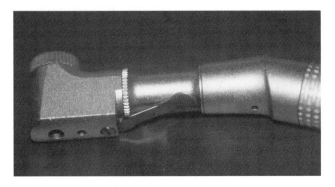

FIGURE 2.123. Contra-angle attachment.

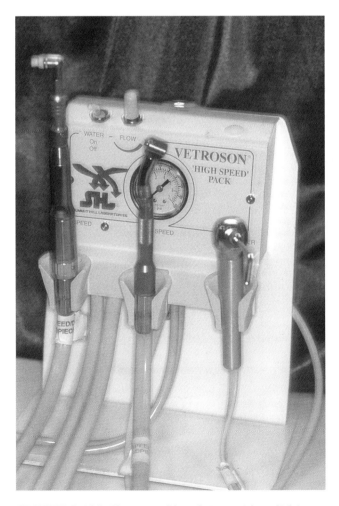

FIGURE 2.120. Slow-speed handpiece with polishing cup attached (on left).

tal bur or other rotary instrument is fitted. Latch-type contra-angles hold the end of the cutting instrument by mechanically grasping a small groove on the end of the instrument shaft. *RA* (right angle) designates latch-type instruments. Friction grip (FG) burs have short, smooth shafts without retention grooves (Figure 2.124).

Contra-angles also are available with reduction gears. A 10:1 gear reduction contra-angle decreases the operational speed ten times. The 10:1 reduction gear is identified by a screw device on the head of the angle (Figure 2.125) (Burns 951-4604, Schein 100-0026):

- The *right (prophy) angle* attaches to a slow-speed straight handpiece to form an extension with a right angle (90°) at the working tip. The right-angle handpiece is used to hold polishing cups, disks, and brushes. There are four types of prophylaxis angles used for polishing teeth:
  - The *metallic prophy angle*, which rotates 360°, might catch and/or pull hair around the animal's lip. Unfortunately, metallic prophy angles are rarely sterilized, predisposing the spread of viral and bacterial infections between patients (951-4635 Burns, iM3 Inc. L6700, Schein 100-7458) (Figure 2.126).
  - The *metallic prophy angle*, which oscillates 90° and reverses, will usually engage less lip hair (Burns 699-3990, iM3 L6970, Schein 928-2280).
  - The *disposable plastic single-use prophy angle* is preferred by the author because of reduced cross-contamination, lack of maintenance, ease of operation, and low expense (Burns 953-2598, Schein 136-2503) (Figure 2.127).
  - The *oscillating disposable prophy angle* rotates 90° and reverses. Advantages of the oscillating disposable prophy angle include decreased heat generated on the tooth surface and less lip hair caught in the polishing cup (Burns 941-2205, iM3 L7465) (Figure 2.128).

There are two ways prophy cups attach to metallic prophy angles:

- The *screw type* holds the polishing cup in place with a threaded shaft.
- The *snap-on type* has a smooth knob for attachment (Figure 2.129).

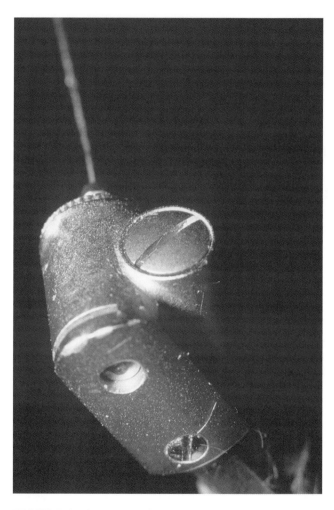

FIGURE 2.125. 10:1 reduction gear contra-angle.

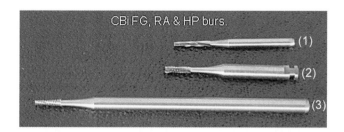

FIGURE 2.124. Friction grip (1), right angle (2), and straight handpiece burs (3).

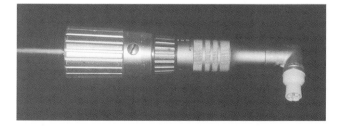

FIGURE 2.126. Metallic right-angled prophy angle attached to a straight handpiece.

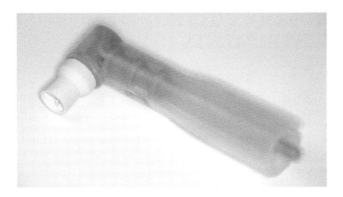

FIGURE 2.127. Disposable polishing angle.

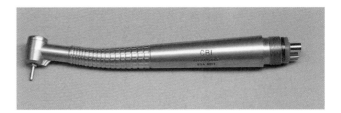

FIGURE 2.130. High-speed handpiece.

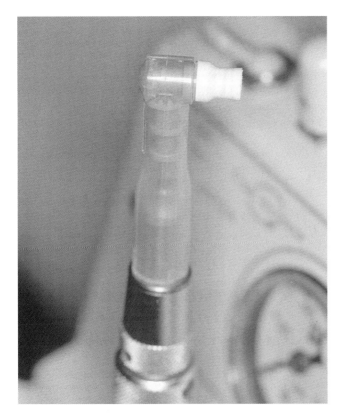

FIGURE 2.128. Oscillating disposable prophy angle (iM3).

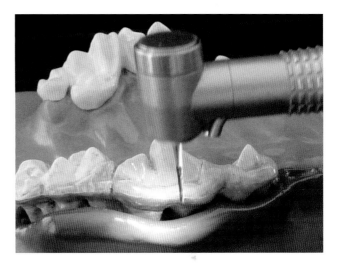

FIGURE 2.131. Fiber-optic illuminated area (CBi)

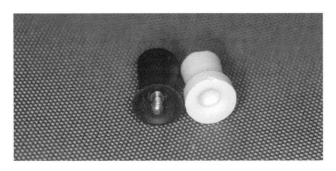

FIGURE 2.129. Screw and snap-on prophy cups.

High-speed handpieces are used when rapid and efficient cutting of the tooth and/or supporting bone is needed. High-speed handpieces are air-powered to 300,000–400,000 RPM. To avoid overheating, an irrigation spray is automatically delivered over the operative field. When choosing the handpiece style, a pediatric head gives the operator improved access in small animals. Some high-speed handpieces have a fiber-optic light built into the head. The light projects a beam from the head of the handpiece directly onto the bur and operative field.

High-speed handpieces use friction grip (FG) burs (iM3 5010 Burns 952-3893, Schein 100-9970) (Figures 2.130, 2.131). Attaching a bur to the high-speed handpiece is an easy procedure. The chuck is tightened by thumb control, built-in lever, or by using a bur inserting/removal tool (Figures 2.132–2.134).

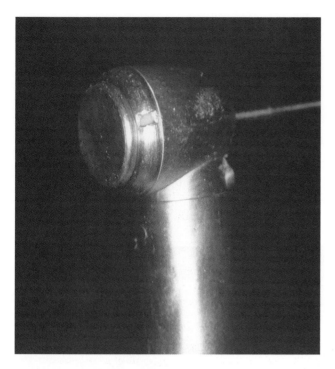

FIGURE 2.132. Thumb control chuck.

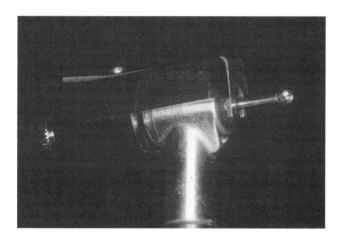

FIGURE 2.133. Bur inserting/removal tool.

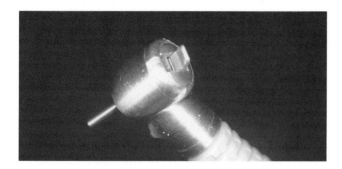

FIGURE 2.134. Lever-controlled bur insertion/removal (iM3).

ROTARY CUTTING INSTRUMENTS

Rotary cutting dental instruments are used to:

- Section multirooted teeth and/or remove part of the buccal alveolus to facilitate extraction.
- Perform alveoloplasty to smooth out sharp projections.
- Provide access points for root canal therapy.
- Provide mechanical retention of restorative material.
- Reduce and reshape teeth for crown preparation.
- Reduce crown height in crown reduction procedures.
- Remove part of the maxilla or mandible.

Burs are instruments placed into the dental hand-piece. Burs consist of two parts:

- The *shaft* fits into the handpiece.
- The *head* is the cutting end.

Operative Bur Types

Carbide steel burs (*carbides*) are used for cutting and are the most commonly used burs.

Diamond points (diamonds) are burs covered with bits of industrial diamonds used for crown preparation, bone smoothing (alveoloplasty), scarification, and shaping teeth (odontoplasty).

Burs have three types of shanks:

- Straight handpiece burs have long *straight shanks.* In dental supply catalogs, they are abbreviated as *SH* or *HP.*
- Latch-type burs have *notched shanks* and are abbreviated as *LA* (latch-type–angle) or *RA* (right-angled).
- Friction grip burs have *smooth shanks,* which are smaller in diameter than HP burs. They are used in high-speed and slow-speed (contra-angle) handpieces. Friction grip burs are identified as *FG, FG:SL,* or *SU* (friction grip surgical), or *FG:SS* (friction grip short shank used for tight areas and restorations). Surgical burs have longer (25 mm) shanks used to reach into deep recesses; restorative burs/shanks are shorter (20 mm).

Bur Shapes and Sizes

Burs come in several sizes, represented by numbers. The lower the number in a series, the smaller the bur head:

- *Round burs* are most commonly used to open the pulp chamber in preparation for endodontic treatment, ans bone smoothing. Their sizes range from

1/4–8 (Burns 952-5100, Schein 100-7205: 1/4; Burns 952-5102, Schein100-3995: 1/2; Burns 952-5108, Schein 100-4907: 1; Burns 952-5110, Schein 100-0288: 2; Burns 952-5116, Schein 100-4535: 4; Burns 952-5122, Schein 100-3220: 6; Burns 952-5126, Schein 100-6131) (Figure 2.135).

- *Pear-shaped burs* sizes 320–343 are used to cut enamel and dentin for cavity preparation, endodontic access, and preparation for restoration retention (Burns 952-5188, Schein 100-8426: 330; Burns 952-5192, Schein 100-1120: 331; Burns 942-5194, Schein 100-5616: 332).
- *Inverted cone burs* are wider at the tip with slightly rounded corners for added protection against chipping. Their sizes range from 33 1/4 to 37L (*L* indicates long). Inverted cones at one time were used to create undercut restoration sites for filling. Unfortunately, inverted cones may leave unsupported enamel at the restoration site (Burns 952-5130, Schein 100-0703: 33 1/2; Burns 952-5132, Schein 100-8454: 34; Burns 952-5134, Schein 100-2484: 35; Burns 952-5138, Schein 100-9299) (Figure 2.136).

- *Fissure burs* have grooved heads and are useful for sectioning teeth and reducing crown height. Sides of the *straight fissure bur* are parallel (Figures 2.137,2.138). The sides of the *taper fissure bur* converge toward the tip. Fissure burs may also contain cross-cuts along the blades (called *cross-cut fissure burs*), which act like sawteeth to allow additional cutting ability (Figure 2.139). Common sizes for

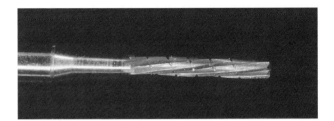

FIGURE 2.137. Straight cross-cut fissure bur.

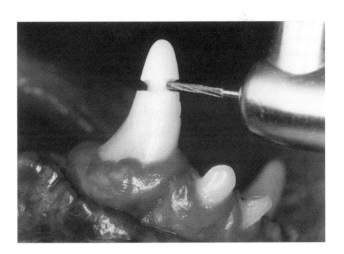

FIGURE 2.138. A straight fissure bur used for crown reduction.

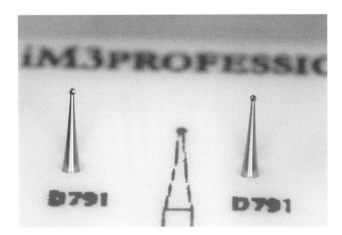

FIGURE 2.135. Round burs (iM3).

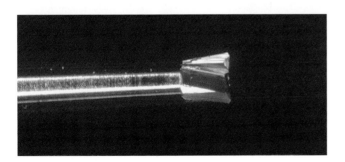

FIGURE 2.136. Inverted cone bur.

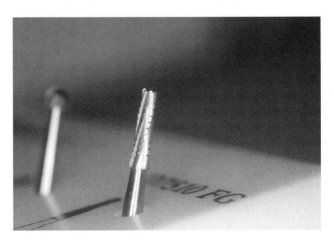

FIGURE 2.139. Tapered cross-cut fissure bur (iM3).

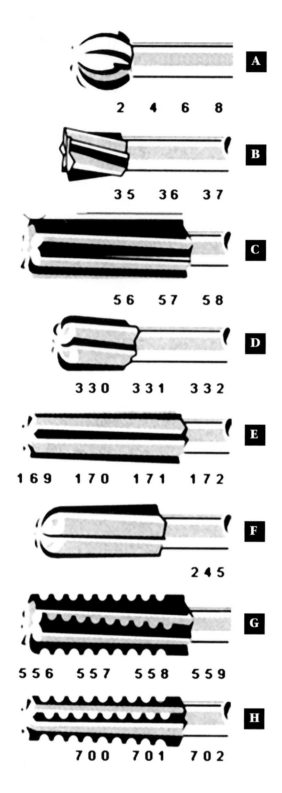

FIGURE 2.140. Bur shapes and common identification numbers: round (A), inverted cone (B), plain cylinder (C), long pear (D), plain taper (E), amalgam prep (F), cross-cut fissure (G), tapered cross-cut fissure (H).

straight fissure burs range from 55–60, 56L–59L. Cross-cut straight fissure burs range from 555–561, 556L–560L. Sizes for taper fissure burs range from 699–703, 699–703L (Burns 952-5210, Schein 100-0281: 556; Burns 952-5204, Schein 100-3307: 557; Burns 952-5210, Schein 100-3104: 558; Schein 100-9613: 699; Burns 952-5224, Schein 100-4546: 701; Burns 952-5236, Schein 100-7228: 701L) (Figure 2.140).

• *Diamond burs* have bits of industrial diamonds embedded into the working surfaces. Diamonds are used in many places that carbides are, and especially in restorative dentistry to prepare crowns for impressions, and to help finish composite restorations (Burns 952-6310, Schein 878-3648 flame diamonds preferred by author for crown preparation) (Figure 2.141).

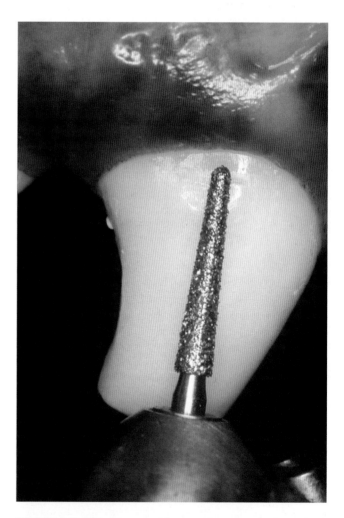

FIGURE 2.141. Diamond bur used to prepare margin line for crown.

- *Trimming* and *finishing burs* are designed for completing restorations, odontoplasty, and alveoloplasty. The more flutes on a finishing bur, the finer the finish (for example, a 30-fluted bur, also know as a *fine finishing bur*, produces a smoother finish than does a 12-fluted bur) (blade trimming and finishing bur kit Burns 952-5234, Schein 100-3833) (Figure 2.142).
- *Stones* are used for polishing and finishing restorations. Stones are mounted on a mandrel (mounting device), which is inserted into the handpiece (Burns 888-3400, Schein 195-4022 Shofu finishing kit-Dura Green and Dura white stones). Stones are identified by color:
  - *White* stone burs are commonly used in veterinary dentistry to finish composite restorations, or to smooth minor enamel defects (Burns 823-1278, Schein 195-1823) (Figure 2.143).
  - *Green* stones are used to finish amalgam and smooth enamel.
  - *Gray* stones, made of carborundum and rubber, are used for polishing fabricated crowns (Burns 823-1256, Schein 195-7905).

- *Discs* are circular cutting instruments made of paper, rubber, diamond chips, or metal used to finish restorations or incise hard tissue (teeth or bone). The disc may be flat, oval, or concave with the abrasive material placed on the inside, outside, or on both sides. *Only a clinician trained in advanced veterinary dentistry should use diamond discs because of their greater potential for patient/surgeon injury.* Carbide or diamond burs are safer and as effective.

Finishing discs are used to shape and smooth restorations. Finishing discs are available in various grades of abrasiveness, from coarse to superfine. They are used sequentially from coarse (to shape restorations) to fine grade (to smooth surfaces). The finest-grade disk is used with a paste (Burns 868-0690, Schein 294-8195 finishing disc kit) (Figures 2.144, 2.145).

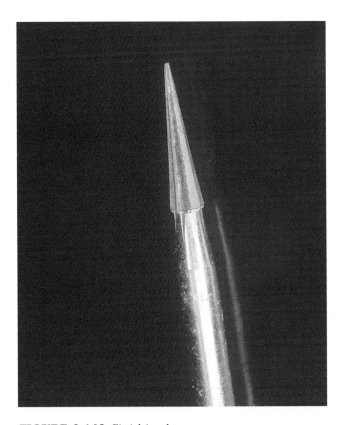

FIGURE 2.142. Finishing bur.

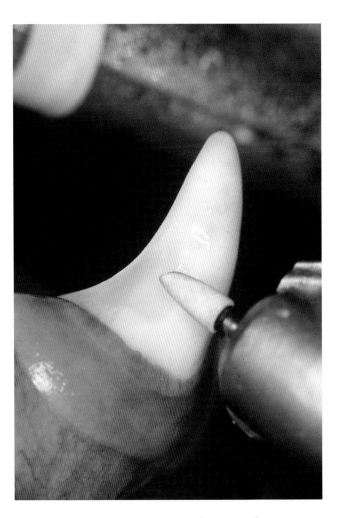

FIGURE 2.143. White stone used to smooth out restoration.

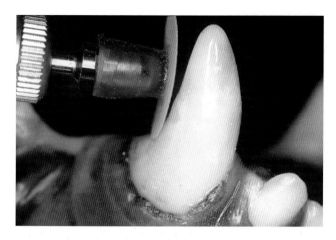

FIGURE 2.144. Finishing disc.

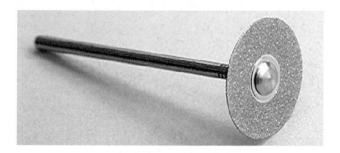

FIGURE 2.145. Diamond disc attached with centered mandrel.

Bur Care

Burs are surgical cutting instruments and should be cleaned and sterilized before each use. To remove debris lodged in the bur head, the bur is removed from the handpiece; rinsed; brushed free of debris with a nylon (Schein 953-9664) or wire (Burns 950-2305, Schein 365-1135) bur brush, or pencil eraser; and soaked in a cold sterile solution for 24 hours or autoclaved.

EQUIPMENT MAINTENANCE

Dental handpieces are precision instruments and must be maintained properly to ensure optimal operation and maximum life. The veterinarian or technician should check with the manufacture's instructions for specific care.

A generic lubrication/sterilization process consists of these steps:

1. At the end of each procedure, scrub the handpiece with gauze, a sponge, or a brush and cleaning solution to remove debris.

2. Following the manufacturer's instructions, rinse the handpiece without immersion.
3. Dry the handpiece with gauze, paper towel, or air from the air/water syringe.
4. For handpieces requiring lubrication, add three drops of lubricant to the smaller of the two large holes (drive air tube) at the connection area. (Figures 2.146, 2.147). Note: some handpieces are lubrication-free and will be destroyed if lubricated; check manufacturer's instructions.
5. Briefly power the handpiece with bur inserted to remove excess lubricant.
6. Place the handpiece in an autoclavable envelope.
7. Sterilize the handpiece in the autoclave.

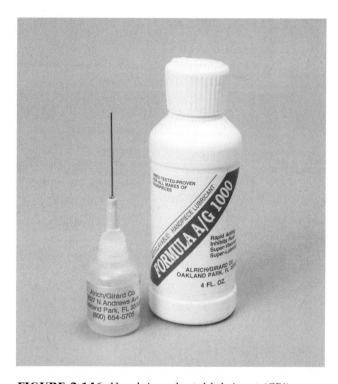

FIGURE 2.146. Handpiece dental lubricant (CBi).

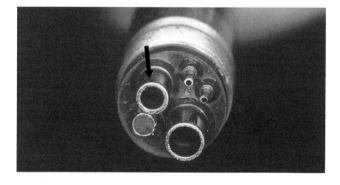

FIGURE 2.147. Arrow pointing to correct hole to apply lubricant.

Replacing the High-Speed Turbine

The turbine is secured in the high-speed handpiece head by a screwed faceplate. After the faceplate is unscrewed using the manufacturer-supplied tool, the turbine can be easily replaced (Figures 2.148–2.152).

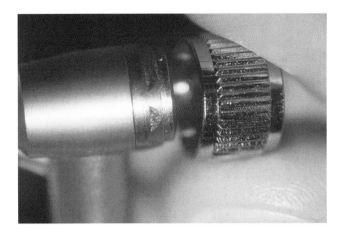

FIGURE 2.148. Turbine removal tool used to unscrew the turbine cover.

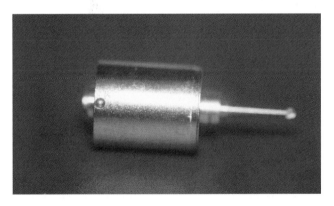

FIGURE 2.149. Canister turbine.

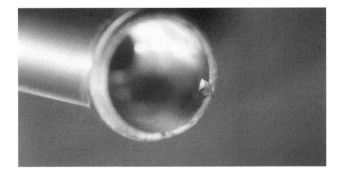

FIGURE 2.150. Handpiece head without turbine (note indented space for turbine).

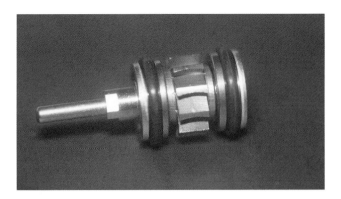

FIGURE 2.151. Open turbine.

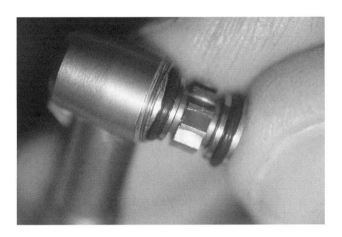

FIGURE 2.152. Snapping turbine into handpiece head.

To clean and lubricate the low-speed handpiece and attachments, use the following steps:

1. Place the working end of the handpiece into a small bottle of handpiece-cleaning solvent (Schein 772-5718, CBi handpiece solvent, Burns 952-1065) (Figure 2.153).
2. Power the handpiece backward and forward for 1 minute (Figure 2.154).
3. Remove the handpiece from the cleaner and wipe dry.
4. Periodically, disassemble the handpiece, using the special wrench furnished by the manufacturer (Figures 2.155, 2.156).
5. Following the manufacture's instructions, place one drop of liquid lubricant on the neck of the head, one drop on each gear of the gear and shaft assembly, and three drops into the back end of the angle. Alternatively, place heavy lubricant (Schein 100-2037) (petroleum jelly) on the gears of the handpiece before reassembly (Burns 952-1057) (Figure 2.157).

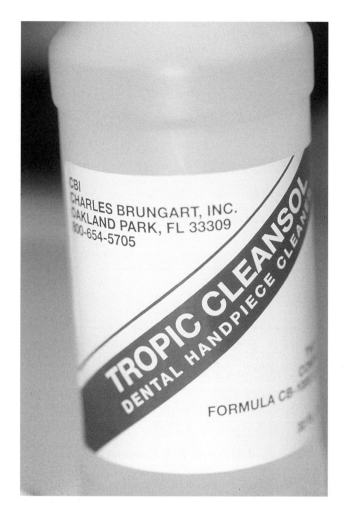

FIGURE 2.153. Handpiece cleaner.

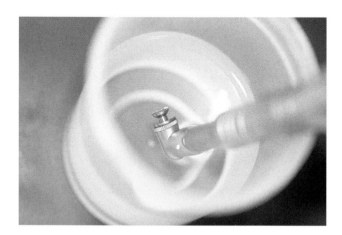

FIGURE 2.154. Polishing angle in container with cleaner.

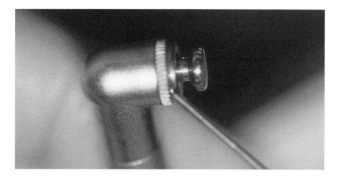

FIGURE 2.155. Tool used to remove polishing angle gear.

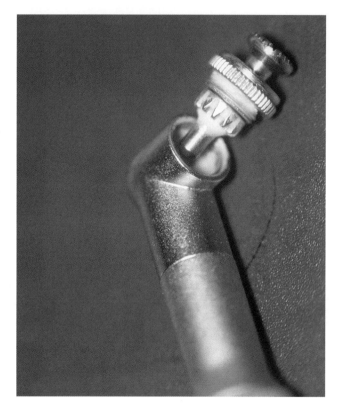

FIGURE 2.156. Removed gear.

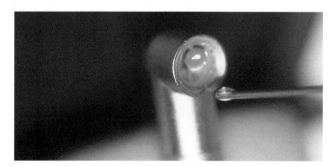

FIGURE 2.157. Application of oil to head of polishing angle.

Compressor Maintenance

OIL LEVEL   Oil-cooled compressors are equipped with a dipstick or view port to monitor the oil level. The owner's manual should be checked for the recommended replacement oil if needed (Schein 100-4746 VetBase oil) (Figure 2.158).

Condensation in the air storage tank accumulates with each use. The accumulated fluid should be drained daily/weekly or monthly depending on use and ambient humidity (Figure 2.159).

Table 2.2 lists the recommended schedule for preventative compressor/storage tank maintenance.

INFECTION CONTROL

Disinfection is the process of destroying microbial life by placing instruments in a solution (Example: Cidex) for a specified period. Chemical disinfection does not eliminate all viruses and spores.

Sterilization kills all microorganisms. The autoclave is a steam chamber for sterilizing instruments. During the sterilization cycle, distilled water flows into the chamber and is heated to create steam. Because the chamber is sealed, pressure increases to approximately

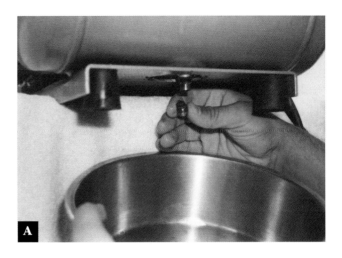

A

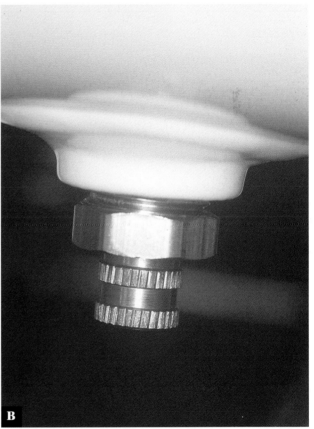

B

FIGURE 2.159. Screw device used to empty condensation from air tank (iM3).

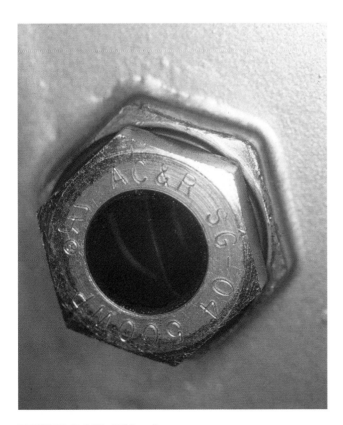

FIGURE 2.158. Oil level gauge.

15 pounds per square inch. The increase in pressure causes the heat of the steam to rise to approximately 250° F. When the instruments are exposed to this high pressure/steam temperature for 15 minutes or more, sterilization occurs. Dental instruments used in the

Table 2.2. Preventative compressor/storage tank maintenance.

	Weekly	Monthly
Check oil level. Do not overfill.	X	
Drain condensation from air storage tank.	X	
Check compressor and air line for leaks.		X
Visually check and wipe unit with soft rag. Dust and dirt prevents cooling. If necessary, use paraffin on rag to remove sticky adhesions.		X
Inspect, clean, or replace intake filter. Hair and dust can clog a filter, forcing the compressor to overwork.		X

mouth should be sterile. After cleaning, instruments can be placed in an autoclavable see-through sleeve and sterilized (Figures 2.160–2.163).

Patient and operator infection control requires the following:

- An individual set of sterilized instruments be used on each patient. High- and slow-speed handpieces should be sterilized before each use.
- Human dentists have developed aggressive infection control procedures in response to spreading HIV and hepatitis among patients and staff. Many of these protocols can be adopted in veterinary hospitals for similar reasons. Viral and bacterial particles may become lodged in the paste remaining on the head of

the prophy angle and transmitted to the next patient even if the prophy cup is changed. Disposable prophy angles or autoclaved metal angles are recom-

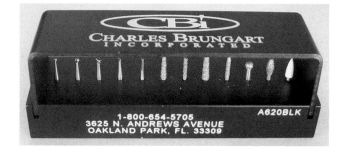

FIGURE 2.161. Burs loaded into bur block before sterilization.

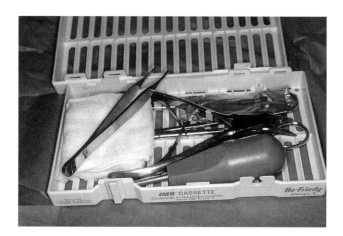

FIGURE 2.160. Extraction pack and dental storage tray before sterilization.

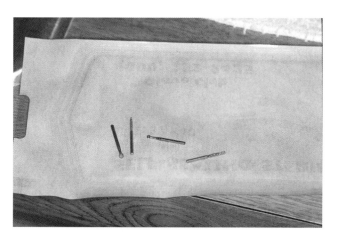

FIGURE 2.162. Sterile burs.

mended for all patients (Burns 951-8500, iM3 L7465, Schein 136-2503).

- A mask, gloves, ear, and eye protection should be worn when performing dental care (Schein 100-7382).
- The oral cavity should be rinsed with a 0.12% chlorhexidine solution before periodontal care to reduce the number of bacteria (Burns 953-2598, iM3 C3130, Schein 277-8728).
- All dental procedures should be performed under general anesthesia with a cuffed disinfected endotracheal tube in place and the oropharynx packed with absorbent material.
- The patient's head should be angled downward to promote drainage.
- High-speed delivery system fluid lines can develop a biofilm of potentially harmful viruses and bacteria. Chlorhexidine can be used to flush the fluid lines decreasing the viral and bacterial load (CLS Flush system iM3 F3130) (Figure 2.164).
- Polishing paste is available in individual cups (Burns

951-8652, Schein 100-9016) or in bulk form in a supply container. When using the bulk container, the paste should be applied with a tongue depressor to avoid contaminating the contents of the container.

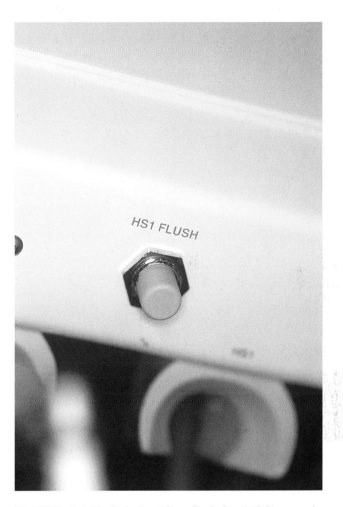

FIGURE 2.164. Chlorhexidine flush for iM3 lines and handpieces.

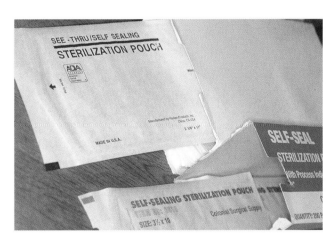

FIGURE 2.163. Sterile pouches.

3
Patient Monitoring

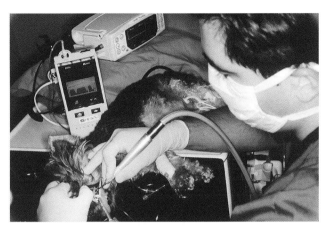

FIGURE 3.1. Pulse oximetry and capnography used to monitor patient receiving dental care.

General anesthesia is required to perform most dental procedures (Figure 3.1). To make the anesthetic event as safe as possible, the veterinarian must be able to work with the following:

- A patient that has been evaluated pre-operatively with a physical examination, as well as hematological, urologic, radiographic, electrocardiographic, and ultrasound examinations where indicated by age and/or condition
- Safe and effective pre-anesthetic and anesthetic agents
- A monitoring and recording system that accurately measures the patient's response to anesthesia
- A veterinary technician to help with anesthesia monitoring while the veterinarian performs the dental procedure

Anesthesia monitoring varies from observing respiration and noting mucous membrane color, to arterial blood gas evaluation. The general practitioner has res-

piratory, electrocardiograph, pulse oximetry, blood pressure, and CO_2 monitors available for periodic and/or continuous noninvasive evaluation of the patient's response to anesthesia. Blood gas measurements provide accurate information about a patient's ventilation, oxygenation, and acid-base status, but are seldom available to the veterinarian in private practice.

ELECTROCARDIOGRAM

Electrocardiogram units include the HESKA Vet/ECG 2000 Monitor (Figure 3.2), PAM from VMS, VetSpecs VSM-4, and Biolog.

ECG evaluations before and during anesthesia give the veterinarian information regarding heart rate, rhythm, and abnormal complexes. Lead 2 is primarily used to monitor rate and rhythm in patients under anesthesia. Continuous monitoring of the ECG pattern allows early recognition of electrical changes associated with disorders of rate, rhythm, and conduction. Handheld units used as part of the pre-operative patient

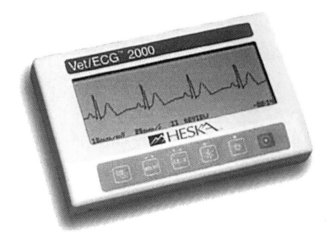

FIGURE 3.2. HESKA handheld ECG monitor.

evaluation can also perform single lead continuous readings during the dental procedure (Figures 3.3,3.4).

Electrocardiograms can also be generated using esophageal probes. While anesthetized, the probe is inserted into the esophagus until the distal electrode reaches the area dorsal to the heart base. If the ECG tracing appears small, the probe may not be inserted far enough. If inserted too deep, the tracing may appear inverted (Figure 3.5).

The electrocardiogram gives minimal information on

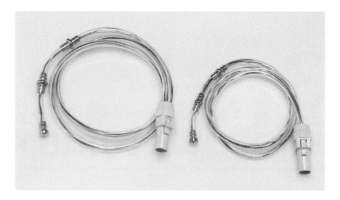

FIGURE 3.5. Esophageal probes used to obtain electrocardiograph during anesthesia.

cardiac contractility and tissue perfusion. Presence of normal-appearing complexes does not indicate that the patient's tissues are adequately perfused. The ECG should be used with another form of monitoring (end tidal CO_2 and/or blood pressure) for patient evaluation during anesthesia.

RESPIRATORY MONITOR

Respiratory monitors include Escort Prism Schein 310-4019, HESKA Vet/Ox 4800 monitor (ECG, respiration, pulse oximetry, temperature), VetSpecs VSM-5.

Respiratory depression—from anesthetic premedication, induction agents, and/or inhalant anesthetics—is common. The effects of these medications are dose-dependent and, when multiple agents are used, may become synergistic.

Apnea monitors alert the clinician when the patient's respiratory rate is depressed or stops. Most respiratory monitors detect exhaled airflow. The sensor is attached between the endotracheal tube and the anesthesia machine's delivery tubes. Every time the animal exhales, the monitor emits an audible sound. When choosing an apnea monitor it is important that the signal be loud enough to easily hear over the ambient noise. The monitor should also be equipped with a sensitivity adjustment.

PULSE OXIMETER

Pulse oximeters include HESKA Vet/Ox G2 digital monitor (Figure 3.6) and VetSpecs VSM-4 (pulse rate and SpO_2).

Hemoglobin travels through the blood in two forms: oxyhemoglobin and reduced hemoglobin. Most oxygen

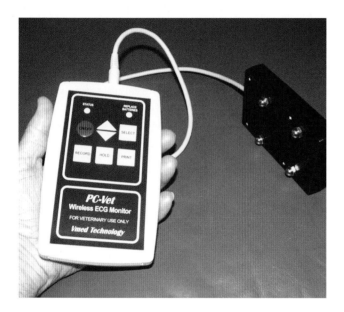

FIGURE 3.3. Battery-operated hand-held lead II ECG recorder (PC-Vet).

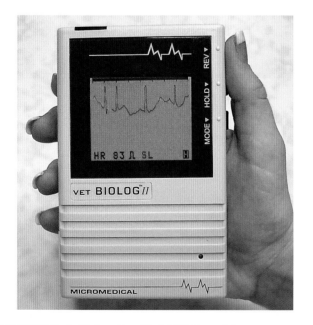

FIGURE 3.4. Biolog Handheld ECG machine.

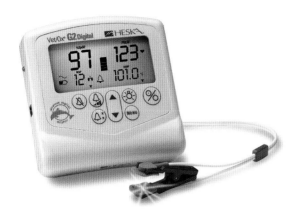

FIGURE 3.6. G2 digital monitor (HESKA).

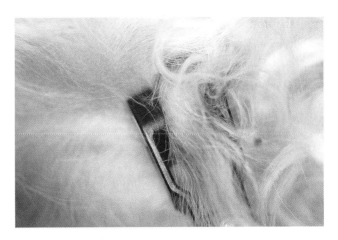

FIGURE 3.8. Application of probe to vulva.

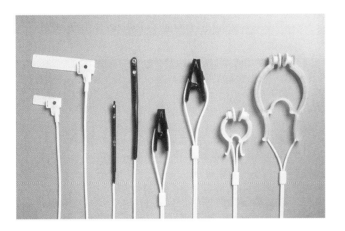

FIGURE 3.7. Oximetry probes (HESKA).

transported to the tissues is carried on the hemoglobin molecule. Pulse oximetry is used for noninvasive oxygen saturation measurement. The pulse oximeter estimates the patient's oxygenation via light absorption measurement of oxygen saturation of arterial hemoglobin.

A probe is used to pass and measure light through pulsating blood vessels. One of the most effective placements of the oximeter probe is on the tongue. Dental procedures by their nature involve movement and instruments in the mouth, which often dislodge the tongue oximeter probe. Other areas for probe placement include the pinna, toe, prepuce, vulva, metacarpus (tarsus), digits, and tail. Rectal probes are also available. Excessive pigmentation and hair usually preclude accurate readings (Figures 3.7,3.8).

Oxygen saturation should be maintained between 95% and 100%, particularly if the animal is breathing 100% oxygen. Saturation readings of 90% or less indicate marked desaturation, hypovolemia, shock, or anemia.

The oximeter measures only the level of oxygen saturation and heart rate, which may be elevated when the patient hyperventilates in response to discomfort. Unfortunately, a hyperventilating patient may also inhale excessive anesthetic gas leading to hypovolemia. Pulse oximeters do not measure how forcefully the heart is beating. Oximetry is not a reliable sentinel for hypovolemia.

BLOOD PRESSURE MEASUREMENT

In human medicine, blood pressure measurement is part of most examinations and constantly evaluated under general anesthesia. In small animal practice, blood pressure measurement is equally important. The mean arterial pressure (MAP) should be greater than 60 mm Hg under anesthesia. If blood pressure drops below this level, the anesthetic concentration should be lowered.

Invasive blood pressure measuring involves placing a catheter into an artery connected to a transducer. Although the procedure may yield accurate results, it is not practical in clinical practice.

Noninvasive blood pressure measurement uses a cuff placed around the patient's limb or tail at the level of the heart. In cats, the tail base may have to be clipped. The cuff diameter should be 40% of the circumference of the limb or tail base (3 cm in cats, 4 cm for small dogs, and 5 cm and up for larger dogs). Normal readings for anesthetized dogs and cats are systolic 90–105

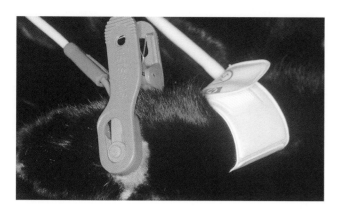

FIGURE 3.9. Application of pressure plethsmography cuff to a cat's carpal joint (VetSpecs).

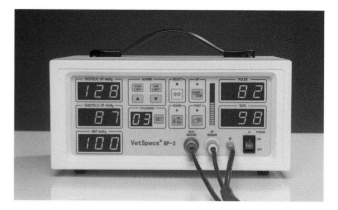

FIGURE 3.11. Blood pressure monitor (VetSpecs).

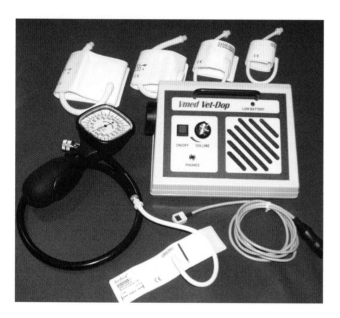

FIGURE 3.10. VetDop battery-operated Doppler blood pressure system for small animals.

mm Hg, diastolic 40–60 mm Hg, and mean 60–70 mm Hg (Figure 3.9).

Commonly used types of noninvasive blood pressure monitors include

• Doppler
• Pressure-plethysmography

Doppler measures systolic arterial pressure. The pitch of the sound reflected from the moving blood cells is proportional to their velocity. A piezoelectric crystal microphone, amplifier, inflatable cuff, manometer, and earphones are used. To use Doppler, an ultrasonic flow detector is placed over an artery and taped in place. A cuff is placed proximal to the crystal and inflated until blood flow is occluded. The cuff is slowly deflated. The pressure at which blood flow becomes audible again is the systolic pressure (Vmed VetDop, Park's Doppler Schein 568-7368) (Figure 3.10).

Pressure-plethysmography provides systolic, diastolic, and mean pressure using an inflatable cuff to occlude blood flow and a sensor placed distal to the cuff to detect arterial pulsation. The cuff is wrapped above the carpus, tail, or below the hock, and the sensor placed on the same limb just below the cuff. Accurate placement over an artery is not essential. The cuff automatically inflates to a pressure, which occludes the underlying arteries, and then deflates gradually. When the cuff pressure is equal to systolic arterial pressure, flow proceeds and arterial pulsation returns. After systolic and diastolic arterial pressures have been determined, the computer calculates the mean pressure (Figure 3.11).

CARBON DIOXIDE MEASUREMENT-END TIDAL CAPNOGRAPHY

Carbon dioxide is produced by animal cells, transported by the circulatory system, and eliminated through the lungs. Alveoli are sites of gas exchange. The highest concentration of carbon dioxide should occur at the end of expiration when the diluted gases from the trachea and primary bronchi are no longer being sampled. Changes in carbon dioxide levels reflect changes in metabolism, circulation, and respiration (Figure 3.12). Expired carbon dioxide or end tidal carbon dioxide (ETCO2) is a measurement of the following:

• CO2 produced in the cells, a function of metabolism

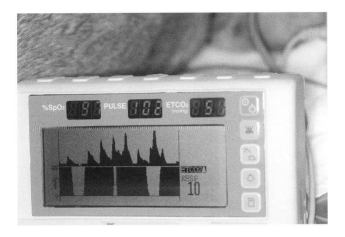

FIGURE 3.12. Carbon dioxide monitor.

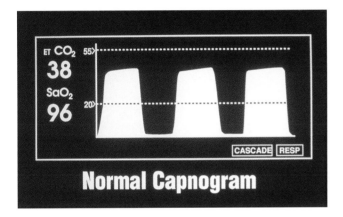

FIGURE 3.13. Normal CO_2 readings.

- CO_2 transported from the cells to the lung, a function of circulation
- CO_2 eliminated by the lungs

Capnography gives a graphic as well as a numerical readout of the carbon dioxide concentration in the patient's exhaled gases. Capnography provides a means to assess ventilation, integrity of the airway, and breathing circuit, as well as cardiopulmonary function. Measuring expired carbon dioxide allows an estimation of arterial CO_2, which lets the operator know whether the anesthetized patient is ventilating adequately.

A capnogram is the graphic portrayal of the changing concentration of exhaled carbon dioxide during the respiratory cycle. P-Q-R-S letters are used to refer to different portions of the waveform. The normal waveform should have a baseline of zero during inspiration (inspiratory baseline). This is followed by an expiratory upstroke (P-Q) that contains little or no CO_2 and moves the curve upward until it levels out at a plateau

(Q-R). Concentration of CO_2 continues to increase until its maximum is reached at point R just before the onset of inhalation (inspiratory down stroke). The height, frequency, shape, rhythm, and baseline position of the waveform are monitored during anesthesia. The concentration of the CO_2 in the sample is reflected by the height of the wave. Changes in the standard waveform should alert the veterinarian to a problem with the patient, the airway, or the anesthetic circuit. Normal readings should be in the 35–45 mm Hg range (Figure 3.13).

Increased CO_2 readings can be seen due to the following (Figure 3.14):

- Mild to moderate airway obstruction
- Hypoventilation
- Faulty check valves
- Exhausted soda lime

Decreased CO_2 readings can be seen due to the following (Figure 3.15):

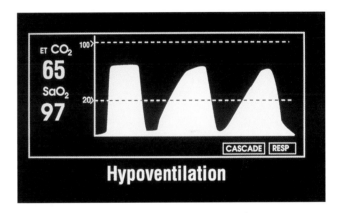

FIGURE 3.14. Increased CO_2 readings.

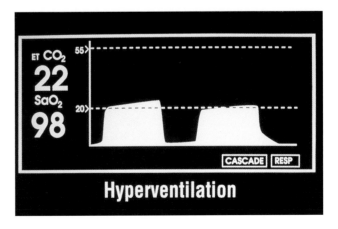

FIGURE 3.15. Decreased CO_2 readings.

- Hyperventilation
- Extubation
- Disconnection from the breathing circuit
- Esophageal intubation
- Cardiac arrest

TEMPERATURE MONITORING

Temperature control and monitoring is important for dental patients. Dental procedures often last hours during which the animal may be exposed to air conditioning and water irrigation. As the patient temperature decreases, so does the blood pressure and heart rate. Temperature monitors can be as straightforward as a technician inserting a rectal thermometer every 15 minutes and recording results, to a real-time constant digital evaluation (Figure 3.16).

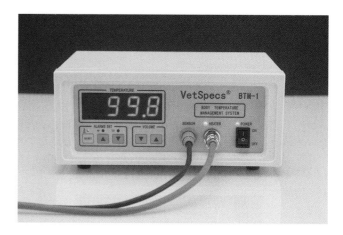

FIGURE 3.16. Constant temperature management system (VetSpecs).

4
Dental Radiography

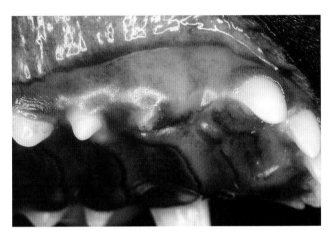

FIGURE 4.1. Right anterior maxilla of 9-month-old dog whose canine is not visually apparent.

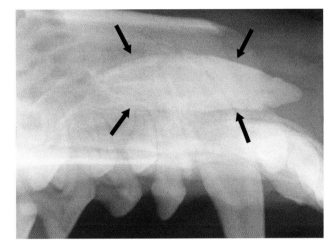

FIGURE 4.2. Radiograph showing "missing" canine located dorsally.

Dental radiology should play an integral part in most dental cases. This chapter covers radiographic indications, equipment, materials, and interpretation of radiographic findings.

Intraoral radiography offers the capability of:

- Viewing lesions below the gingiva and inside the tooth (Figures 4.1,4.2).
- Evaluating an area where the teeth are not clinically apparent (Figures 4.3,4.4).
- Determining, in some cases, the cause of chronic nasal discharge.
- Documenting the presence of lesions to support treatment decisions (Figures 4.5,4.6).
- Evaluating tooth vitality.
- Evaluating pre-operative, intra-operative, and post-operative endodontic treatment (Figure 4.7).
- Following the progression of pulpal pathology and/or periodontal disease (Figures 4.8,4.9).

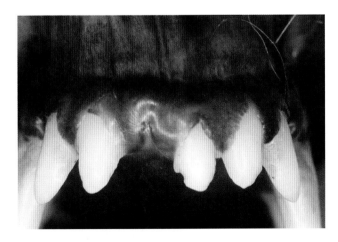

FIGURE 4.3. Clinically missing right first maxillary incisor.

Glossary

Alveolar bone encases and supports the tooth structure.

Alveolar bone loss radiographically appears as decreased bone surrounding the tooth roots in the maxilla or mandible.

Alveolar margin is the most coronal portion of alveolar bone located between the teeth. The alveolar margin is composed of dense cortical bone.

Bisecting angle is a radiographic technique in which the central x-ray beam is positioned perpendicular to the line that bisects the angle formed by the long axis of the tooth and film packet.

Buccal object rule allows localization of superimposed dental structures or foreign objects viewed on a radiograph using parallax shift.

Cementoenamel junction (CEJ) is the area where the cementum and enamel meet.

Chairside processor is a portable light-safe box with developer, fixer, and distilled water in small containers used to develop exposed dental radiographs.

Condensing osteitis appears as a well-circumscribed radiopaque focal lesion adjacent to the tooth's apex in response to chronic inflammation.

Contrast is the relative difference in densities between adjacent areas on a radiograph.

Control panel is the part of the radiograph unit that controls exposure settings.

Density is the overall darkness or blackness of a radiograph.

Elongation is a radiographic image error resulting from insufficient tube head vertical angulation. Elongated teeth on the film appear longer than their actual length.

External resorption is the cementoclastic and dentinoclastic action that takes place on a root.

Foreshortening is a radiographic image error resulting from excessive vertical angulation. Foreshortened teeth on the film appear shorter than their actual length.

Furcation is the anatomic area of a multirooted tooth where the roots diverge.

Horizontal bone loss is the full thickness loss of alveolar crestal bone parallel to the cementoenamel junction.

Internal resorption is a lesion originating from the pulp extending to the adjacent dentin usually caused by previous trauma.

Interproximal refers to an area between two adjacent tooth surfaces within the same arch.

Lamina dura is the radiographic term for the cribiform plate and dense alveolar bone surrounding a root. The lamina dura appears as a dense white line adjacent to the periodontal ligament space.

Mental foramina are radiolucent openings (holes) in the bone located on the lateral surface of the mandible in the region of the first three mandibular premolars.

Overdeveloped film is a dark film resulting from excess development time, an inaccurate timer, or hot developer solution.

Overexposed film is a dark film that results from excessive exposure time, kilovoltage, or milliamperage.

Parallel technique places the film parallel to the long axis of the tooth with the central x-ray beam positioned perpendicular to the film.

Periapical refers to an area around the tooth apex.

Periodontal ligament space is the radiolucent area between the root of a tooth and the lamina dura.

Position indicating device (PID) is the cone portion of the x-ray tube head.

Underdeveloped film appears light from too little time in the developer, cool developer solution, or stale developer.

Underexposed film is a light film that results from inadequate exposure time, kilovoltage, or milliamperage.

Vertical bone loss is destruction of periodontal support adjacent to the tooth root, with normal or near normal crestal bone height.

- Evaluating the number of permanent teeth present in a puppy or kitten as part of a detailed soundness examination before they erupt. Some breeds must have a minimum number of teeth to be accepted in the show ring.
- Anatomical orientation and documentation of root structure before extraction.
- Post-operative evaluation after extraction to confirm all root fragments were removed. (Figures 4.10, 4.11).
- Pre-operative evaluation of gross tumor margins to help plan surgery (Figure 4.12).
- Treatment planning when periodontal disease is present anywhere in the mouth (gingival bleeding on probing, tooth mobility, gingival recession, furcation exposure, increased probing depths).
- Evaluating feline odontoclastic resorptive lesions (FORLs).
- Evaluating mandibular and maxillary fractures.
- Evaluating tooth support before and after orthodontic care.
- Evaluating oral and facial swellings.
- Obtaining baseline records for comparison with future radiographic studies.

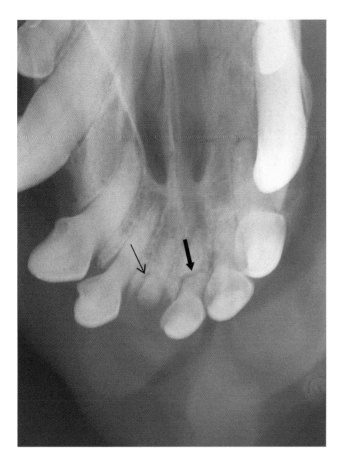

FIGURE 4.4. Radiograph showing incisor root fragment (thin arrow) plus fractured adjacent incisor (bold arrow).

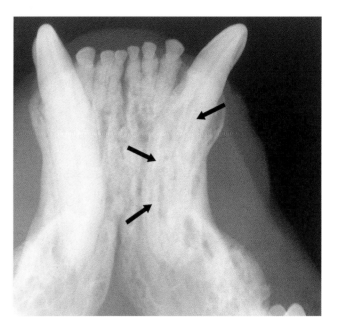

FIGURE 4.6. One mandibular canine appears normal on this 8-year-old feline but the other canine root shows radiographic evidence of internal resorption requiring extraction.

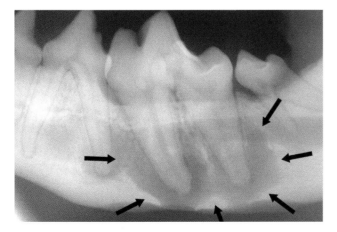

FIGURE 4.5. The crown of the mandibular fourth premolar and first molar appears normal but the roots have periapical radiolucencies requiring extraction.

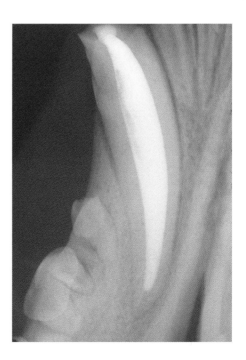

FIGURE 4.7. Proper root canal fill in a 1-year-old dog treated with conventional endodontics.

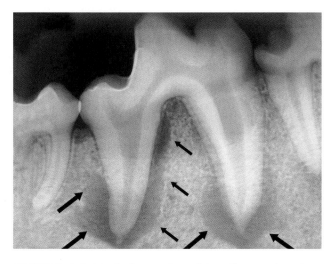

FIGURE 4.8. Marked periodontal (small arrows) and apical (large arrows) radiographic lesions in a fractured tooth that is also affected with periodontal disease.

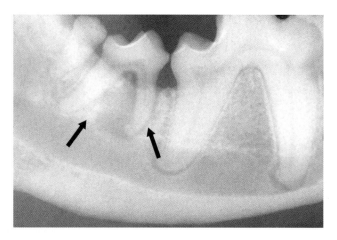

FIGURE 4.10. Pre-operative radiograph showing root structure of mandibular second molar to be extracted.

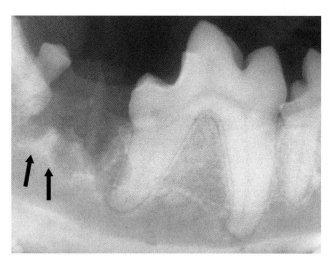

FIGURE 4.11. Intra-operative radiograph revealing root fragments to be removed.

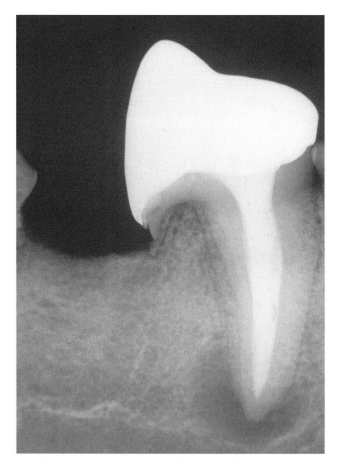

FIGURE 4.9. Six-month follow-up after hemisection and root canal therapy of the tooth in figure 4.8, showing bone regrowth and partial resoluton of radiographic endodontic and periodontic lesions.

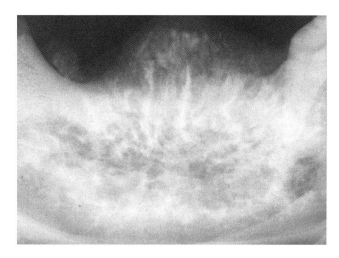

FIGURE 4.12. Pre-operative radiograph of a mandibular tumor for evaluation of surgical margins.

INCORPORATING DENTAL RADIOGRAPHY INTO A GENERAL PRACTICE

Periodontal disease is the most common ailment affecting small animals. Frequently, patients presented for "routine teeth cleaning and examination" have periodontal disease. The decision to extract, perform flap surgery, apply local antibiotics, or only clean and polish, is made by visual examination, probing depths, and radiographs.

Logistically, when the patient is admitted to the hospital for dental evaluation and care, the pet owner cannot receive an accurate treatment plan until a thorough tooth-by-tooth assessment is conducted. The client is encouraged to return to the office or call at a preset time, or is paged usually 2 or 3 hours later to discuss the treatment plan based on clinical exam and radiographic findings while the patent is still anesthetized. After the therapy plan and fees are approved, the patient is treated.

The following is a sample timeline for one patient (additional patients are fitted into the schedule depending on availability of anesthesia units and staff):

- 9:00 a.m.: The patient is examined or left for an examination. The owner is advised to call the office or come back at noon for dental examination and radiograph findings, while the animal is still anesthetized.
- 9:30–10:30: Preoperative laboratory and electrocardiograph evaluation. An intravenous catheter is placed.
- 10:30–11:45: The patient is anesthetized, teeth cleaned, mouth probed charted, and radiographs taken by staff. A treatment plan is formulated by the veterinarian and fees calculated.
- 12:00 p.m.: The client calls or returns to the office. The veterinarian discusses exam findings, treatment plan, and fees while the technician is completing the teeth cleaning procedure.
- 12:10: When the treatment plan is approved, additional therapy begins.
- 2:00: Therapy completed (time depends on procedure).
- 5:00–6:00: The patient is released to its owners.

THE RADIOGRAPH UNIT

Although the veterinarian may choose to use a conventional radiograph unit, delivery of *efficient* dental imaging necessitates the use of the dental radiograph unit (Figure 4.13).

Advantages of using the conventional radiograph unit include the following (Figure 4.14):

- The veterinarian does not need to spend additional money to purchase more equipment.
- The conventional radiograph unit can expose quality films.

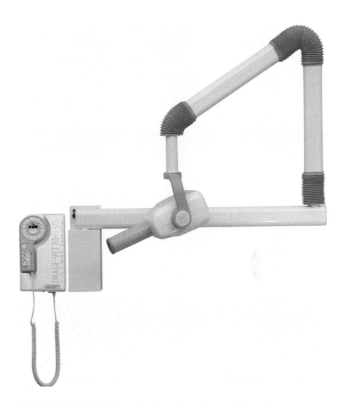

FIGURE 4.13. Dent X dental radiograph unit.

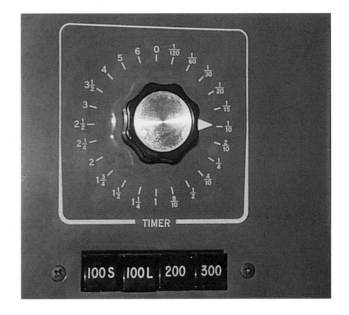

FIGURE 4.14. Standard radiograph unit set for dental film exposure.

Advantages of using the dental radiograph unit include the following:

• Most dental units cost between $3,000 and $5,000 U.S., so they are economical.
• Shorter film focal length and fixed collimation results in less scattered radiation and radiation exposure to the patient and operator.
• Extension arms of various lengths allow vertical, horizontal, and rotational movement, resulting in less patient repositioning.
• The long arm can reach closely located operatory areas.
• Radiographs can be obtained on the dental operatory table rather than moving the patient to radiography area.

Anatomy of a Dental X-ray Unit

The *position indicating device (PID)* is an extension placed on the tube head at the collimator attachment. To minimize the amount of radiation exposure, the PID is lead-lined. (*Note:* older units were not lead-lined.) The shape of the PID may be circular or rectangular (Figure 4.15).

The *arm* connects the radiograph tube and the control panel.

The *control panel* contains the timer, kilovoltage, (kV) and/or milliamperage (mA) regulators (Figure 4.16). Most machines have a fixed mA (7–15) and kV (50–120). The only variable parameter is duration of the exposure in fractions of seconds or pulses.

The *exposure timer* regulates the time an exposure lasts. The timer is engaged only while the switch is depressed and automatically cuts off the electric current at the end of the preset exposure. The timer resets after each exposure.

Most American dental units use 110V, 60Hz AC electricity. A separate dedicated electrical circuit is recommended.

The *kilovoltage peak* (kVp) determines the penetrating power or quality of radiation produced. Kilovoltage affects the contrast (shades of gray). The higher the kVp setting, the higher photon energy that strikes an area. To penetrate larger teeth, a higher kilovoltage is required to produce a diagnostic film. When using ultra speed D film, the kV setting varies from 40–70 depending on the tooth and animal size. Low kVp techniques are recommended.

The *speed (exposure time)* is measured either in fractions of a second or pulses. A *pulse* is 1/60 or .016 of a second. Thirty pulses equal 1/2 second. When using a standard veterinary radiography unit, the speed is commonly set to 1/10 second.

*Milliampere (*mA) settings affect the number of electrons produced. Changing the mA setting increases or decreases the intensity of the x-ray beam affecting density of the radiograph. The milliampere number is usually preset between 7 and 15 mA. When using standard veterinary radiograph machines, 50 or 100 mA is commonly used.

The *mA and exposure times* have a direct effect on the quantity of photons produced in an x-ray beam. The mAs (milliampere seconds) is the product of milliamperage times seconds of exposure; mAi (mAimpulses) is the product of milliamperage times the impulses of energy. If the product is the same, the quantity of radi-

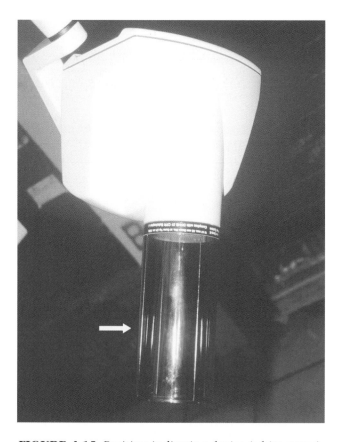

FIGURE 4.15. Position indicating device (white arrow).

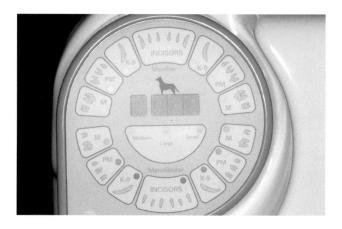

FIGURE 4.16. Handheld control panel (AFP Imaging).

ation produced is essentially the same.

When using a conventional radiograph unit and intraoral film, the following values can be used as starting points:

- Small dogs and cats: 40–50 kVp and 8–10 mAs (100 mA times 1/10 second equals 10mAs))
- Medium-sized dogs: 50–65 kVp and 10 mAs
- Large dogs: 65–75 kVp and 10 mAs

The *film focal distance (FFD)* is another variable to consider when acquiring an image. The x-ray generator is located inside the tube head. The FFD is measured from the film to the x-ray tube. Moving the tube closer or farther away from the patient affects radiation intensity. The exposure needed to produce diagnostic films increases with greater distance by the inverse square law. As the distance doubles, the exposure must be increased four times; as distance triples, exposure must increase by nine times to produce similar films.

When using a dental radiograph unit, the PID should be placed on the skin or within inches of the patient's maxilla or mandible. When using a standard veterinary radiography machine, the tube head (without a cone) should be placed 12–16 inches from the area of interest.

Dental lead-lined cones are available in a variety of lengths from 4–16 inches. The end of a 4 inch cone may be 8 inches from the x-ray generator. An 8 inch extension (using a 4 inch cone) is referred to as *short cone technique*; longer extensions result in a *long cone technique*. Exposure adjustments are necessary to accommodate different cone lengths. Generally, short cone technique, which produces more magnification, is preferable because it uses less exposure and is easier to position. The long cone technique, however, produces films with increased detail (Figure 4.17).

Exposure Factors Affecting Film Quality

- kVp setting (usually preset)
- mA setting (usually preset)
- Exposure time setting
- Film focal distance (FFD)
- Long or short cone technique (related to FFD)

DIGITAL DENTAL IMAGING

Digital imaging is a technical advancement in dental radiography. Instead of film, an electronic sensor pad is placed against the teeth, which accepts the image and transfers it to a computer screen where it can be enhanced, enlarged, printed, or archived (Figures 4.18, 4.19).

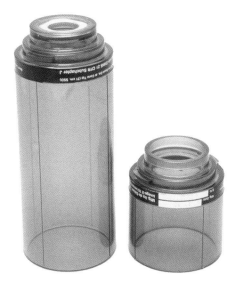

FIGURE 4.17. Long and short cone attachments.

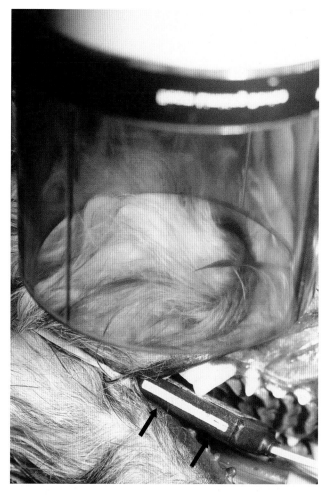

FIGURE 4.18. Digital sensor placed against the maxillary fourth premolar.

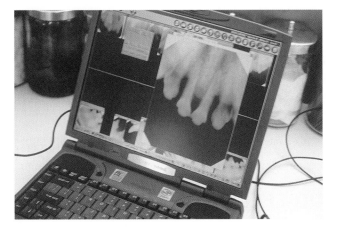

FIGURE 4.19. Digital image displayed on computer screen in the dental operatory.

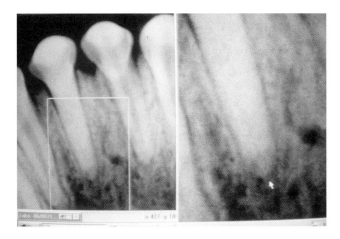

FIGURE 4.20. Digital image enlarged.

A dental radiograph unit is still needed to expose the sensor. Approximately 1/10–1/2 of the nondigital exposure is needed to obtain a diagnostic image. Because of low time exposure settings of 0.1–.05 seconds, older dental radiograph machines may not have fast enough timers to produce digital images.

Advantages of digital imaging include:

- 50–90 percent reduction in radiation needed to expose an image, compared to Ektaspeed or Ultraspeed film; 30% less exposure than Insight film
- Instant image production, eliminating processing chemicals and anesthetic time
- The ability to retake images immediately if the results are not diagnostic
- The ability to enlarge the entire image or certain sections, adjusting contrast and brightness, enhancing the margins, inversing and rotating images (Figures 4.20–4.23)
- The ability to measure the distance between two points, which helps estimate endodontic working file lengths (Figure 4.24)
- The ability to measure tooth densities for evaluating Stage 1 or 2 feline odontoclastic resorptive lesions
- Instant progress evaluation during endodontic and oral surgery procedures
- Electronic transfer of radiographs to the patient file, consultant, or referring veterinarian

Disadvantages of digital dental imaging include the following:

- $6,000–$15,000 U.S. expense in addition to the dental radiography unit
- Occlusal size (number 4) sensors are not currently available, necessitating multiple exposures with smaller sensors

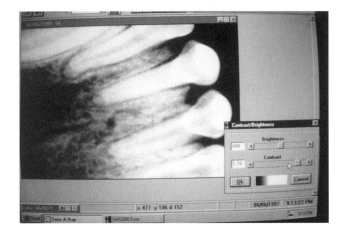

FIGURE 4.21. Digital image contrast adjustment.

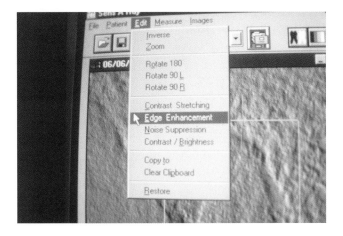

FIGURE 4.22. Highlighted digital enhancement of periodontal ligament.

- Possibility of sensor damage because of animal or operator trauma, necessitating costly replacement
- Extra time needed for computer patient input
- Need for a computer in the dental operatory

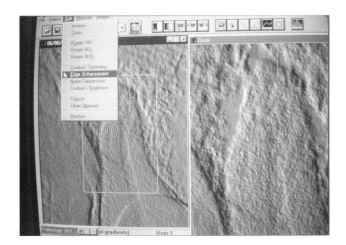

FIGURE 4.23. Enlarged digital enhanced area.

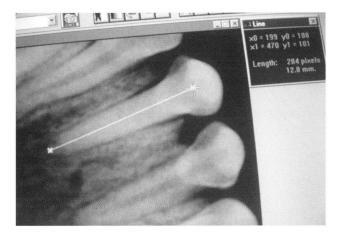

FIGURE 4.24. Digital radiography used for measurement of root canal for endodontic care.

RADIATION SAFETY

The ALARA Principle

Radiation exposure should be *"as low as reasonably achievable" (ALARA)*. This concept endorses the use of the least possible exposure of the patient (and operator) to radiation to produce a diagnostically acceptable radiograph.

Staff of the veterinary facility must be protected against excessive radiation exposure. X-ray aprons, gloves, and thyroid shields should be worn when exposing films. Preferably the operator is able to leave the radiograph area.

Veterinarian responsibilities include the following:

- Prescribe only radiographs that are clinically necessary.
- Install and maintain the radiographic equipment in safe working condition.

- Adequately train, supervise, and monitor personnel who expose radiographs.

Two types of radiation apply to operator safety:

- *Primary radiation* comes from direct exposure from the x-ray beam. The veterinarian or staff should never hold film or digital sensors in the patient's mouth with bare or gloved fingers. Film or sensors can be positioned in the mouth using the endotracheal tube, clay encased in a plastic bag, gauze, thin wash cloth, or crumpled newspapers, decreasing operator exposure.
- *Secondary (scatter) radiation* reflects from areas that have been irradiated by the primary beam. Protective aprons must be worn for shielding.

Personnel Monitoring

A film badge service is used to provide radiation monitoring for all members of the office staff functioning near radiation exposure. The dosimeter badge should be worn at all times in the veterinary office. It measures the amount and type of radiation an individual is exposed to in the working environment. The badge should not be worn outside the office. The periodic radiation monitoring report should be evaluated and saved indefinitely.

FILM

Intraoral, non-screen film is primarily used in small animal dental radiography. It is inexpensive, flexible, and provides superb diagnostic detail.

Individual dental films are packaged in a light-safe packet made of either soft plastic or paper material. The back of the packet has a tab opening used to remove the film for processing. The tabbed side is placed away from the radiation beam. Inside the packet, film is positioned between two sheets of black paper. Lead foil, which protects film from secondary backscatter radiation, is located next to the tab opening (Figure 4.25).

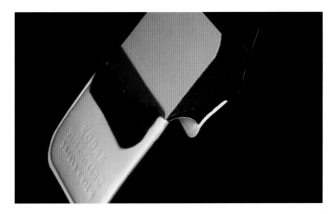

FIGURE 4.25. Opened film packet.

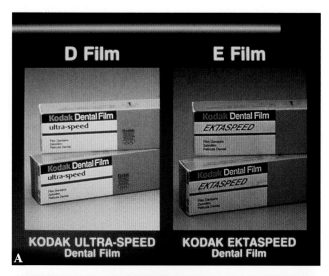

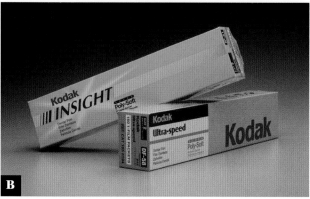

FIGURE 4.26. Samples of Kodak film: (A) Ultra-Speed and Ektaspeed film; (B) InSight and Ultra-speed film.

Intraoral dental film is packaged with one or two films per packet. The practitioner may use the second film to give to the client or referring veterinarian, or to archive interesting cases.

Film Speed

The efficiency with which a film responds to x-ray exposure is known as film sensitivity or speed:

- *D speed* (Ultraspeed, Kodak) provides high contrast and fine detail. Ultraspeed is the most popular film used for veterinary dentistry.
- *E speed* (Ektaspeed, Kodak) requires 25% less exposure time, compared to D speed film, with minimal loss of contrast (Figure 4.26).
- *F speed* (InSight, Kodak) requires 60% less exposure time than D speed film, and 20% less than E speed film.

Table 4.1. Color-coded film packages.

Speed	Single Film	Double Film
Ultraspeed	Green	Grey
Ektaspeed	Blue	Mauve
InSight	Lavender	Tan

Kodak film packet backs are color-coded to indicate film speed and number of films in the packet (Table 4.1).

Film Sizes

Four sizes of dental film commonly used in veterinary dentistry (Figure 4.27):

- *Child periapical (size 0)* measures 7/8 x 1 5/8 inches. Size 0 is used mostly in cats, exotics, and small dogs (Burns 833-0709, Schein 111-8895).
- *Adult bitewing (size 2)* measures 1 1/4 x 1 5/8 inches and is the most commonly used size in veterinary dentistry. Size 2 fits into 35 mm slide mounts for use in presentations (Burns 833-1135, Schein 111-2875).
- *Bitewing (size 3) film* measures 1 1/16 by 2 1/8 inches. Size 3 films adapt well to the mandibular cheek teeth (Burns 833-0692, Schein 111-3261).
- *Occlusal (size 4) film* measures 2 1/4 x 3 inches. Occlusal film is used to radiograph larger teeth, survey studies, and maxillary occlusal views in dogs and cats (Burns 833-0702, Schein 111-1262).

Film Dot

Most dental films are embossed with a raised dot (or dimple) in one of the corners (Figure 4.28). The raised

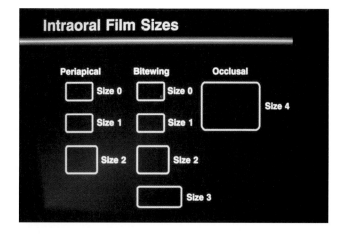

FIGURE 4.27. Intraoral film sizes.

(convex) side of the dot indicates the side to be positioned toward the radiation beam. The dot is used to identify right from left.

There are many methods for using the film dot for tooth identification. One method places the raised dot against the occlusal or cutting edge of the teeth and toward the tube head. Using this system to determine whether a processed film is from the right or left side, the progression of the teeth from molars to incisors is identified, as well as the location of the raised film dot. With this method the "apple" and "par" rule can be applied. *Apple* stands for *a*nterior to *p*osterior = *l*eft. *Par* stands for *p*osterior to *a*nterior = *r*ight side when the film dot is positioned toward the occlusal surface (Figures 4.29–4.34; film dot artificially highlighted).

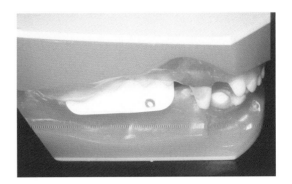

FIGURE 4.30. Film dot position for right maxillary premolar exposure.

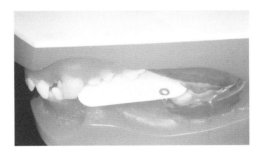

FIGURE 4.31. Film and dot position for left maxillary premolar exposure.

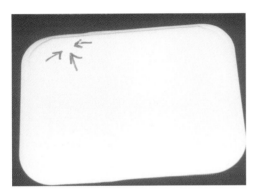

FIGURE 4.28. Embossed film dot (arrows).

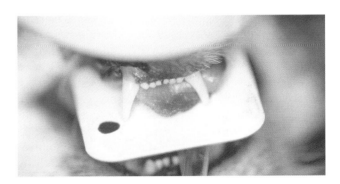

FIGURE 4.32. Film and dot position for mandibular incisors.

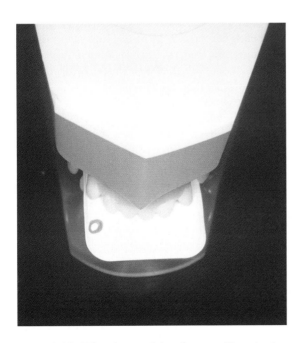

FIGURE 4.29. Film dot position for maxillary incisor exposure.

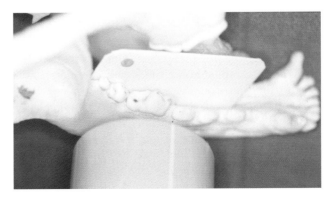

FIGURE 4.33. Film and dot position for right mandibular premolars/molars.

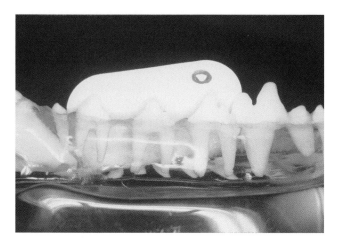

FIGURE 4.34. Film and dot position for left mandibular premolars.

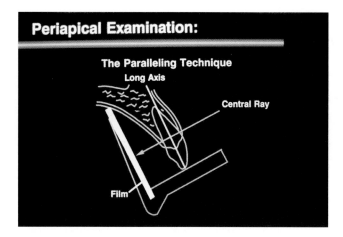

FIGURE 4.35. Parallel technique.

An alternative system positions the dot on the right side of the radiographed object. When reading the radiograph, if the dot is in the "air" it is the right side. If it is in the "bone" it is the left side.

Intraoral Film Placement and Angulation of the Primary Beam

The film should be placed inside the mouth, as parallel as possible to the long axis of the tooth roots to be radiographed. The non-tabbed side faces the tube head. The film can be held in position by the endotracheal tube, wadded-up newspaper, gauze, hair curler devices, lead x-ray gloves (without fingers inside), sponges, clay encased in plastic bags, or by commercial holding devices. Operators must not use their fingers to hold film during exposure.

Vertical angulation refers to the up-and-down movement of the PID. Vertical angulation determines how accurately the length of the object being radiographed is reproduced.

Horizontal angulation refers to back-and-forth movements on a plane that is parallel with the floor. Proper horizontal angulation produces normal interproximal anatomic representation of the teeth without overlapping.

Parallel technique places the film parallel to the tooth, and the radiograph beam is positioned perpendicular to the film, creating a nondistorted image. Only the mandibular cheek teeth allow the film to be placed lingually (parallel) in the flexible intermandibular soft tissue parallel to the roots (Figures 4.35, 4.36).

Parallel technique is not usually feasible for most studies. Instead, the *bisecting angle technique* is used. Imaginary lines are drawn along the long axis of the

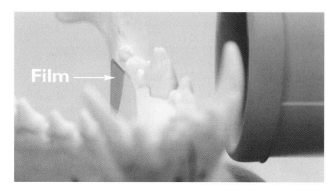

FIGURE 4.36. Placing the film parallel to the roots of the mandibular cheek teeth.

tooth and the plane of the film. The point where these two lines meet creates an angle. Instead of aiming the central beam perpendicular to the film, as in the parallel technique, the central beam is aimed perpendicular to the imaginary line that bisects the angle formed by the plane of the film and the long axis of the tooth (Figures 4.37, 4.38).

The *SLOB rule* (same *l*ingual, opposite *b*uccal—also called the buccal object rule) is a tube-shift technique that helps identify the relative bucco-lingual location of objects in the oral cavity. When two roots of a triple-rooted tooth (maxillary fourth premolar and molars in the dog) are superimposed on the radiograph, it is sometimes difficult to distinguish the individual roots. Defining which root is which is important during root canal therapy and with pathology associated with advanced periodontal disease. To visualize the roots, two radiographs are taken at oblique angles, fixing the vertical position and moving the tube horizontally. Horizontal tube shift will result in a film with the overlapped roots moved apart. When the root "moves" in

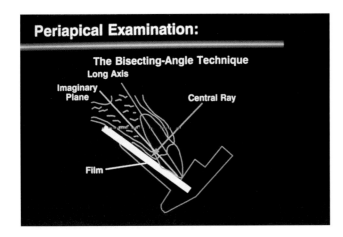

FIGURE 4.37. Bisecting-angle technique.

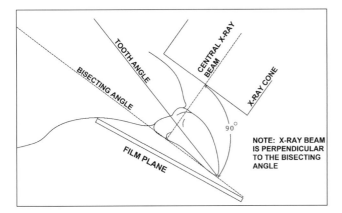

FIGURE 4.38. X-ray beam is perpendicular to the bisecting angle.

an opposite direction to the horizontal shift of the tube, the root is buccal. For example, when the tube head is moved rostrally, the palatal root of the maxillary fourth premolar will be the most rostral root on the radiograph, and the mesiobuccal root will be distal to the palatal root. When the root "moves" in the same direction as the tube, it is lingual or palatal.

Tube/Film/Patient Positioning

A radiographic dental survey consists of a minimum of eight views:

- Rostral maxilla
- Lateral left canine
- Lateral right canine
- Rostral mandible
- Right maxillary cheek (premolars and molars) teeth
- Left maxillary cheek teeth
- Right mandibular cheek teeth
- Left mandibular cheek teeth

In the maxillary views, the patient is positioned in sternal recumbency with a support placed under the chin at a height where the muzzle is parallel to the table-top:

- *Incisors:* Place the film packet toward the tube head against the incisors and palate. Position the PID perpendicular to an angle bisecting the film and teeth planes (Figures 4.39, 4.40).
- *Canine:* Place the film packet facing the tube, between the tongue and maxilla and beneath the canine tooth root. Center the PID over the mesial root of the second maxillary premolar, dorsally or laterally depending on the view needed. Determine the angle between the plane of the canine root and

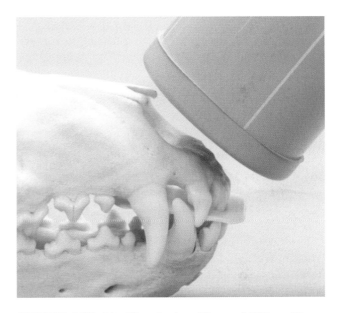

FIGURE 4.39. Maxillary incisor film and PID position.

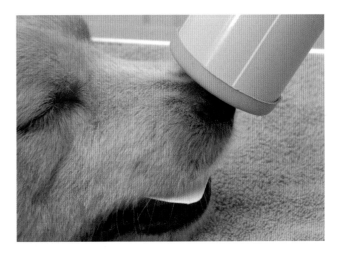

FIGURE 4.40. PID perpendicular to an angle bisecting the film and teeth planes.

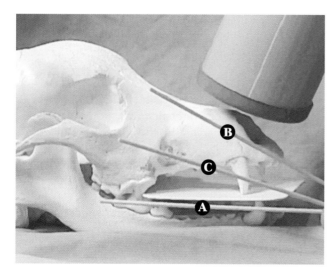

FIGURE 4.41. Bisecting-angle technique with markers demonstrating: (A) place of film, (B) plane of the canine root, and (C) the bisected angle. (Courtesy AFP imaging)

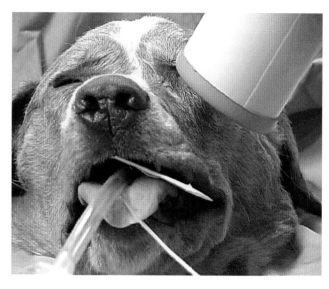

FIGURE 4.43. Maxillary premolar film and PID position.

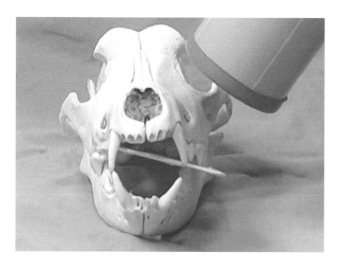

FIGURE 4.42. Maxillary premolar film and PID position (skull).

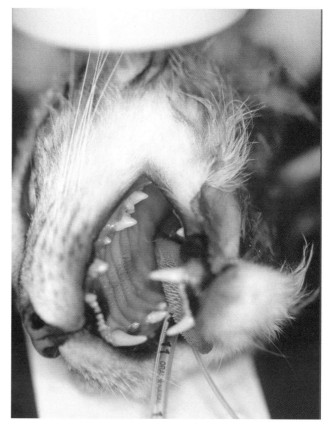

FIGURE 4.44. Extraoral technique used in exposing feline maxillary premolars.

the plane of the film. Position the cone perpendicular to the bisected angle (Figure 4.41).

- *Premolars:* Place the film packet as close as possible to the inner surface of the cheek teeth. Aim the PID at the roots of the premolars at approximately 45°. The maxillary fourth premolar has three roots (mesiobuccal, mesiopalatal, and distal). To avoid overlap of the mesial buccal and palatal roots, position the PID 20° in the rostral horizontal plane (rostral oblique) in the medium- to long-muzzled dog, and in the caudal horizontal plane (caudal oblique) in brachycepahlic breeds (Figures 4.42, 4.43). In cats, the zygomatic arch is superimposed over the maxillary fourth premolar root. To avoid the arch, use a

rostral oblique bisecting angle projection, aimed at the premolar roots with the PID positioned just ventral to the arch. Alternatively, the extraoral near-parallel technique may be used to visualize the maxillary cheek teeth (Figures 4.44, 4.45).

- *Molars:* Place the film packet against the maxilla beneath the molar teeth. Aim the PID at the eye and film in a caudoventral direction (Figure 4.46).

When radiographing the mandible: Place the patient in ventral or lateral recumbency with support under the neck to place the muzzle parallel to the tabletop.

- *Incisors:* Position the film packet toward the tube head against the incisors and the lingual frenulum. Position the PID perpendicular to the bisecting angle (Figures 4.47, 4.48).
- *Canine:* Place the patient in ventral recumbency. Position the film between the tongue and mandible, pushing the lingual frenulum distally. To obtain a lateral view, position the PID approximately 45° toward the canine (Figures 4.49, 4.50).

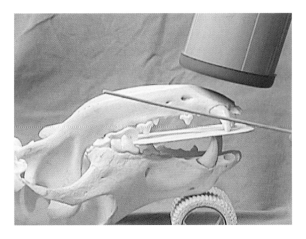

FIGURE 4.47. Mandibular incisor film and PID position.

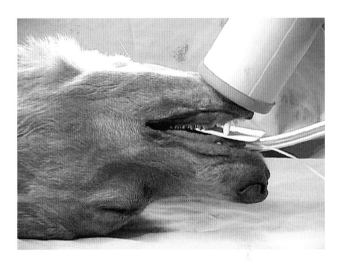

FIGURE 4.48. Mandibular incisor PID and film positions.

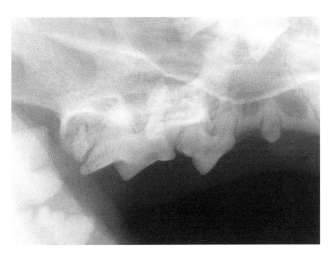

FIGURE 4.45. Radiograph results of extraoral maxillary premolar technique.

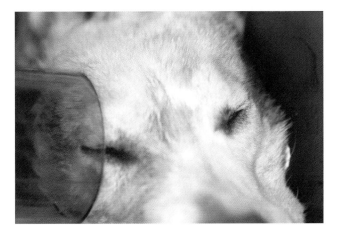

FIGURE 4.46. Maxillary molar PID positioning.

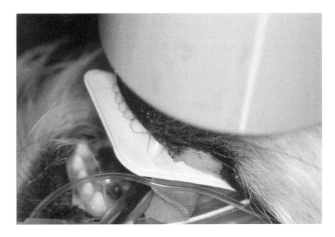

FIGURE 4.49. Mandibular canine film and PID position.

- *Anterior premolars:* Place the patient in lateral recumbency, with the film against the anterior premolars to include the periapical area. Aim the PID at

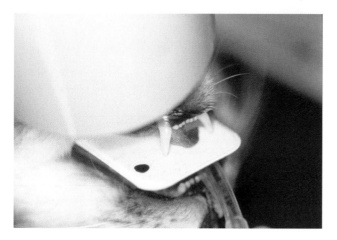

FIGURE 4.50. Left mandibular canine PID and film position.

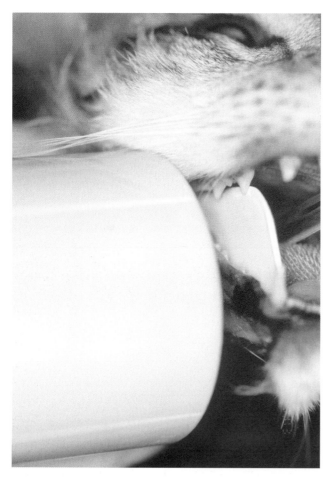

FIGURE 4.51. Feline mandibular film and PID premolar positioning.

the apex of the first premolar 20° to the ventral border of the mandible (Figure 4.51).

- *Posterior premolars and molars:* Place the patient in lateral recumbency. Position the film at the floor of the mouth lingual to the premolars. Place gauze or a hemostat to help depress the film into the floor of the mouth. Aim the PID perpendicular to the tooth roots and film (parallel technique) (Figures 4.52, 4.53).

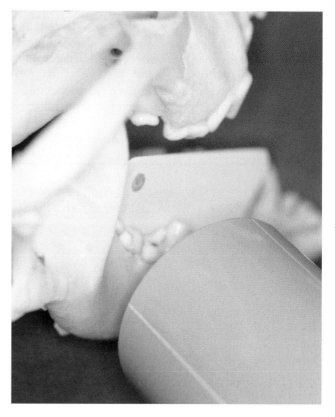

FIGURE 4.52. Posterior mandibular premolars and molars positioning.

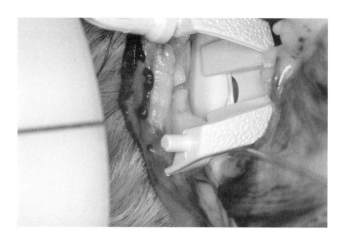

FIGURE 4.53. Feline mandibular positioning using a film-holding device.

Extraoral technique can be used to examine any teeth. Unfortunately, because of the difficulty of patient and x-ray beam positioning, extraoral technique is rarely used. Placing the film on the outside of the mouth is helpful when radiographing feline maxillary cheek teeth, removing the superimposition of the zygomatic arch over the maxillary premolars.

When using the extraoral technique to radiograph the maxillary cheek teeth, the film is placed under the arch to be examined. Extraoral technique requires positioning the dog or cat's mouth obliquely, held open with a mouth prop or cut syringe casing.

The x-ray beam is centered on the arcade nearest the film. The endotracheal tube should be diverted away from the beam.

The *temporomandibular joint (TMJ)* is formed from the condyloid process of the mandible and the mandibular fossa of the temporal bone. The joint may be affected by congenital defects (TMJ dysplasia, craniomandibular osteopathy), trauma (luxation, condylar fracture, zygomatic process fracture), infection (septic arthritis, degenerative joint disease), or neoplasia. Imaging of the TMJ can be difficult. Intraoral or extraoral techniques can be used to view the joint.

Using intraoral technique, number 2 or number 4 films can be placed in the oropharynx wedged against the endotracheal tube, in the area of the TMJ. The PID is placed against the horizontal ear canal.

Alternately, extraoral technique can be used. The dorsal ventral position usually gives the most information concerning the TMJ. Lateral oblique can be exposed with the PID position at 45° in the dog and 20° in the cat.

FILM PROCESSING

Processing Fundamentals

- Active fresh solutions
- Standardized method of processing
- Light secured area

Film may be developed in the following ways:

- *Manually*, using developer, water, and fixer solutions in the practice darkroom.
- With the *chairside darkroom*, a portable light-safe box containing developer, distilled water, and fixer in small containers placed in the dental operatory. The chairside darkroom is covered with a Plexiglas safe-

light filter, which enables operators to see their hands while handling the film(s). The filter is either amber (when D speed film is exposed), or red (for E or F speed film). Processing time from opening the film packet to initial examination of a rinsed film takes approximately 2 minutes (Burns 951-1423, Schein 189-4677) (Figure 4.54).

Developer and fixer jars in the chairside darkroom should be covered when not in use. Depending on the chemical manufacturer, number of films processed, and environmental conditions, the fixer and developer remain usable for 2 days to 2 weeks. To maximize the life of the developer, marbles can be placed in lidded cups to displace air, decreasing oxidation. Stock solutions can be stored in a refrigerator to prolong shelf life. The developer and fixer should be brought to room temperature before use (Burns 952-1160, Schein 189-4910).

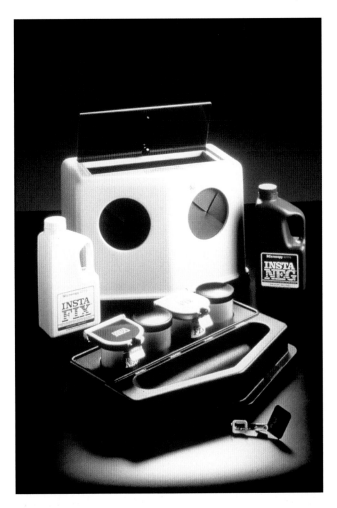

FIGURE 4.54. Chairside darkroom with instant chemicals (Microcopy).

Manual processing includes the following steps:

1. After exposure, carry the film into the practice darkroom or chairside darkroom for processing. Slide the film packet tab down to present film, cardboard, and lead blocker. The film will feel firm to the touch, compared to the other film pack contents.
2. A film hanger is attached to the film edge. Touch only the sides of the film with fingers. Apply a gentle tug to make certain the film is firmly attached to the clip (Burns 951-2350, Schein 100-0921) (Figure 4.55).
3. Place the film in prestirred developer solution for the specified time recommended by the manufacturer (Kodak Rapid Access Chemistry: 15 seconds at 68°). Note: an alternative method starts manual film processing with water immersion for 5 seconds to soften the emulsion before placement in the developer (Figure 4.56).

4. After removal from the developer, rinse the film in fresh distilled water (wash) for 10–15 seconds. Rinsing removes the alkaline developer from the film surface, preventing mixture with the acid fixer.
5. Place the film in the prestirred fixing solution for at least 2 minutes. Fixer removes the unexposed or underdeveloped silver halide crystals and rehardens the emulsion.
6. Rinse the film for 30 seconds in distilled water.
7. After viewing, place the film back in the fixer for 5 minutes, followed by distilled water rinse for 10 minutes.
8. When rinsing is complete, attach the radiograph to a clip on the drying rack (Figure 4.57).

With a standard automatic film processor:

- The dental film can be attached to a larger film with silver photographic tape. This procedure is discouraged because small dental films might become lost in the processor, and/or the tape might harm the processor's rollers.

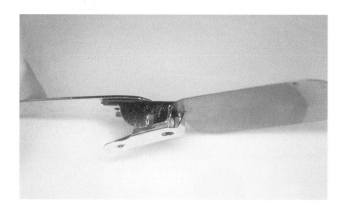

FIGURE 4.55. Film hanger attached to film.

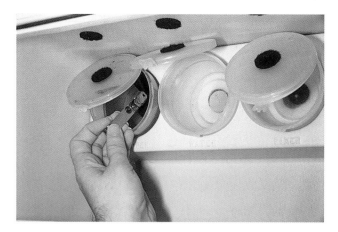

FIGURE 4.56. Looking down into the chairside darkroom, exposed film is manually inserted in developer container.

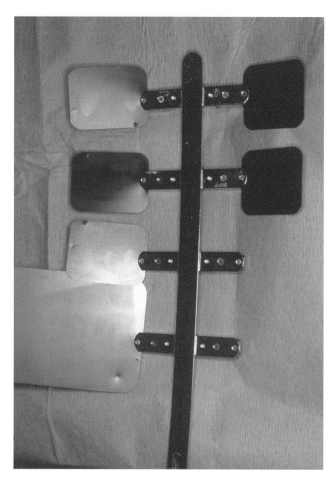

FIGURE 4.57. Film drying rack.

- The film can be attached to a film holder (Film Tran carrier, Bisco International, Inc.) to carry the film through the standard automatic film processor on a cardboard sheet. Film holders permit transport of number 2 and 4 dental films. The sheet is developer- and fixer-resistant.

The technique for using a film holder includes the following steps:

1. Remove the film wrapper in the darkroom.
2. Remove the protective liner from the carrier window, exposing adhesive.
3. Place the film into the window frame and press firmly around the edges.
4. Feed the carrier through the processor.

An automatic dental film processor can be located chairside or in the darkroom.

Exposed dental film(s) are inserted at one end of the automatic dental processor and exit fully developed,

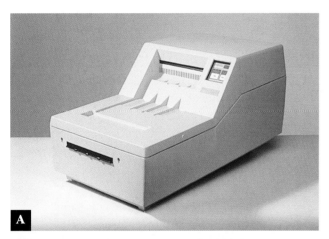

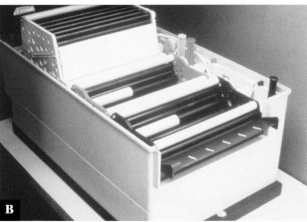

FIGURE 4.58 Developing exposed film: (A) automatic dental processor; (B) automatic dental processor rollers.

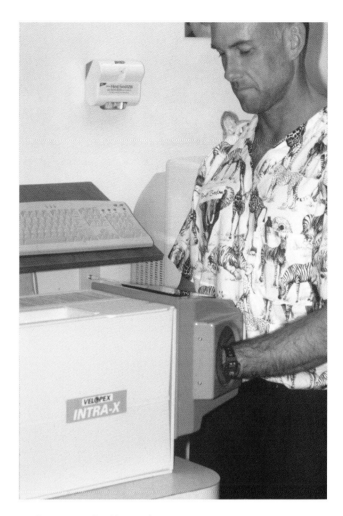

FIGURE 4.59. Chairside automatic processor.

fixed, and dried in 5–7 minutes (or in 2 minutes, rapid cycle, for endodontic intraoperative films not fully fixed) (Figures 4.58, 4.59):

1. Remove all wrappers around the film in the darkroom.
2. Insert the film into the film processor.

QUALITY CONTROL

A good radiograph is useless unless it is read accurately, and a poor radiograph cannot be read accurately.

Daily, a quality assurance film should be exposed to verify that all parts of the dental radiography system are working properly. Use of an aluminum *step wedge* helps accomplish this goal. The step wedge is composed of graduated pieces of aluminum placed to produce a step effect (Burns 998-6484, Schein 263-3389) (Figure 4.60).

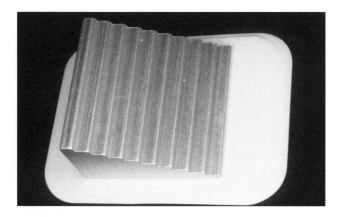

FIGURE 4.60. Step wedge on top of dental film.

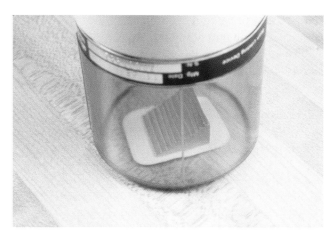

FIGURE 4.61. PID position for exposing quality assurance films.

To use a step wedge to establish a control radiograph:

1. Lay a dental film tab-side–down on a flat surface.
2. Place a step wedge over the film.
3. Use medium-dog technique to expose the film (Figure 4.61).
4. Process the film using new chemicals in a light-secured area.

The processed image should show 10 shades of varying densities, from light gray to black. Using fresh chemicals, if all 10 steps are not apparent, adjust the exposure up or down until all can be distinctly seen. If the lightest steps (from the thickest part of the wedge) are indistinct, the exposure is increased. If the darkest steps (from the thinnest part of the wedge) are indistinct, the exposure is decreased. When the correct exposure is determined, this becomes the *control film*. Thirty reference films are exposed but not processed. Reference films should be stored in a refrigerator (Figure 4.62).

The control film is placed on the view box. Every day, one of the pre-exposed reference films is developed to confirm that the density (overall darkness of the image) and contrast (number of visible steps of the wedge) remain constant when compared to the baseline film. If they are not identical, the correct processing time and temperature are verified. If more than two steps are lighter than the control film, and other variables have not changed, the developing and fixing solutions should either be replenished or changed (Figure 4.63).

Film quality encompasses many variables:

- *Detail* is the delineation of minute structure. kVp and the developing process control detail.

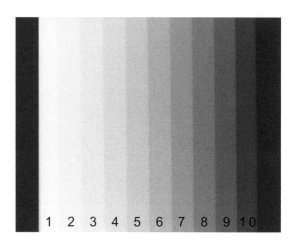

FIGURE 4.62. Control film processed with new chemicals—all steps identified.

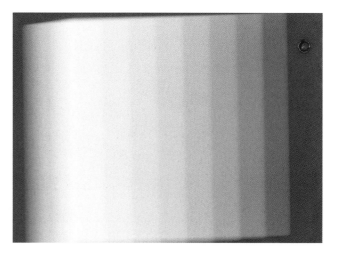

FIGURE 4.63. Example of film processed in exhausted chemicals—cannot identify all steps.

- *Definition* is the distinctness and demarcation of the detail that makes up the radiographic image. For example, adequate definition is present when the apical lamina dura, periodontal ligament space, and individual trabeculae can be clearly demarcated around a healthy tooth. Definition is controlled by distance, focal spot size, type of film, and motion.
- *Density* is the degree of blackness created on film. Density is controlled predominantly by mAs. Settings of 10–12.5 mAs provide proper density.
- *Contrast* is the relative difference between densities. High-contrast film appears black and white. Low-contrast films demonstrate many shades of gray. Contrast is controlled by kVp (normally between 40–75) and processing variables (temperature, development time, light leaks, and inherent characteristics of film).

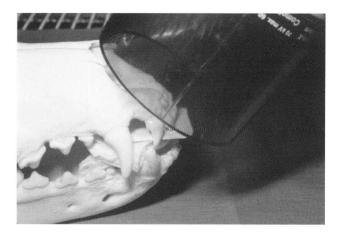

FIGURE 4.64. Proper PID angulation for maxillary incisors.

Troubleshooting: Common Causes for Repeated Films

- Incorrect film/tube head positioning
- Movement of tube head or patient during exposure
- Incorrect exposure setting
- Placing film in the mouth upside-down (lead foil side toward the tube head)
- Exposing film twice
- Processing errors

Tube Head Positioning Errors

FORESHORTENED IMAGE   The exposed dental image should be approximately the same size as the patient's tooth (figures 4.64, 4.65). Foreshortened images, caused by excessive vertical angulation, appear shorter than the patient's normal anatomy. To correct a foreshortened image, the vertical angulation is reduced (Figures 4.66, 4.67).

ELONGATED IMAGE   Elongated images, caused by too little vertical angulation, appear longer than the actual tooth. To correct an elongated image, vertical angulation is increased (Figures 4.68, 4.69).

Film Errors

FILM FOGGING   Film fogging appears as a gray or dark film, and can have several causes:

- The film was not placed in fixer for a sufficient length of time (most common reason). To correct this

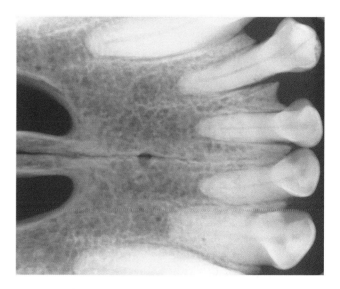

FIGURE 4.65. Proper angulation results in diagnostic film.

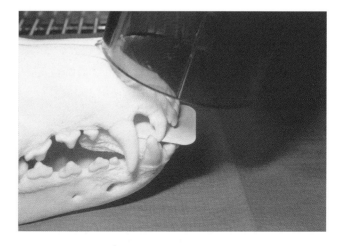

FIGURE 4.66. Excessive vertical angulation results in a foreshortened image.

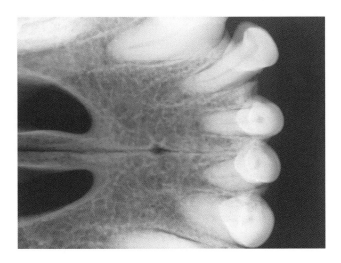

FIGURE 4.67. Foreshortened image.

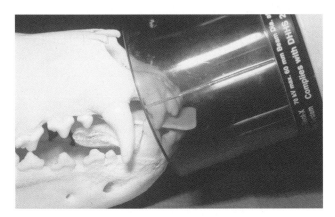

FIGURE 4.68. Too little angulation results in an elongated image.

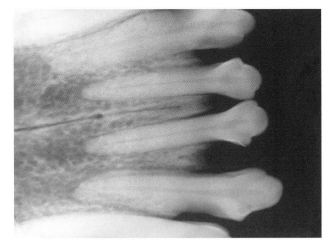

FIGURE 4.69. Elongated image.

fault, immerse the film in the fixer for an additional 5 minutes.

- The processing chemicals were exhausted.
- The film was outdated.
- Light leaks occurred from the film packet or processing area. To evaluate whether the processing area was at fault, place a coin on top of an open unexposed film packet in the dark room for 10 minutes. Then process the film. If an outline of the coin shows, there is a light leak in the darkroom.
- The film was processed in fixer contaminated with developer solution.
- The film was exposed to excessive heat.

NO IMAGE   If there is no image:

- The film was immersed in the fixer before the developer.
- The film was not exposed (either due to poor PID or packet placement, or failure to engage the timer).

LIGHT IMAGE   If the film image is light:

- The exposure time was insufficient.
- The kilovoltage was insufficient.
- The developer was weak or contaminated.
- The time in the developer was insufficient.
- The film was placed in the mouth upside-down (stippling pattern on film).

DARK IMAGE   If the film image is dark:

- The exposure was excessive.
- The kilovoltage was excessive.
- The exposure time was excessive.
- The film was in the developing solution too long.
- The developer was too warm (ideal temperature, 68° F.).

If the film is black, it has been exposed to light before processing.

BLURRED IMAGE   Blurred image results from motion of the patient, film, and/or PID during exposure (Figure 4.70).

PARTIAL IMAGE   If the image is only partial:

- The film was partially immersed in the developer.
- While in the developer, the film became attached to other films or the side of the container.
- The film or tube head was incorrectly positioned, creating cone cutoff (Figure 4.71).

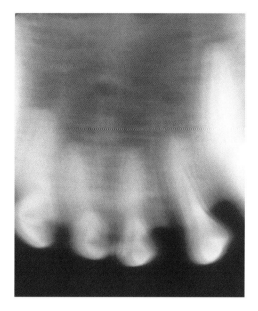

FIGURE 4.70. Blurred image secondary to either patient, film, or tube movement.

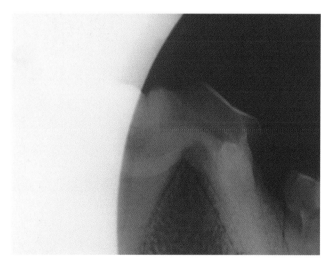

FIGURE 4.71. Partially exposed film from cone cutoff.

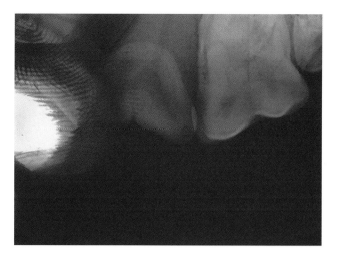

FIGURE 4.72. Fingerprints on processed film.

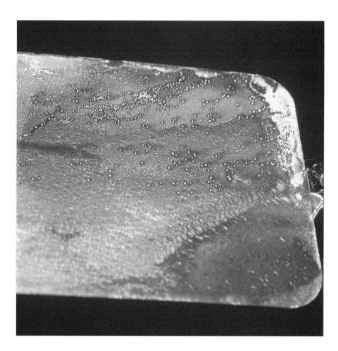

FIGURE 4.73. Frosty film due to improper washing/fixing technique.

FINGERPRINTS   Fingerprints occur from poor handling while processing. The film should be handled only by the edges (Figure 4.72).

FROSTY FILMS   Frosty films occur from insufficient removal of fixer when rinsing manually processed films. The remaining residue dries on the film leaving a frosty finish. Rinsing a processed film with fresh distilled water for sufficient time easily prevents frosty films (Figure 4.73).

STREAKED FILMS   Streaked films might occur when the film is insufficiently developed, fixed, rinsed or if the processing solutions are contaminated. (Figure 4.74).

CRESCENT-SHAPES   Crescent-shaped lines occur when the film packet is sharply bent (Figure 4.75).

TIRE TRACKS   Low-density tire tracks or geometric patterns on the film occur as the result of directing the x-ray through the lead foil side of the film packet (Figure 4.76).

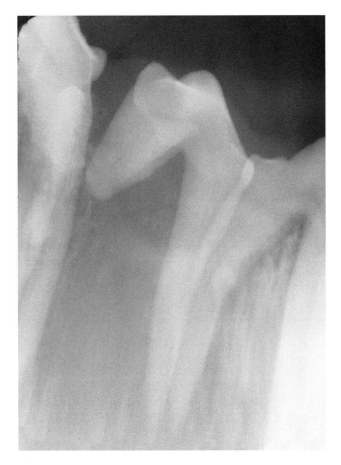

FIGURE 4.74. Streaked film.

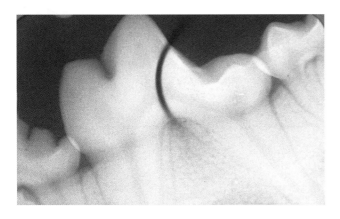

FIGURE 4.75. Crescent line artifact from bent film packet.

BLACK DOTS OR SPOTS   Black dots or spots on the developed film are caused by moisture from improper film storage.

DOUBLE IMAGES   Double images occur when the film is exposed twice (Figure 4.77).

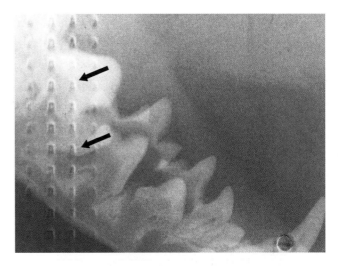

FIGURE 4.76. Tire-track artifact due to upside-down placement of film packet.

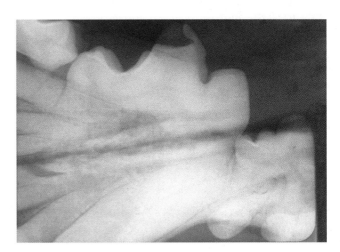

FIGURE 4.77. Double exposure.

RADIOGRAPHIC LANDMARKS

It is important to be able to look at a film and anatomically identify the area exposed:

- The *maxillary incisor area* contains a radiodense (white) area distal to the incisors, with two ovals representing the palatine fissures (Figures 4.78, 4.79).
- The *mandibular incisor area* has a linear radiolucent (black) area representing the mandibular symphysis, separating the right and left mandibular bodies (Figures 4.80, 4.81).
- The *maxillary premolar and molar area* contains a radiodense fine line apical to the roots, representing the line of conjunction between the vertical body of the maxilla and its palatine process (Figures 4.82, 4.83).

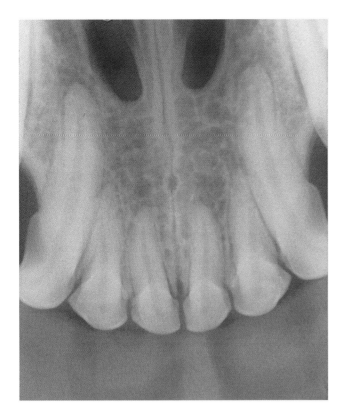

FIGURE 4.78. Canine maxillary incisors.

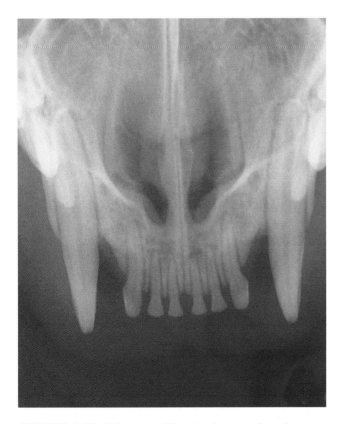

FIGURE 4.79. Feline maxillary incisors and canines.

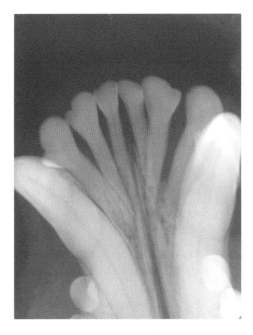

FIGURE 4.80. Canine mandibular incisors with bone loss secondary to periodontal disease.

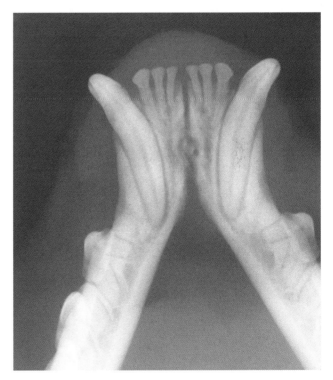

FIGURE 4.81. Feline mandibular incisors, canines, and premolars.

- The *mandibular premolar and molar area* has radiolucent (black) areas above and below the mandibular ramus (Figures 4.84, 4.85).

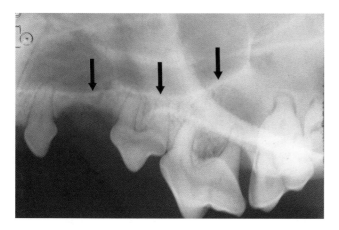

FIGURE 4.82. Canine maxillary premolars (crown of second premolar absent). Arrows mark the fine radiodense line consistent with maxillary radiograph.

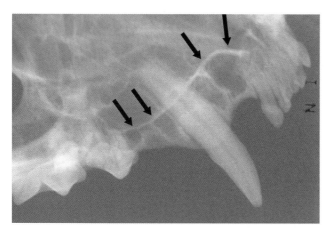

FIGURE 4.83. Feline maxillary incisors, canine, and premolars. Fine radiodense line consistent with maxillary radiographs (arrows)

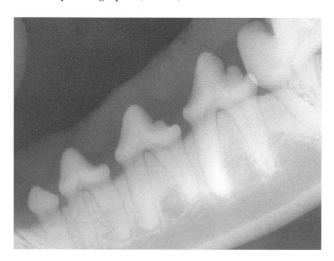

FIGURE 4.84. Canine mandibular premolars and the mesial root of the first molar. Note radiolucent areas above and below the body of the mandible.

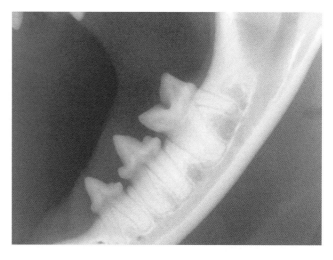

FIGURE 4.85. Feline mandibular premolars and molar.

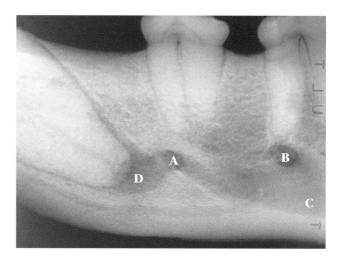

FIGURE 4.86. Radiograph showing middle (A), caudal mental foramina (B), the mandibular canal (C), periapical endodontic lesion (D).

Mental foramina are normal radiolucent anatomical structures that may be confused as lesions. Dogs and cats have three mental foramina:

- The *rostral mental foramen* is usually located distal to the incisor apices near the symphysis.
- The *middle mental foramen* is usually located ventral to the mesial root of the second premolar in the dog and distal to the apex of the canine tooth in the cat. The middle mental foramen may radiographically appear as a periapical radiolucency suggesting endodontic disease. If in doubt, the tooth can be radiographed in an oblique angle, which will show that the foramen is not connected to the tooth's apex.

• The *caudal mental foramen* is usually located ventral to the mesial root of the mandibular third premolar.

The *mandibular canal* appears as a radiolucent tubular structure parallel to the ventral border of the mandible. The mandibular canal may be superimposed on the apices of the mandibular cheek teeth, giving the appearance of periapical disease (Figure 4.86).

FILM MOUNTING AND IDENTIFICATION

Film mounts are used to organize and store radiographs. Mounts are available in a variety of styles, materials, and sizes of windows (openings), to accommodate the patient's radiographic survey. All the radiographs in a single series should be in the same mount and labeled with the patient's name and date of the study (Burns 952-2800, Schein 100-0920, Universal film mounts) (Figures 4.87–4.89).

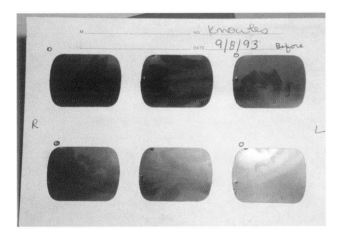

FIGURE 4.87. Cardboard film mount.

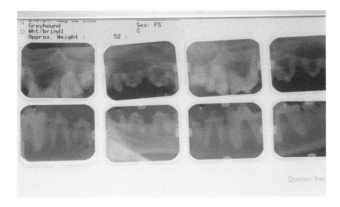

FIGURE 4.88. See-through film mount.

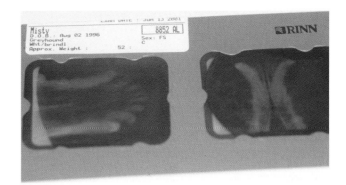

FIGURE 4.89. Large film mounts for size number 4 films.

There are two common methods used to mount films. Both rely on the knowledge of the normal radiographic anatomical landmarks for each region of the mouth, tooth morphology (shape and form), and identification of the embossed corner dot.

Labial mounting (nose to nose) arranges the film with the raised dots facing the clinician. The radiographs are examined as if the viewer is looking directly at the patient nose to nose; the patient's left side is on the viewer's right side, and the patient's right side is on the viewer's left side. For labial mounting:

• All radiographs of the dental survey are placed on a flat view box with the convex side of the dot toward the operator.
• The radiographs are arranged anatomically—maxilla above, mandible on the bottom.
• The patient's right side should be placed on the left side of the box.
• The maxillary radiographs are positioned with the crowns of the teeth facing the bottom of the view box.
• The mandibular radiographs are rotated until the coronal portions of the teeth are directed toward the top of the view box.
• The films are placed into the mount as positioned on the view box. The rostral maxillary and mandibular views are mounted in the upper and lower center mount openings.

Lingual mounting (sitting on the tongue) arranges the film in the mount with raised dots facing away from the clinician. In this method, radiographs are viewed as if the viewer is inside the patient's mouth looking out; the patient's left side is on viewer's left side.

INTERPRETING DENTAL RADIOGRAPHS

Dental radiographs, when correlated with clinical examination and case history, are important diagnostic aids available to the veterinary dentist.

Periodontal Radiographic Anatomy

The *alveolar margin* is the cortical border of the alveolar process positioned approximately 1–2 mm apical to the cementoenamel junction (CEJ) in the dog and 1/2–1 mm in the cat. The shape of the alveolar margin varies from pointed to flat. The rostral alveolar margins appear sharply pointed. Normal cheek teeth alveolar margins appear parallel or flat between adjacent cementoenamel junctions (Figure 4.90A).

The *lamina dura* is a radiographically visible, thin radiopaque line that represents a layer of compact bone lining the alveolus. The lamina dura is not a structure in its own right, but represents dense cortical bone continuous with the alveolar margin. Lamina dura appears dense and uniform in the younger animal, becoming ill-defined in the aged patient or in various disease states (Figure 4.90B).

The lamina dura of each tooth should be inspected to see whether it is continuous or interrupted (indicating pathology). A complete lamina dura generally indicates good periodontal health. In cases of early and established periodontal disease, the coronal lamina dura appears radiographically indistinct, irregular, and fuzzy. Resorption of the alveolar bone with advanced stages of periodontal disease leads to widening of the periodontal ligament space and loss of the lamina dura.

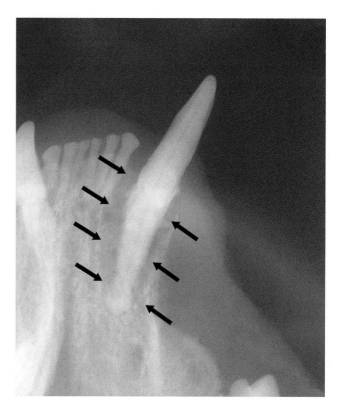

FIGURE 4.91. Loss of lamina dura from tooth affected by periodontal disease.

The *periodontal ligament,* composed mostly of collagen, appears radiographically as a radiolucent space between the lamina dura and tooth root. The periodontal ligament space (PDLS) is normally wider in younger animals and narrows with advancing age (Figure 4.90C). The PDLS also appears wider due to tooth mobility in the presence of periodontal disease. With disease, the periodontal ligament space varies, indicating that involvement is not consistent around the entire root (Figure 4.91). When viewing the lamina dura and the periodontal ligament, only the interproximal portions are visible. The buccal and lingual areas are not seen in the radiograph.

Radiologic Interpretation of Periodontal Disease

STAGES OF PERIODONTAL DISEASE Periodontal disease can be classified from Stages 1 to 4 based on severity of radiographic and clinical signs. Normally, interdental bone appears 1–2 mm apical to the cementoenamel junction.

The bone level in periodontal disease decreases as inflammation extends and bone is resorbed. *Forty per-*

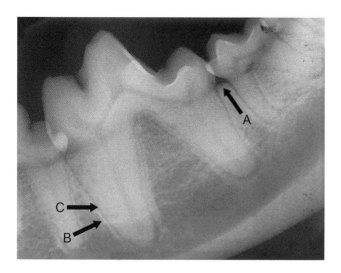

FIGURE 4.90. Periodontal anatomy: (A) alveolar margin ; (B) lamina dura; (C) periodontal ligament.

cent of the bone has to be destroyed before bone loss can be radiographically visualized. The radiograph is used indirectly to determine amount of bone loss. Distribution of bone loss is classified as either *localized* or *generalized*, depending on the number of areas affected. Localized bone loss occurs in isolated areas. Generalized bone loss involves the majority of the crestal bone.

Stage 1, gingivitis, occurs when the gingiva appears inflamed. In Stage 1 disease there is no periodontal support loss or radiographic changes.

Stage 2, early periodontitis, occurs when attachment loss is less than 25%, as measured from the CEJ to the apex. Clinically, early periodontitis is typified by pocket formation or gingival recession. Radiographically, Stage 2 disease appears as blunting (rounding) of the alveolar margin. There may also appear to be a loss of continuity of the lamina dura at the level of the alveolar margin (Figure 4.92).

Stage 3, established periodontitis, is diagnosed when 25–50% of attachment loss occurs.

The direction of bone loss may be *horizontal* or *vertical* (angular) (Figure 4.93):

• Horizontal bone loss radiographically appears as decreased alveolar marginal bone around adjacent teeth. Normally, the crestal bone is located 1–2 mm apical to the cementoenamel junction. With horizontal bone loss, both the buccal and lingual plates of bone, as well as interdental bone, have been resorbed. Clinically, horizontal bone loss is typified by *suprabony* pockets, which occurs when the epithelial attachment is coronal to the bony defect (Figure 4.94).

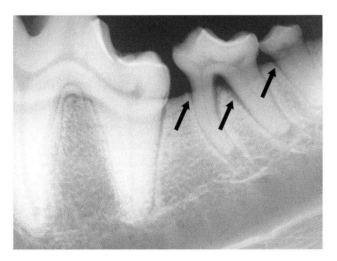

FIGURE 4.92. Loss of the normally sharp angles between the lamina dura and the alveolar margins and vertical bone loss of a dog's second mandibular molar.

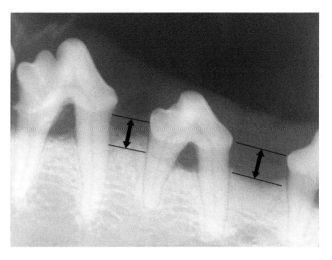

FIGURE 4.93. 25–40% horizontal bone loss around the second and third mandibular premolar tooth roots.

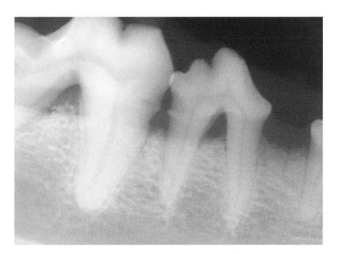

FIGURE 4.94. Horizontal bone loss around the mandibular fourth premolar and first molar.

• Vertical bone loss, resulting from infrabony (intrabony if three-walled) defects, occurs when the walls of the pocket are within a bony housing. Periodontal disease may cause a vertical defect to extend apically from the alveolar margin. At first, the defect is surrounded by three walls of bone: two marginal (lingual or palatal and facial) and a hemisepta (the bone of the interdental septum that remains on the root of the uninvolved adjacent tooth). As disease progresses, two-, one-, and no-walled (cup) defects may occur. Radiographically, vertical bone defects are generally V-shaped and are sharply outlined (Figure 4.95).

Stage 4, advanced periodontal disease is typified by deep pockets and/or marked gingival recession, tooth

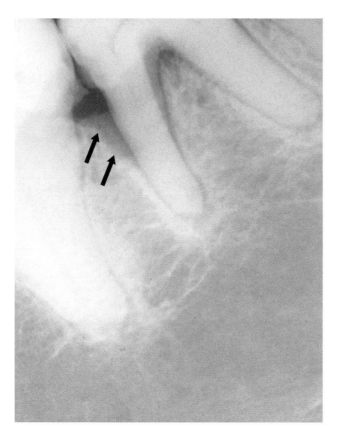

FIGURE 4.95. Vertical bone loss along distal root of the mandibular second molar.

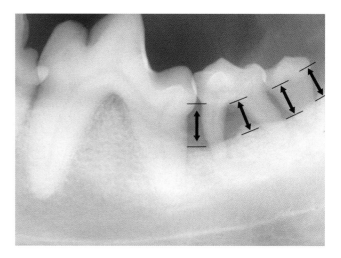

FIGURE 4.96. Stage 4 periodontal disease with greater than 50% bone loss around the second and third mandibular molars.

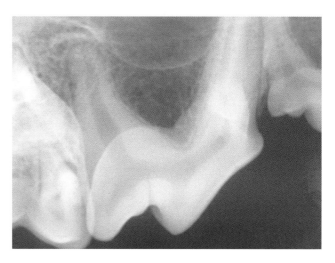

FIGURE 4.97. Normal appearance of the furcation of the maxillary fourth premolar.

mobility, gingival bleeding, and purulent discharge. Attachment loss is greater than 50% of the root height (Figure 4.96).

FURCATION EXPOSURE   Furcation exposure results from intraradicular bone loss due to advanced periodontal disease. It is sometimes difficult to determine radiographically whether the intraradicular space is involved unless there is a radiolucent area in the region of the furcation. Lack of radiographically detectable furcation involvement is not confirmation of the absence of periodontal destruction (Figure 4.97). Advanced furcation exposures, where both cortical plates are resorbed, are easily recognized on radiographs.

Class I (incipient) furcation involvement exists when the tip of a probe can just enter the furcation area. Bone partially fills the area where the roots meet. Radiographically, there is a decreased density of the bone at the furcation (Figure 4.98).

Class II (definite) furcation exposure exists when the probe tip extends horizontally into the area where the roots diverge, but does not exit on the other side.

Radiographically, there will be bone loss at the furcation (Figure 4.99).

Class III (through-and-through) exposure lesions exist secondary to advanced periodontal disease with extensive osseous destruction. Alveolar bone has resorbed to a point that an explorer probe passes through the defect unobstructed. Radiographically, there will be an area of complete bone loss (Figure 4.100).

ALVEOLAR DEHISCENCE   Alveolar dehiscence is a defect of the buccal alveolar bone plate involving the alveolar margin. Radiographically, there is loss of the lamina dura, periodontal ligament space, and alveolar bone surrounding the affected root (Figures 4.101, 4.102).

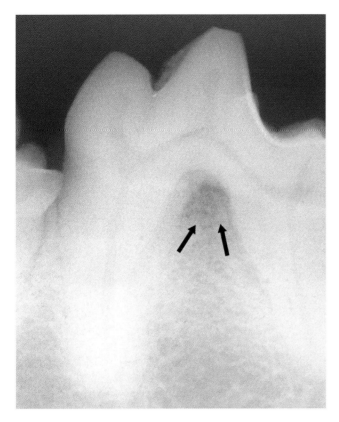

FIGURE 4.98. Radiograph of class I furcation involvement.

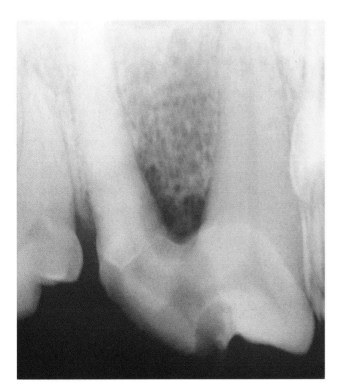

FIGURE 4.99. Radiograph of an advanced class II furcation exposure.

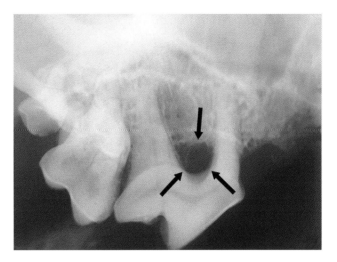

FIGURE 4.100. Radiograph of a class III furcation exposure.

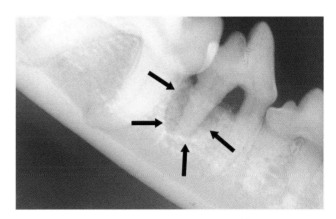

FIGURE 4.101. Radiograph showing total loss of attachment around the distal root of the mandibular fourth premolar.

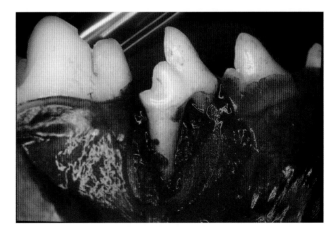

FIGURE 4.102. Surgical exposure of the mandibular fourth premolar portrayed in figure 4.101 (note the loss of alveolar bone around the distal root).

FELINE CHRONIC ALVEOLAR OSTEITIS Feline chronic alveolar osteitis (buccal bone expansion) clinically appears as bulging alveoli around one or both maxillary and/or mandibular canines. Radiographically, this lesion appears as bone loss around the root and expansile alveolar canine bone growth (Figures 4.103, 4.104).

FELINE SUPERERUPTION Feline supereruption (extrusion) occurs when one or more of the canine teeth appear longer than normal. Radiographically, the affected teeth have marked loss of periodontal support.

HYPERCEMENTOSIS Hypercementosis appears as increased thickness of cementum, usually at the apical third of the root in response to chronic inflammation or excessive occlusal forces.

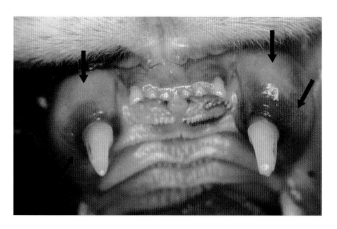

FIGURE 4.103. Bulging areas around the maxillary canines caused by feline chronic alveolar osteitis.

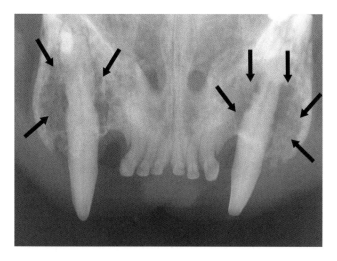

FIGURE 4.104. Radiographs showing bone loss around the canine roots caused by feline chronic alveolar osteitis and root resorption.

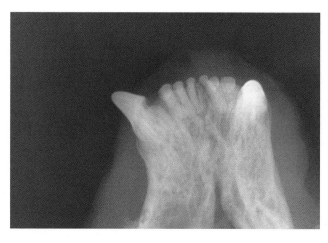

FIGURE 4.105. Ankylosis of the mandibular canines and root resorption.

ANKYLOSIS Ankylosis is the union of cementum with the alveolar bone through calcification of the periodontal ligament. The tooth root becomes fused to the alveolar wall. Radiographically, there will be no periodontal ligament space (Figure 4.105).

Radiologic Interpretation of Endodontic Disease

Radiography is essential for evaluation of a tooth affected by endodontic disease. The pulp is contained within the pulp cavity of the tooth. Pulp tissue appears radiolucent. Radiographs of an endodontically affected tooth are examined for the following:

- Radiographic apical closure necessary for conventional endodontic therapy
- Fractures
- Abnormalities in the canal, such as obstruction (pulpal stones) or resorption
- Periapical lesions, widened periodontal ligament space at the tooth's apex, and periapical radiolucency secondary to bone resorption
- Relative canal widths compared to adjacent or contralateral teeth (Figure 4.106).

PERIAPICAL DISEASE Periapical disease is a pathologic process surrounding the apex of one or more roots that occurs as an extension of periodontal disease, inflammation, or necrosis of the dental pulp from trauma or infection. Radiographic appearance of periapical disease includes the following:

- *A thickening of the apical periodontal ligament* with minimal alveolar bone resorption typical of a granulomatous lesion (Figure 4.107)

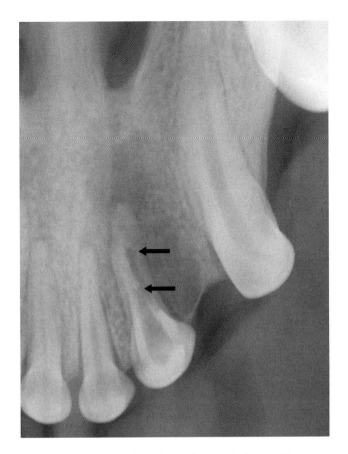

FIGURE 4.106. Widened canal of endodontically affected maxillary second incisor compared to normal first incisor.

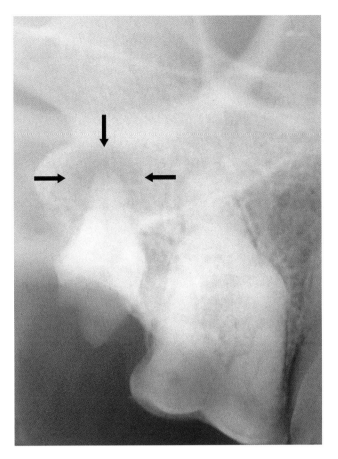

FIGURE 4.107. Radiograph of a periapical granuloma affecting the second maxillary molar.

- *A homogeneous radiolucency at the apex* or a dark halo in the periapical tissues probably caused by an abscess (Figure 4.108)
- *Sharply outlined circumscribed radiolucent areas* probably caused by a periapical cyst (most apical cysts arise from preexisting granulomas) (Figures 4.109, 4.110)

EXTERNAL ROOT RESORPTION   External root resorption may result from periapical inflammation, excessive occlusal forces, or from unknown stimuli. Radiographically, external resorption will appear as irregular loss of root structure, which can occur in any area of the root surface (Figures 4.111–4.113).

ENDODONTIC-PERIODONTIC LESIONS   Class I endoperio lesions are primary endodontic lesions which exhibit a radiolucent halo that extends coronally from the root apex eventually reaching the gingival sulcus, causing a secondary periodontal lesion. The pattern of bone loss often resembles a *J* shape (Figure 4.114).

Class II periodontic-endodontic (perioendo) lesions

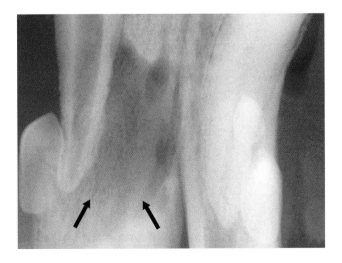

FIGURE 4.108. Radiograph of a mandibular canine periapical abscess.

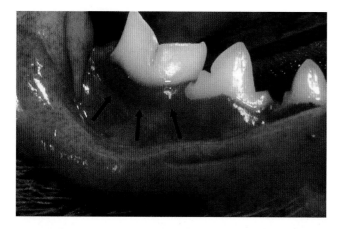

FIGURE 4.109. Inflammation of the attached gingiva around the mandibular first molar.

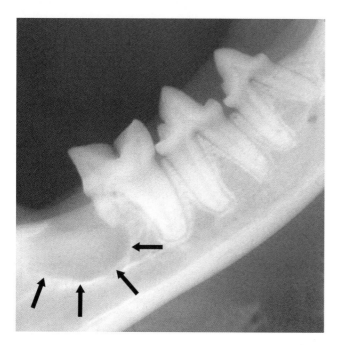

FIGURE 4.110. Radiograph revealing a probable peri-apical cyst.

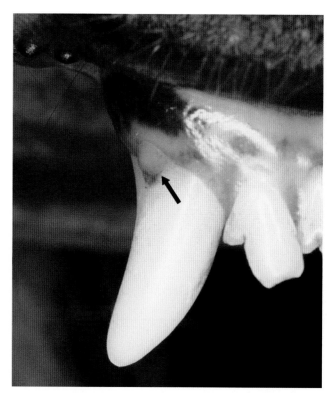

FIGURE 4.111. Gingiva filling enamel and dentin resorption at the CEJ.

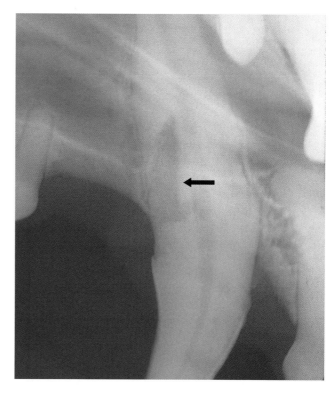

FIGURE 4.112. Radiograph showing lesion extending subgingivally.

occur when the loss of attachment extends uniformly apically to a lateral canal or to the apical delta leading to pulpal necrosis. Class II perioendo lesions often affect the mandibular first molar and appear as one "floating" root without alveolar support, with a periapical endodontic lesion affecting the other tooth root (Figure 4.115).

Class III periodontic-endodontic lesions are true combined separate endodontic and periodontal lesions, which have coalesced (Figure 4.116).

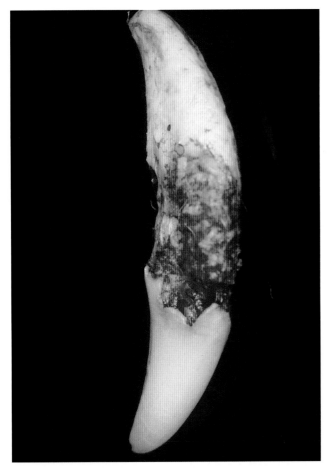

FIGURE 4.113. Extracted canine tooth affected by external resorption.

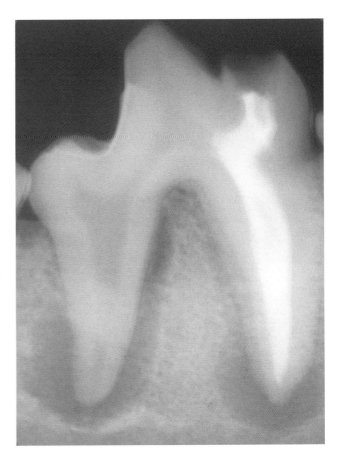

FIGURE 4.114. Class I endoperio lesion in a mandibular first molar tooth after standard root canal therapy of one root canal before hemisection of the distal root.

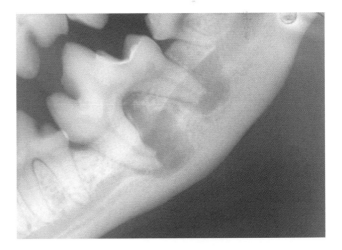

FIGURE 4.115. Class II perioendo lesion.

INTERNAL RESORPTION Internal resorption arises from the pulp. The cause is unknown, but trauma or pulpal death from anachoresis (bacteria gaining access to the injured pulp through vascular channels) are believed to be contributing factors. Often, it is difficult to determine whether a lesion is due to internal or external resorption. If a normal-appearing root canal is visualized radiographically, the lesion is considered external in origin (Figures 4.117–4.120).

CONDENSING OSTEITIS *Condensing osteitis* occurs in response to low-grade infection. It appears as a radiodense area around the apex of a tooth (Figure 4.121).

FELINE RESORPTIVE LESIONS Radiographic findings of feline odontoclastic resorptive lesions (FORLs) include:

- Class 1 FORLs rarely show radiographic changes.

- Class 2 FORLS extend through the enamel or cementum into the dentin, and may appear radiographically as a focal decreased dentin density in the affected areas (Figures 4.122, 4.123).

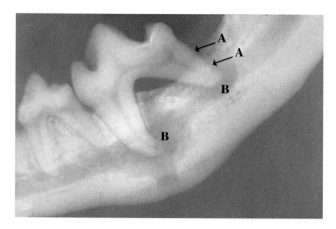

FIGURE 4.116. Class III combined lesion: (A) area of periodontal support loss; (B) endodontic disease.

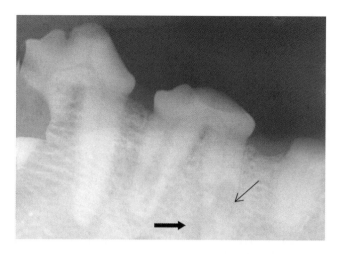

FIGURE 4.118. Radiograph confirming pulpal exposure, internal resorption (thin arrow), and periapical disease (bold arrow).

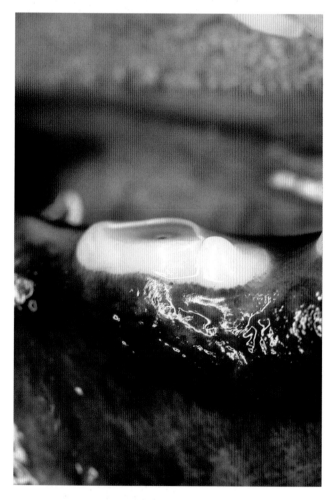

FIGURE 4.117. Pulpal exposure in a mandibular premolar due to tennis ball chewing.

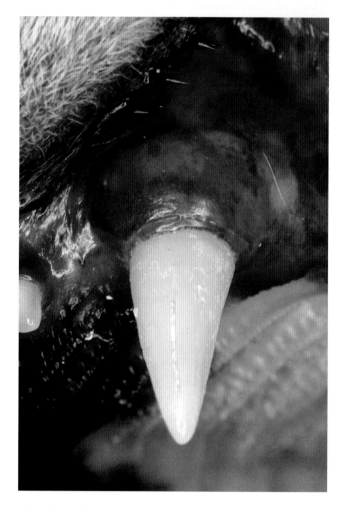

FIGURE 4.119. Clinically normal-appearing canine in a 4-year-old cat.

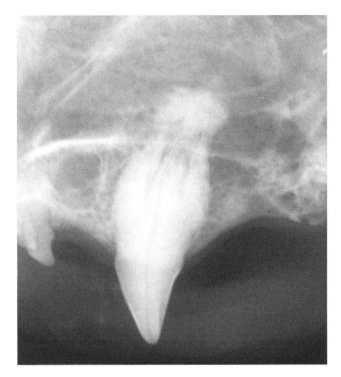

FIGURE 4.120. Radiograph revealing marked internal and external resorption.

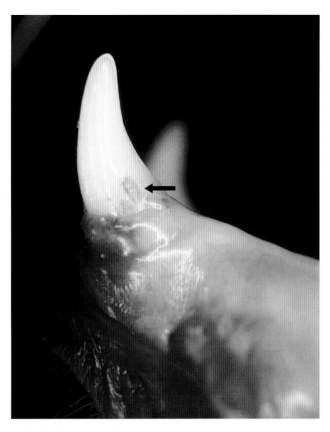

FIGURE 4.122. Class 2 FORL.

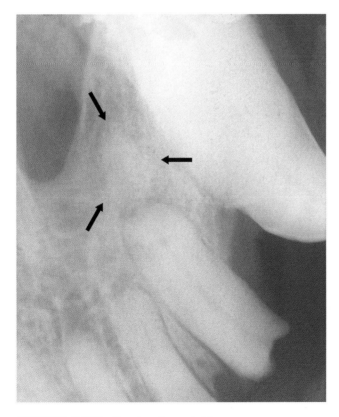

FIGURE 4.121. Condensing osteitis.

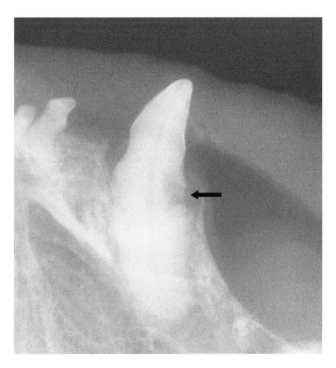

FIGURE 4.123. Radiograph showing Class 2 FORL extending through the dentin into the enamel.

- Class 3 lesions enter the pulp. Radiographically, pulpal penetration may be noted, or the normally uniform pulp chamber may show evidence of internal or external resorption (Figure 4.124).
- Class 4 lesions show extensive structural damage.
- Class 5 lesions have complete crown loss, with part of the root(s) present subgingivally in varying stages of ankylosis and resorption (Figures 4.125, 4.126).

RENAL SECONDARY HYPERPARATHYROIDISM
Renal secondary hyperparathyroidism (rubber jaw) appears radiographically as if the teeth are floating in the jaw without surrounding bone (Figure 4.127).

NEOPLASIA Neoplasia appears as destruction and/or increased production of all tissues around the tooth. Occasionally, the teeth will appear to be floating. (Figures 4.128–4.133).

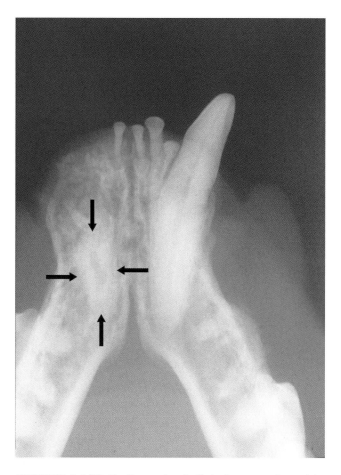

FIGURE 4.126. Radiograph of clinical case portrayed in figure 4.125 revealing tooth root located subgingivally.

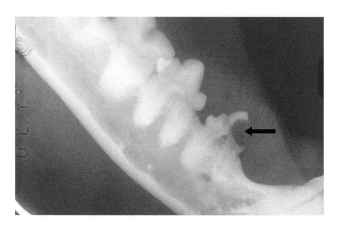

FIGURE 4.124. Radiograph of a class 3 FORL penetrating the enamel, dentin, and pulp of a mandibular third premolar.

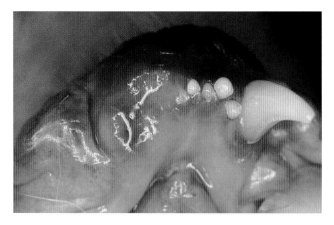

FIGURE 4.125. The left mandibular canine crown is not apparent visually in this 6-year-old feline.

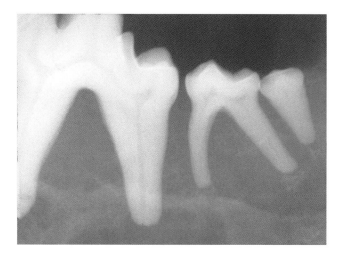

FIGURE 4.127. Radiograph of mandible affected by renal secondary hyperparathyroidism.

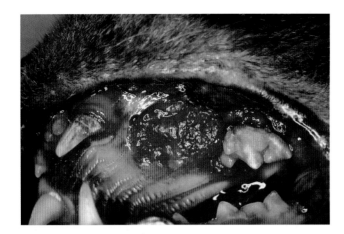

FIGURE 4.128. Squamous cell carcinoma.

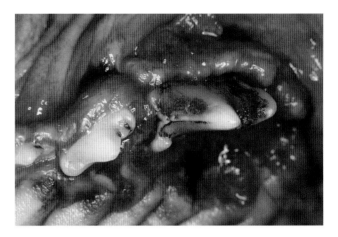

FIGURE 4.130. Squamous cell carcinoma invading a canine's maxilla.

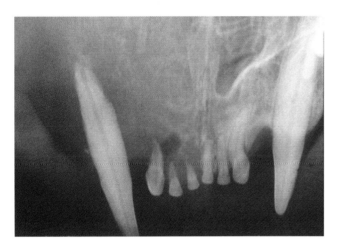

FIGURE 4.129. Radiograph of feline squamous cell carcinoma displayed in figure 4.128 destroying all visible tooth support.

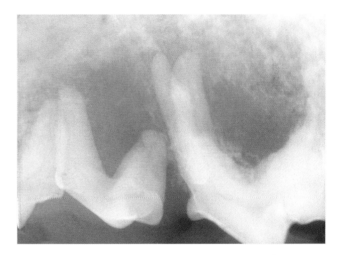

FIGURE 4.131. Radiographic appearance of canine squamous cell carcinoma in figure 4.130 destroying tooth support.

AMELOBLASTOMA Canine acanthomatus ameloblastoma (acanthomatus epulis) appears as multilocular honeycombed bone with an indistinct border (Figures 4.134, 4.135).

FOREIGN BODIES Foreign bodies can cause oral swellings and nasal discharge (Figure 4.136).

DENTIGEROUS CYST A dentigerous cyst appears as a fluid-filled swelling that contains an embedded tooth (Figure 4.137).

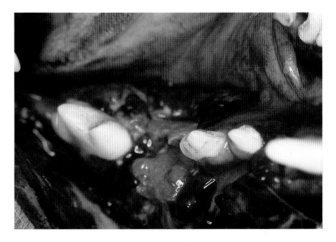

FIGURE 4.132. Canine oral melanoma invading the mandible.

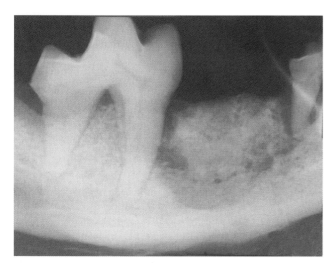

FIGURE 4.133. Radiographic appearance of sequestered bone secondary to canine oral melanoma as portrayed in figure 4.132.

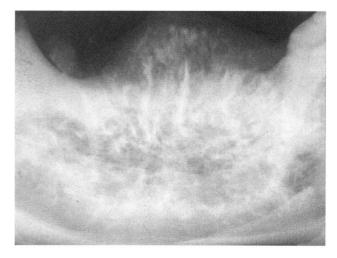

FIGURE 4.135. Radiograph of acanthomatus ameloblastoma regrowth 2 years after en bloc removal showing bone production and destruction.

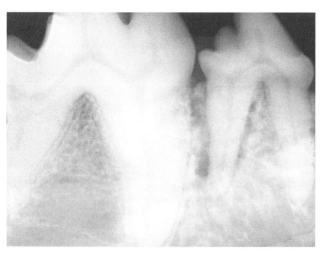

FIGURE 4.134. Radiograph of acanthomatus ameoblastoma of the mandible; note honeycombed appearance of bone between the mandibular fourth pre-molar and first molar.

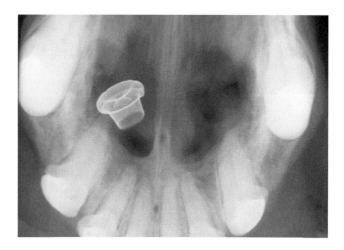

FIGURE 4.136. Metallic foreign body in nasal cavity of a dog with a 1-year history of nasal discharge.

JAW FRACTURES   Jaw fractures should be evaluated radiographically to help evaluate a therapy plan. Often the fracture line will include a tooth that should be extracted. *Normal* breed (brachycephalics) and age variations of the mandibular symphysis should not be confused with a fracture that needs therapy (Figures 4.138, 4.139).

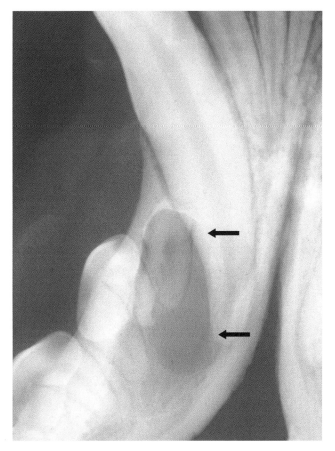

FIGURE 4.137. Radiograph of dentigerous cyst.

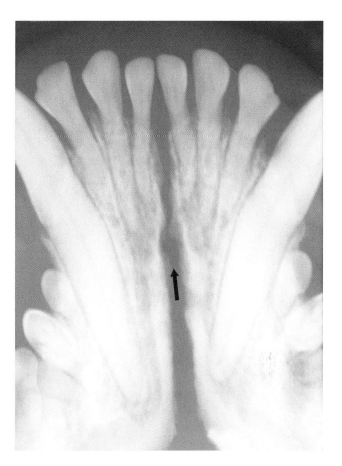

FIGURE 4.139. Normal appearing mandibular symphysis space in a pug dog.

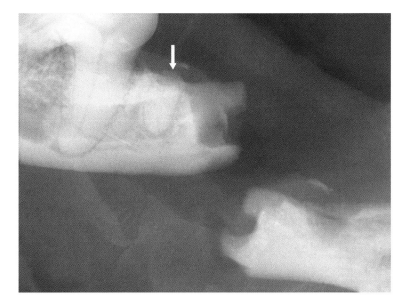

FIGURE 4.138. Mandibular jaw fracture with distal fourth premolar root remnant.

5
Local and Regional Anesthesia and Pain Control

A similarity exists between the way dogs, cats, and humans feel dental pain. Local anesthetics are agents that, when injected or topically applied, decrease or halt nerve conduction in a circumscribed area of the body for a period of time.

The trigeminal nerve (CNV) is responsible for the sensory innervation of the oral cavity. The maxillary teeth, as well as maxillary soft and hard tissues are innervated by the maxillary nerve, a branch of CNV, which branches into the infraorbital nerve. The mandibular nerve, a branch of CNV, branches into the lingual nerve, which innervates the tongue and the inferior alveolar nerve, which branches into the mental nerves.

Mode of Action

Local anesthesia occurs after depositing an anesthetic agent in close proximity to a nerve innervating the area intended for dental treatment. Following the injection, anesthetic molecules move by diffusion into the nerve, blocking its normal action.

To obtain complete anesthesia following an injection, the nerve must be permeated by a sufficient concentration of the anesthetic base to inhibit conduction in all fibers. *Induction* is the length of time from the deposition of the anesthetic solution to complete and effective conduction blockage. The action of a local anesthetic continues until the concentration is carried away by the blood stream. *Duration* is the length of time from induction until the reversal process is complete.

The following are benefits of local and regional anesthesia:

- Decreased pain during and after surgical procedures
- Decreased risk of vagally mediated reflex bradycardia

- Lower inhalant anesthetic requirement; decreased minimum alveolar anesthetic concentration (MAC) needed to provide analgesia
- Less post-operative analgesic medication needed
- Improved level of anesthesia; eliminates the variation of anesthetic depth when painful stimulation occurs

Indications for local and regional anesthesia include the following:

- Surgical and nonsurgical extractions
- Root canal therapy
- Mandibulectomy, maxillectomy
- Mandibular or maxillary fracture repair
- Vital pulpotomy
- Periodontal procedures—flaps, root planing, gingivectomy
- Oronasal fistula repair
- Oral mass incision or excision

Contraindications for local and regional anesthesia include the following:

- Local anesthetic agents may not be effective when injected into a region of increased acidity, due to infection.
- If halothane is used for anesthesia, epinephrine containing local anesthetic should not be injected.
- Epinephrine-potentiated local anesthetics should not be used in cardiac or hyperthyroid patients.

Materials

Bupivacaine is the most commonly used local anesthetic in veterinary dentistry.

Potency

Local anesthetic potency is measured by lipid solubility (Table 5.1).

Table 5.1. The relationship between lipid solubility and relative potency.

Agent	Lipid Solubility	Relative Potency
	(Partition coefficient)	
Procaine	0.6	1
Mepivicaine	0.6	2
Lidocaine	2.9	2
Bupivacaine	27.5	8
Tetracaine	80.0	8
Etidocaine	141.0	8

Duration

The action of a local anesthetic will continue until the concentration is carried away by the blood stream to other tissues. Local anesthetics are metabolized primarily in the liver and excreted through the kidneys.

Anesthetic duration is related to the amount of medication bound to proteins in the nerve membrane. The greater the binding affinity to nerve proteins, the longer duration of action. For example, the increased protein binding of bupivacaine compared with mepivacaine causes a two- to fourfold increase in bupivacaine's duration. A similar relationship exists between lidocaine and its longer-acting analogue etidocaine. Local anesthetics that have the greatest potency usually exhibit the longest duration of action (Table 5.2).

Vasoconstriction

Local anesthetics are vasodilators due to their low pH. Their injection into tissue generally increases blood flow at the injection site. Unfortunately, the action of local anesthesia is reversed as the bloodstream carries away the solution. Vasoconstrictors (epinephrine) incorporated into the local anesthetic solution:

- Enhance the duration and effectiveness of anesthesia.
- Decrease systemic toxicity by lowering the blood concentrations of the anesthetic.
- Decrease local bleeding at the injection site.

LOCAL ANESTHESIA EQUIPMENT

Local anesthetic solutions are available as:

- Filled sterilized glass cartridges with rubber stoppers at one end and aluminum caps with a rubber diaphragm at the other end. The cartridges are stored at room temperature and protected from direct sunlight. The cartridge container and/or rubber stopper is color-coded indicating the epinephrine ratio of the solution. After the needle and syringe have been assembled, the cartridge must either be used or discarded (Figure 5.1).
- A multidose vial (Figure 5.2)

Syringes

Syringes and needles are used to administer local anesthesia:

Table 5.2. Anesthethic duration in humans.

Agent	Pulpal Duration (min)	Soft Tissue Duration (min)
2% lidocaine (Schein 465-5161)	5–10	60–120
2% lidocaine and 1:100,000 epinephrine (Xylocaine) (Burns 951-5510, Schein 465-1150)	60–90	180–240
3% mepivicaine (Carbocaine HCL 3%) (Burns 951-6215, Schein 467-0350)	20–40	120–180
3% mepivicaine and 1:100,000 epinephrine	45–60	180–240
0.5% bupivacaine (Marcaine HCL 0.5%) (Burns 216-060, Schein 258-6105) and 1:200,000 epinephrine (Schein 258-3172)	90–180	240–540

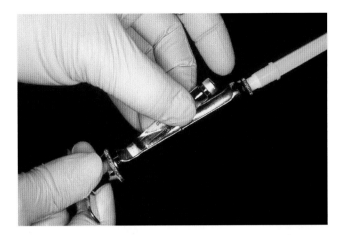

FIGURE 5.1. Local anesthetic syringe and cartridge.

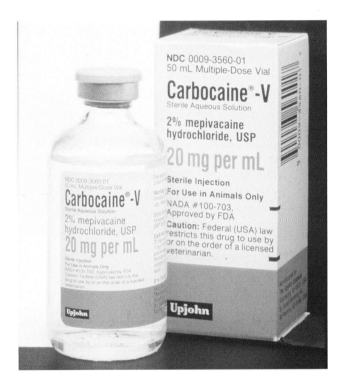

FIGURE 5.2. Mepivicaine multidose vial.

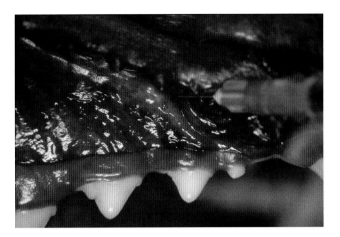

FIGURE 5.3. Tuberculin syringe and needle used to administer local anesthetic.

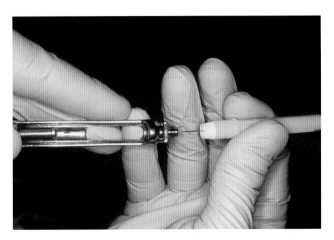

FIGURE 5.4. Dental local anesthetic administration syringe.

- Disposable 1 cc tuberculin syringes equipped with a 3/4- or 1.5-inch 27 gauge needle are most commonly used (Figure 5.3). Disposable 3 cc syringes can also be equipped as above.

- Dental local anesthetic administration syringes, pre-loaded cartridges, and a 30 gauge needle, preferred by the author, allow one-hand aspiration to help ensure that the medication is not administered within the blood vessel (Figure 5.4)—N-tralig (Miltex Instrument Company) (Burns 950-1595, Schein 100-4612).

The technique for using a local anesthetic administration syringe employs the following steps:

1. Select an anesthetic cartridge.
2. Select the appropriate disposable needle.
3. Hold the syringe in the left hand and insert the thumb into the ring to pull back the plunger.
4. Hold the syringe and cartridge in the left hand, while using the right hand to load the local anesthetic syringe. Use the left hand to apply firm pressure until the harpoon is engaged into the rubber stopper. To check that the harpoon is securely in place, gently pull back the plunger.
5. Attach a disposable needle without removing the needle guard from the injection end of the needle.
6. Remove the needle guard. Check anesthetic flow by expelling a small amount of solution.

Needles

Syringe needles that attach to the dental local anesthetic syringe are available in two lengths: 1-inch or 1 5/8-inch. The most commonly used gauges are 27 and 30. The 1-inch "short" needle is used for local infiltration of anesthesia and the 1 5/8-inch "long" needle is used for deeper block anesthesia. The tip of the needle is beveled. During injection, the bevel is turned toward the periosteum to deposit the solution accurately (Burns: 30 g short 953-2460, 25 g long 253-2455, 27 g long 953-2355, 27 g short 953-2350, 27 g short; Schein: 25 g short 194-9510, 25 g long 194-6120, 27 g short 194-1613, 27 g long 194-0506, 30 g short 194-1753, 30 g long 194-5141).

Alternatively, many practitioners use standard veterinary 23-27 g 1- to $1\frac{1}{2}$-inch needles attached to tuberculin or 3 cc syringes for local anesthesia administration.

Dosage

Bupivacaine hydrochloride (Marcaine) with epinephrine is commonly used in veterinary dentistry. The maximum recommended dosage for dogs and cats is 2 mg/kg (total dosage divided over the number of sites that need to be anesthetized). While the recommended volume for local anesthesia is 0.1-0.5 ml per site in the canine, and 0.1-0.3 ml per site in the feline, an extra 0.1-0.2 ml can be injected for the infraorbital block to anesthetize the caudal superior alveolar nerve branches.

General Injection Precautions

Injection into a blood vessel can alter cardiac function. To be certain that the solution is not being injected into a vessel, the veterinarian needs to aspirate before injecting.

LOCAL ANESTHESIA PROCEDURE

Infiltration (Periodontal Ligament Injection) Anesthesia

Infiltration anesthesia is a technique where the anesthetic solution is injected under pressure directly into the periodontal ligament and surrounding tissues. This may be done using either a conventional syringe or a periodontal ligament injection syringe. Infiltration is most effective in areas of thin cortical bone such as the maxillary teeth and mandibular incisors (Figure 5.5).

Intraosseous injection

The interdental septum and the alveolar bone have

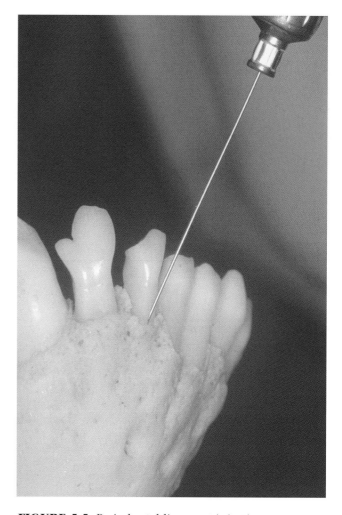

FIGURE 5.5. Periodontal ligament injection.

numerous perforations and porosities containing blood vessels, lymphatics, and nerve fibers, which account for the manner in which the anesthetic deposited into the alveolar bone finds its way to the vessels of the root bed.

A specially designed 1/8-inch long 30 guage needle, which is reinforced with a strong plastic sheath, allows direct injection into the interproximal bone without bending or breaking. The needle should enter tissue perpendicular to the cortical plate. Local anesthetic is injected into the coronal cortical bone mesial and distal to the tooth to be anesthetized.

The technique for the intraosseous block employs the following steps:

1. Insert the needle to a depth of 1-2 mm perpendicular to the tissue surface into the interproximal gingiva midway between the teeth.
2. Aspirate the needle in two planes to make sure the tip is not located intravascular.
3. Inject slowly.

teeth. The rostral superior alveolar nerve branches off the infraorbital nerve just before it exits from the infraorbital canal. These branches supply innervation to the maxillary canine teeth and incisors. The infraorbital artery and vein travel with the infraorbital nerve within the canal and should be avoided when injecting a local anesthetic solution.

For medium and large dogs, 0.25-0.5 ml of bupivacaine is injected. The *infraorbital foramen* can be palpated as a depression in the alveolar mucosa usually found apical to the distal root of the maxillary third premolar. The distal extent of the infraorbital canal can be estimated by palpating the caudal ventral margin of the bony orbit. The needle is placed rostrocaudal (horizontal) to the entrance of the foramen. Before injection, the syringe is aspirated in several directions to make sure the tip is not intravascular (Figures 5.7-5.10).

Local anesthetic diffusion at the *maxillary foramen* desensitizes all maxillary teeth on the same side as the

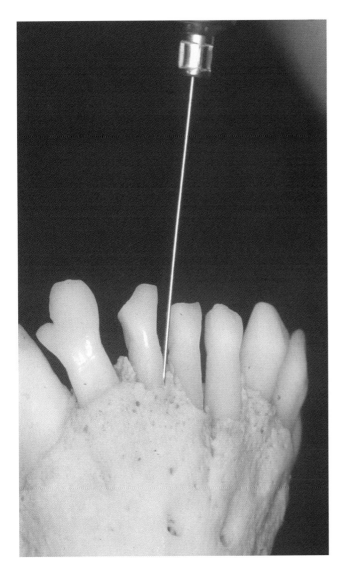

FIGURE 5.6. Interosseus block location.

4. Repeat steps 1 through 3 at the distal papilla (Figure 5.6).

Anesthesia Regional

Desensitization of the teeth occurs through the pulp. Block or regional anesthesia is obtained by injecting the anesthetic solution in the proximity of the nerve trunk.

Maxilla

INFRAORBITAL   Branches of the infraorbital nerve supply sensory innervation to the maxillary dental arcade. Branches from the caudal superior alveolar nerve arise from the infraorbital nerve before it enters the infraorbital canal, innervate the caudal maxillary teeth. Within the infraorbital canal, the middle superior alveolar nerve branches supply the maxillary cheek

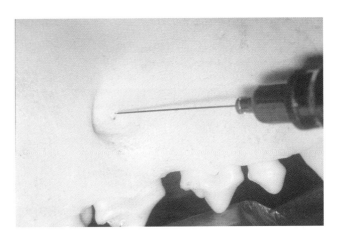

FIGURE 5.7. Canine skull showing syringe tip placement next to the infraorbital foramen.

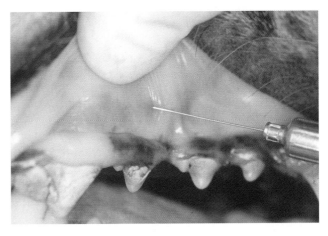

FIGURE 5.8. Infraorbital injection site in the canine cadaver specimen.

injection. The injection is made by advancing a 1-inch needle in the dog and 5/8-inch needle in the cat several millimeters into the infraorbital foramen. Fifty percent more anesthetic (not to exceed 2 mg/kg) is slowly injected into the caudal infraorbital canal. After injection, digital pressure is applied over the foramen for 1 minute to force the agent to diffuse caudally (Figure 5.11).

MAXILLARY The *maxillary nerve block* desensitizes the palatal soft tissue, dentition, lip, and bone on the injected side of the maxilla. The caudal superior alveolar nerve innervates the maxillary fourth premolar.

The procedure employs the following steps:

- Intraorally palpate the depression distal and buccal to the last maxillary molar, adjacent to the zygomatic arch.
- Walk the needle along the caudal aspect of the depression perpendicular to the horizontal plane of the palate at the root tip level.
- Aspirate the needle and slowly inject the anesthetic agent (Figure 5.12).

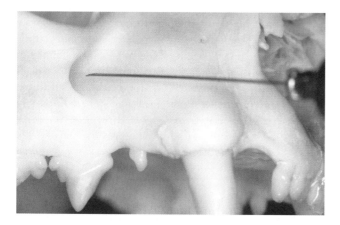

FIGURE 5.9. Feline skull showing infraorbital foramen.

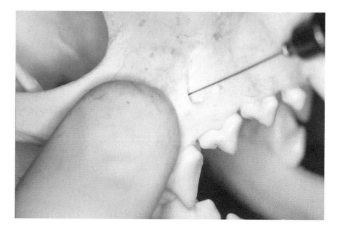

FIGURE 5.11. Needle inserted into the infraorbital canal to deliver anesthetic caudally.

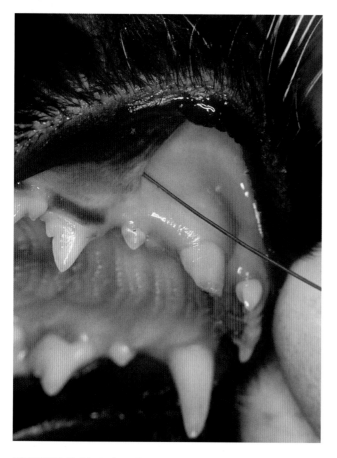

FIGURE 5.10. Infraorbital injection site in the feline.

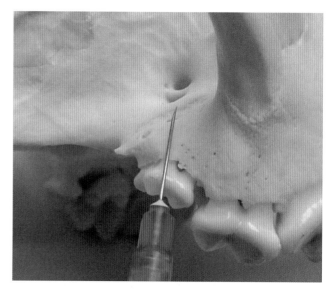

FIGURE 5.12. Canine skull showing maxillary foramen.

Mandible

MENTAL BLOCK   The mental block anesthetizes the lingual and buccal soft tissue of the mandibular incisors and canine on the side injected, as well as the first two premolars.

Use the following technique:

- In dogs, palpate the middle mental foramen (largest of the three mental foramina) intraorally ventral to the mesial root of the second premolar. Position the needle two-thirds of the distance ventral and buccal to the dorsal mandibular border just caudal to the mandibular labial frenulum. The needle may be inserted several millimeters into the canal before anesthetic injection (Figures 5.13, 5.14).
- In cats, locate the middle mental foramen in the center of the space between the mandibular canine and third premolar, half the distance between dorsal and ventral borders of the mandible (Figures 5.15, 5.16).

MANDIBULAR INFERIOR ALVEOLAR BLOCK The mandibular branch of the trigeminal nerve exits the foramen ovale, dividing into the anterior and posterior branches. The posterior divides into the lingual and inferior alveolar nerves. The inferior alveolar nerve enters the mandibular foramen on the medial side of the ramus just rostral to the angle of the mandible to occupy the mandibular canal.

The inferior alveolar nerve can be anesthetized by intraoral or extraoral techniques. The foramen is easily palpated from inside the mouth lingually, just caudal to the last molar. The foramen in dogs is 1/2 to 1 inch and in cats is 1/2 inch from the ventral surface of the mandible. When anesthetized, the inferior alveolar will

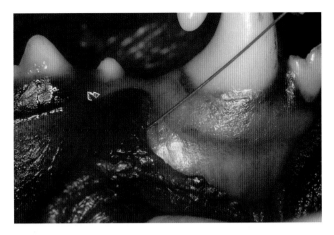

FIGURE 5.14. Placement of needle for injection of the middle mental foramen in the dog.

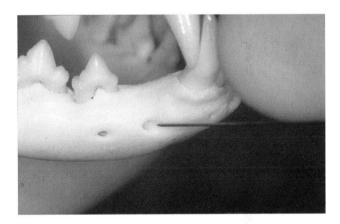

FIGURE 5.15. Feline middle mental foramen location on skull.

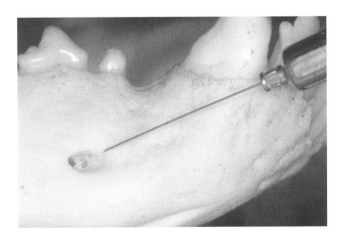

FIGURE 5.13. Canine skull showing middle mental foramen.

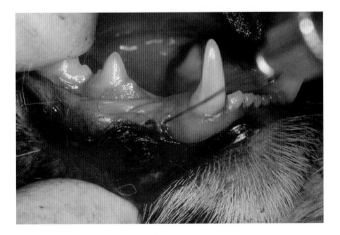

FIGURE 5.16. Placement of needle for injection of the middle mental foramen in a feline patient.

desensitize the body of the mandible and lower portion of the ramus, all mandibular teeth on the same side, the floor of the mouth, the rostral tongue innervated by the lingual nerve, the gingiva on the lingual and labial surfaces of the mandible, and the mucosa and skin of the lower lip and chin.

When the author-preferred *transcutaneous (extraoral) approach* is chosen, a small area of skin ventromedial to the angle of the mandible just rostral to the angular process is clipped and prepped. The mandibular foramen is transorally palpated with the index finger of one hand while the needle is introduced through the skin toward the lingual surface with the other. The syringe is aspirated and anesthetic injected caudal to the foramen (Figure 5.17).

In cats, the needle in inserted at a point ventral to the lateral canthus, and directed medially along the border of the mandible (Figure 5.18).

When using the *intraoral approach*, the mandibular inferior alveolar nerve is infiltrated where it enters the mouth at the angle of the jaw. The needle is gently "walked" along the medial border of the mandible just caudal to the last molar. The needle is then advanced toward the angular process to an area half the dorsoventral width of the mandible. The syringe is aspirated and anesthetic delivered at the location of the mandibular foramen (Figure 5.19).

MANDIBULAR BUCCAL NERVE BLOCK The mandibular buccal nerve block anesthetizes soft tissue buccal to the mandibular premolars and molars. It can be used in addition to the inferior alveolar block.

The needle is placed in the submucosa, buccal and apical to the mandibular second molar (Figure 5.20).

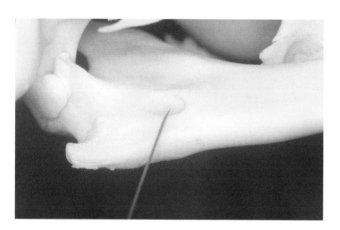

FIGURE 5.17. Extraoral position of needle for mandibular inferior alveolar block in a feline skull.

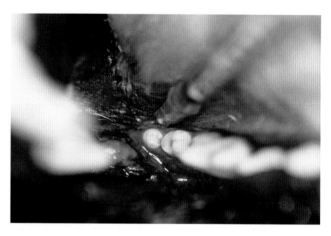

FIGURE 5.19. Placement of needle at the mandibular foramen area in the canine patient.

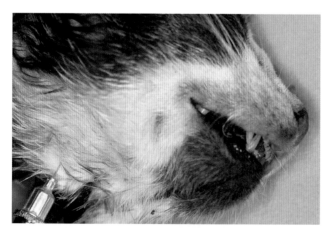

FIGURE 5.18. Syringe placement for extraoral infiltration of the feline inferior alveolar nerve in a non-prepped cadaver specimen.

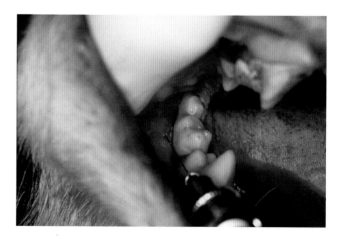

FIGURE 5.20. Placement of needle at the angle of the dog jaw for the mandibular buccal nerve block.

Dispensable Pain Relief Medication

Post-operative oral surgery pain must be controlled. Oral medications used to control pain include NSAIDs, opioids, and opioid/acetaminophen preparations.

Transdermal analgesic preparations are available which can be placed on a clipped region. The Duragesic (Fentanyl) patches are especially effective in cats to con-trol pain. The patch can be applied the evening before surgery to ensure serum levels are appropriate pre-oper-atively.

Tables 5.3 through 5.5 list non-steroidal anti-inflam-matories (NSAIDs), opioid preparations, and opioid/acetaminophen preparations (for dogs only), respectively.

Table 5.3. Non-steroidal anti-inflammatories (NSAIDs).

NSAID	Dog	Cat
Aspirin tablets 65, 325 mg	10–25 mg/kg q12h	10–20 mg/kg q48–72h
Carprofen (Rimadyl) 25, 75, 100 mg	2.0 mg/kg q12h	1.0 mg/kg PO 1–2 doses only (extra label)
Ketoprofen (Orudis)	25, 50.75 mg 2.0 mg/kg loading dose, then 1.0 mg/kg q24h (5 days maximum)	Same dosage as dog
Etodolac (Etogesic)	150, 300 mg 10–15mg/kg q25h	—
Meloxicam (Metacam oral suspension) 1.5 mg/ml	0.2 mg/kg loading dose, then 0.1 mg/kg q24h	0.2–0.3 mg/kg loading dose, then 0.1 mg/kg q24h 2–3 days, not approved for cats in the U.S.
Acetaminophen tablets 235, 500 mg or elixir 160 mg/5ml	15mg/kg q8h	Toxic to cats

Table 5.4. Opioid preparations.

Opioid	Dog	Cat
Buprenorphine	0.01–0.02 mg/kg q12h, IV, IM, SC	0.005–0.01 IV, IM
Butorphanol (Torbutrol) 1, 5, 10 mg	0.2–1.0 mg/kg q1–4h	0.2–1.0 mg/kg PO q4h
Codeine tablets 30, 60 mg	1.0–2.0 mg/kg PO q6–8h	0.1–1.0 mg/kg q4–8h
Morphine tablets 10, 15, 30 mg	0.3–1.0 mg/kg PO q4–8h	—
Hydromorphone	0.08–0.3 mg/kg IV, IM, SC q2–6h	0.08–0.3 mg/kg IV, IM, SC q2–6h

Table 5.5. Opioid/acetaminophen preparations (for dogs only).

Preparation	Dosage
Codeine 60 mg + acetaminophen 300 mg (Tylenol with codeine #4 tablet)	Dose based on codeine at 1–2.0 mg/kg PO q6–8h
Codeine 2.4 mg/ml + acetaminophen 24 mg/ml (Tylenol with codeine elixir)	Dose based on codeine at 1.0–2.0 mg/kg PO q6–8h
Oxycodone 5 mg + acetaminophen 325 mg (Percocet)	Dose based on acetaminophen at 10–15.0 mg/kg PO q8–12h

6
Periodontal Equipment, Materials, and Techniques

Periodontal inflammation is the most common disease affecting small animals. The dedicated veterinarian and dental team can make a lifelong difference in patient health by concentrating on periodontal health. Periodontal care includes supragingival and subgingival scaling, application of local medication, bone graft implants, periodontal surgery, tooth resection, extraction, and home care.

TISSUES OF THE PERIODONTIUM

The term *periodontium* is used to describe tissues that surround and support the teeth, and includes the gingiva, alveolar bone, periodontal ligament, and cementum. Understanding the normal features and appearance of the periodontium is essential to appreciating the pathologic changes that occur with gingival and periodontal infections (Figure 6.1).

The oral cavity is lined with keratinized, parakeratinized, and nonkeratinized mucosa. *Attached gingiva* refers to the tissues covering the alveolar process surrounding the teeth. The gingiva includes oral, sulcular, and junctional epithelium. Normal gingiva appears coral pink, firm, and stippled, with knife-edged margins. Pigment is normally present. The *marginal gingiva* is the most coronal (toward the crown) aspect of the gingiva. Marginal gingiva is not attached to the tooth, but lies passively against it. The space between the tooth and the marginal gingiva is the *gingival sulcus* or *crevice*. The normal depth of the sulcus is 0.5–1 mm in cats and 1–3 mm in dogs. The *free gingival margin* is the coronal edge of the marginal gingiva. Free gingiva is distinguished from attached gingiva by the *free gingival groove*, a slight depression on the coronal gingiva corresponding to normal sulcus depth (Figures 6.2A, 6.2B).

In the dog, the healthy free gingival margin of premolars and molars is 1–3 mm coronal to the *cemento-*

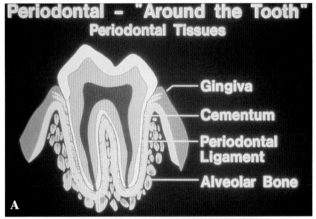

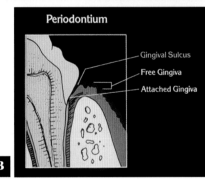

FIGURE 6.1. (A) Tooth and surrounding peridontium; (B) gingival sulcular structures.

enamel junction (CEJ), where root cementum meets the coronal enamel. The free gingival margin of the canine teeth is 1–3 mm coronal to the CEJ. In the feline, the free gingival margin is .5–1 mm coronal to the CEJ.

The *attached gingiva* is located apical to the marginal gingiva and normally is tightly bound to the alveolar margin and the periosteum of alveolar bone. The width of the attached gingiva varies in different areas of the mouth. Attached gingiva is keratinized to withstand the stresses of ripping and tearing (Figure 6.2C).

Glossary

Alveolar bone, alveolar process is part of the mandible and maxilla that surrounds the roots of erupted teeth forming the sockets.

Alveolar margin is the most coronal edge or portion of the alveolar bone, terminating at and parallel with the contours of the cementoenamel junction.

Alveolar mucosa (lining mucosa) is the mucous membrane that covers the alveolar process and extends from the mucogingival line into the vestibule, covering the inside of the lips, cheeks, soft palate, and ventral surface of the tongue.

Alveoloplasty (AP) is a surgical procedure used to recontour the alveolar bone.

Alveolus, alveolar socket is the bony cavity within the alveolar process in which the root of a tooth is held by the periodontal ligament.

Attached gingiva is that portion of the masticatory mucosa firmly attached to the underlying teeth and alveolar process. Attached gingiva is bound coronally by the free gingival groove and apically by the mucogingival junction.

Attachment apparatus consists of the alveolar bone, cementum, and periodontal ligament, which support the teeth.

Attachment loss (attachment level) is measured from the CEJ to the depth of the periodontal pocket. Attachment loss is the combination of the pocket depth and gingival recession measurements.

Biofilm is a well-oganized community of symbiotic micro-organisms.

Bone grafting is a surgical procedure using a variety of materials in an effort to actively induce bone formation, deposit new bone, or act as a scaffolding for bone formation.

Bone loss is a reduction in the height of alveolar bone due to periodontal disease.

Buccal mucosa lines the oral cavity facing the cheeks.

Calculus or tartar is comprised of multiple mineralized layers of plaque adherent to the tooth's surface. Calculus is inert, but provides a rough surface for plaque accumulation.

Cementoenamel junction (CEJ) is a line between the anatomical root and crown where the enamel ends and the cementum covering the root begins.

Cementum is avascular calcified mesenchymal tissue, which forms the outer covering of the roots. The periodontal ligament fibers (Sharpey's fibers) anchor into the cementum.

Cleft is a longitudinal fissure or opening of the marginal gingiva, exposing the underlying tooth root.

Cribriform plate is the dense inner bony wall of the alveolus, consisting of cancellous bone.

Dental prophylaxis is the use of appropriate dental procedures and/or techniques to prevent dental and oral disease.

Disclosing solution is a coloring agent applied to the teeth to reveal dental plaque.

Envelope flap is a section of gingiva raised with a horizontal releasing incision for exposure.

Flap is a section of gingiva and/or mucosa surgically separated from the underlying tissues to provide visibility and access to the underlying bone and root surfaces.

Free (marginal) gingiva is the most coronal unattached portion of the gingiva that encircles the tooth to form the gingival sulcus.

Free gingival graft is utilized to increase the zone of gingiva at the buccal or lingual aspects of a single tooth or group of teeth.

Frenectomy is the excision of the frenulum, a thin muscle tissue that attaches the upper or lower lips to the gingiva, or tongue to the floor of the mouth.

Full-thickness flap (mucoperiosteal) is a surgical procedure used to access roots, which include the periosteum.

Furcation is the anatomic area of a multirooted tooth where the roots diverge.

Furcation exposure occurs when both cortical walls of a double- or triple-rooted tooth are exposed.

Furcation involvement occurs where one, or a portion of one, wall remains around a double- or triple-rooted tooth root trunk.

Gingiva is the part of the oral mucosa that covers the alveolar process.

Gingival curettage is the scraping of the gingival wall of a periodontal pocket to remove diseased soft tissue.

Gingival hyperplasia is the proliferation of the attached gingiva.

Gingival recession is the exposure of tooth root(s) caused by the retraction of the gingiva secondary to periodontal disease (apical migration), abrasion, or surgery. Gingival recession can be measured from the cementoenamel junction to the free gingival margin.

Gingival sulcus or crevice is a normal space between the free gingival margin and the epithelial attachment. The floor of the gingival sulcus is the most coronal aspect of the junctional epithelium.

Gingivitis is the reversible inflammation of the gingival tissues.

Guided tissue regeneration (GTR) is a procedure that uses a barrier placed on top of a periodontally treated area to protect the area while it heals and prevents unwanted cells from migrating into the wound.

Infrabony (intrabony) pocket is a periodontal defect wherein the epithelial attachment is apical to the level of the adjacent alveolar bone.

Junctional epithelium attaches to the tooth at the base of the gingival sulcus or pocket.

Masticatory mucosa is the parakeratonized or keratinized mucosa covering the hard palate and gingiva.

Modified Widman flap uses an internally beveled, scalloped mucoperiosteal surgical incision made to gain access for root treatment.

Molt surgical curette is used as a periosteal elevator to separate the periosteum from the underlying bone.

Mucogingival defects consist of pockets extending to or beyond the mucogingival junction, absence of attached gingiva without pocket formation, and/or isolated areas of gingival recession.

Mucogingival flap is a surgical procedure of incising the gingiva and alveolar mucosa.

Mucogingival Junction (MGJ) is a line that separates the thick protective attached gingiva from the alveolar mucosa.

Operculum is the hood or flap of thick fibrous gingiva over an unerupted or partially erupted tooth.

Partial- (split-) thickness flap contains mucosa and connective tissue avoiding the periosteum.

Pellicle is a 0.1–1.0 micron thin film of salivary protein found on the tooth that forms within 1 hour of teeth cleaning and adheres to the exposed tooth surfaces.

Periodontal debridement is the treatment of gingival and periodontal inflammation through mechanical removal of tooth and root surface irritants to the extent that the adjacent soft tissues maintain or return to a healthy, noninflamed state.

Periodontal ligament attaches the cementum of the root to the alveolar socket.

Periodontal pocket is a pathological condition created when the depth of the sulcus exceeds 3 mm in the dog and 1 mm in the cat.

Periodontitis is an inflammation of the periodontium.

Periodontium (attachment apparatus) consists of the gingiva, cementum, periodontal ligament, and alveolar bone.

Plaque is the transparent adhesive fluid on the surface of teeth comprised of salivary glycoproteins, extracellular polysaccharides, and bacteria.

Pocket depth (absolute pocket depth) is the distance from the free gingival margin to the base of a gingival crevice, measured in millimeters.

Root planing is the process of using a curette to remove subgingival calculus and altered cementum from the root surface.

Scaling is the removal of plaque and calculus from the teeth.

Split-thickness flap contains mucosa and connective tissue, but does not include the periosteum.

Subgingival refers to the area located apical to the free gingival margin.

Suprabony pocket is a periodontal defect where the epithelial attachment is located coronal to the alveolar crest.

Supragingival is the area located coronal to the free gingival margin.

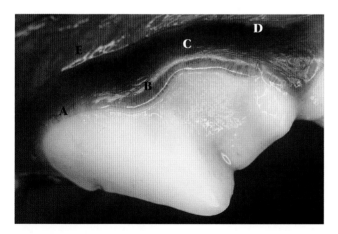

FIGURE 6.2. (A) Marginal gingiva; (B) free gingival groove; (C) attached gingiva; (D) mucogingival junction; (E) alveolar mucosa.

The connection of firm attached gingiva with loose alveolar mucosa is the *mucogingival junction (MGJ),* also called the *mucogingival line (MGL)*. The mucogingival junction remains stationary throughout life although the gingiva around it may change in height due to hyperplasia, recession, or attachment loss (Figure 6.2D).

The *alveolar (oral) mucosa* is loosely attached nonkeratinized tissue apical to the mucogingival junction Figure 6.2E).

The *gingival epithelium* can be divided into three zones:

- The *oral epithelium,* also called *the outer gingival epithelium,* covers the oral surface of the attached gingiva and papillae. The oral epithelium is keratinized or parakeratinized.
- The *sulcular epithelium* is a nonkeratinized extension of the oral epithelium into the gingival sulcus.
- The *junctional epithelium* separates the periodontal ligament from the oral environment. The junctional epithelium attaches to the root cementum immediately apical to the cementoenamel junction. When

probed, the gingival sulcus floor is located on the most coronal junctional epithelial cells:

- The *periodontal ligament* attaches cementum to the alveolar bone by collagen fiber bundles (Sharpey's fibers). The periodontal ligament acts as a suspensory cushion for occlusal forces and as an epithelial attachment to keep debris from entering deeper tissues.
- *Cementum* surrounds the tooth root and serves as an attachment area for the periodontal ligament. Cementum anchors teeth and provides a seal for the dentinal tubules.

The *alveolus* or *alveolar socket* is the bony opening within the alveolar process in which the root of a tooth is held by the periodontal ligament (Figure 6.3). The *alveolar bone height* exists as an equilibrium between bone formation and bone resorption. When bone resorption exceeds formation, the alveolar bone height is reduced (Figure 6.4).

PERIODONTAL DISEASE

Within 20 minutes after teeth cleaning, a glycoprotein layer (acquired pellicle) attaches to the exposed crown. Within 6 hours, bacterial colonization (*plaque*) forms on the glycoprotein layer. In some patients, plaque irritates the gingiva, allowing pathogenic anaerobic Gram-negative bacteria to survive subgingivally. By-products of these bacteria stimulate the host's immune response to release cytokines and prostaglandins that weaken and destroy the tooth's support structure. The progression rate of periodontal disease is dependent on the complex regulatory interaction between bacteria and immune modulators of the host response (Figures 6.5, 6.6).

Bacteria (Gram-positive, nonmotile aerobic cocci) naturally occupy the sulcus. As periodontal infection progresses, the number of bacteria increases at the gingival margin, decreasing the subgingival oxygen. The

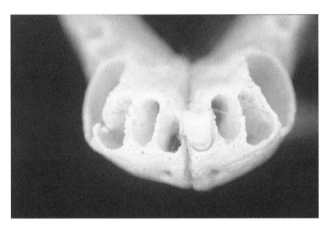

FIGURE 6.3. Alveoli of the mandibular incisors and canine teeth.

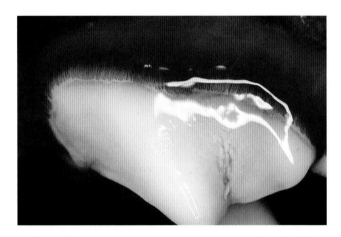

FIGURE 6.5. Plaque accumulation on buccal surface of the maxillary fourth premolar.

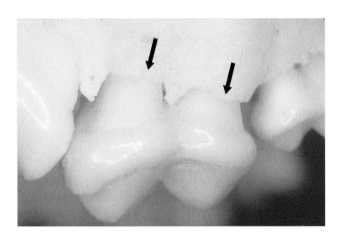

FIGURE 6.4. Buccal alveolar height resorption secondary to periodontal disease.

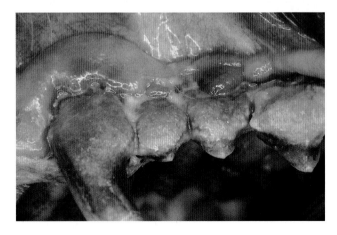

FIGURE 6.6. Plaque-covered calculus and periodontal disease.

anaerobic conditions allow Gram-negative, motile, anaerobic rods and spirochetes to predominate.

Periodontal infection is a multifactorial disease. Many variables influence why some animals develop disease and others do not. Animals that have compromised health often cannot fight periodontal pathogens. Examples of some syndromes that predispose a dog or cat to periodontal disease include diabetes, hypothyroidism, hyperadrenocorticism, pemphigus, lupus, FIV, and FeLV.

Toy canine breeds are prone to developing periodontal disease because:

- Smaller dogs have larger teeth relative to their jaw size, leaving less room for bone support.
- Smaller dogs tend to live longer than larger breeds. The longer an animal lives, the more time periodontal disease has to cause damage.
- Smaller dogs are more prone to dental malocclusions. Crowding abnormalities decrease the normal self-cleaning process, predisposing the animal to periodontal disease.

Genetic factors are also responsible for periodontal disease in some greyhounds, schnauzers, Maltese dogs, and Abyssinian cats.

Plaque and calculus appear as:

- *Supragingival plaque* forms on the coronal tooth surface within hours after a professional teeth cleaning.
- *Subgingival plaque* occurs after microorganisms penetrate and colonize the gingival sulcus. Supragingival and subgingival bacteria form microenvironments of bacterial colonies called *biofilms*, separated from the junctional epithelium by a wall of neutrophils. Toxins produced by biofilm bacteria cause prostaglandin stimulation and lysosome release, which can damage this neutrophil wall, allowing invasion of the junctional epithelium.
- *Supragingival calculus* is mineralized plaque, food debris, calcium, and phosphate (Figure 6.7).
- *Subgingival calculus* is preceded by supragingival plaque, which loosens the seal between tooth and gingiva. Calculus is always covered with bacteria (Figure 6.8).

Calculus plays a role in maintaining and accelerating periodontal disease by keeping plaque in close contact with gingival tissues, decreasing the potential for repair and new attachment. The therapeutic importance of removing all calculus cannot be overemphasized.

Appreciating the difference between gingivitis and periodontitis is important. *Gingivitis* is an inflammatory process affecting the gingiva only. This process does not clinically extend into the alveolar bone, periodontal ligament, or cementum. *Periodontitis* is inflammation involving the periodontal ligament, alveolar bone, and cementum. Periodontal disease can be further classified as *active* or *quiescent*, based on evidence of inflammation.

Gingivitis can be present without periodontitis. Periodontal disease can also exist without gingivitis in an area of periodontitis that has been treated and controlled, relieving inflammation but not attachment loss.

Table 6.1. Plaque index (PI).

Rank	Plaque
0	No plaque
1	Thin film of plaque along the gingival margin
2	Moderate accumulation, plaque in sulcus
3	Large amount of plaque in sulcus

Table 6.2. Calculus index (CI).

Rank	Calculus
0	No calculus
1	Supragingival calculus
2	Moderate amount of supragingival and/or subgingival calculus
3	Large amount of supra- and/or subgingival calculus

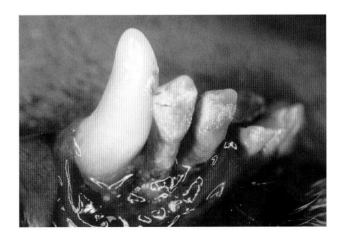

FIGURE 6.7. Subgingival and supragingival plaque and calculus on mandibular canine tooth and incisors.

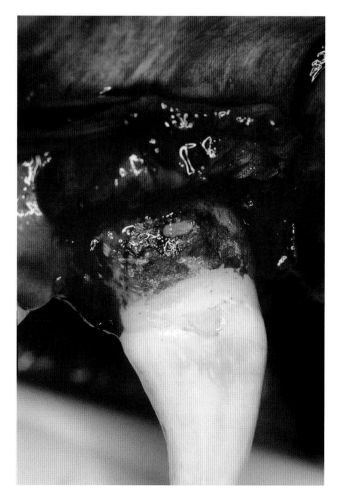

FIGURE 6.8. Subgingival calculus visualized with flap exposure on a "cleaned" maxillary canine tooth of a dog.

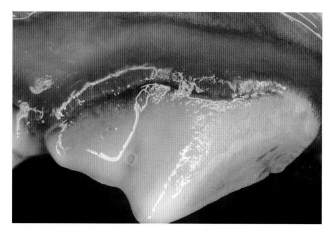

FIGURE 6.9. Stage 1 gingivitis affecting the canine maxillary fourth premolar.

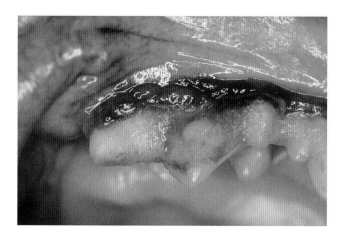

FIGURE 6.10. Stage 1 advanced gingivitis affecting the gingiva overlying a feline maxillary fourth premolar.

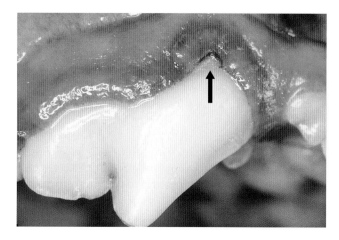

FIGURE 6.11. Gingival recession in stage 2 early periodontitis.

THE FOUR STAGES OF PERIODONTAL DISEASE

There are numerous grading systems used to classify gingivitis and periodontal disease. Generally, gingivitis is used to describe soft tissue inflammatory changes. Periodontitis is diagnosed when attachment loss has occurred. The patient can be "graded" by the worst tooth (i.e., if there is one stage 4 area, the patient has stage 4 disease). After the disease has been treated, the patient can be reclassified.

- *Stage 1 (gingivitis)* appears as gingival inflammation at the free gingival margin. As gingivitis progresses, *advanced gingivitis* appears as gingival inflammation, edema, and bleeding on probing. Advanced gingivitis is limited to the epithelium and gingival connective tissue. There is no tooth mobility or attachment loss. Gingivitis is reversible with proper therapy and aftercare at home (Figures 6.9,6.10).

- *Stage 2 (early periodontitis)* occurs when there is apical migration of the junctional epithelium, resulting in a deeper sulcus called a *pocket,* or *gingival recession.* In stage 2 disease, up to 25% attachment loss occurs (Figure 6.11).
- *Stage 3 (established periodontitis)* is present when 25–50% attachment loss exists around a root. Slight tooth mobility often occurs in single-rooted teeth. Early furcation exposure and/or gingival recession may or may not exist (Figure 6.12).
- *Stage 4 (advanced periodontitis)* presents when marked (greater than 50%) attachment loss occurs. Stage 4 periodontal disease can appear as furcation exposure, abscess formation, tooth mobility, deep pockets, and/or gingival recession (Figures 6.13–6.16).

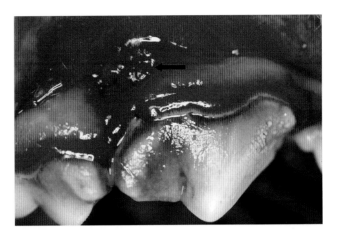

FIGURE 6.14. Periodontal fistula (arrows) secondary to stage 4 periodontal disease of the maxillary fourth premolar in a dog.

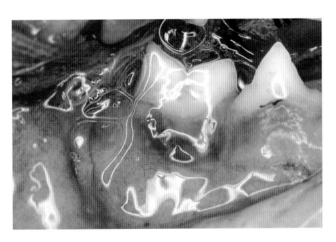

FIGURE 6.12. Stage 3 established periodontitis in the mandibular molar of a cat.

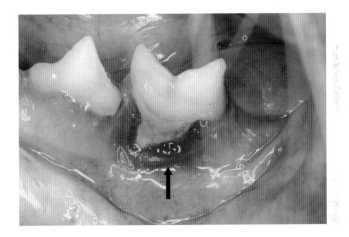

FIGURE 6.15. Stage 4 periodontal disease gingival recession of the mandibular molar in a cat.

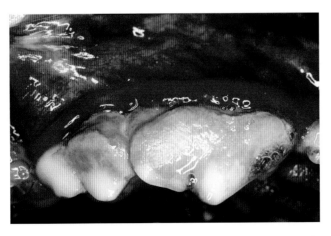

FIGURE 6.13. Stage 4 periodontal disease of the maxillary fourth premolar and first molar of a dog.

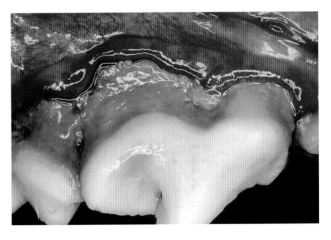

FIGURE 6.16. Stage 4 periodontal disease resulting in gingival recession of the maxillary fourth premolar and first molar in a greyhound dog.

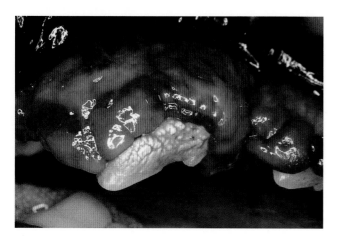

FIGURE 6.17. Gingival hyperplasia.

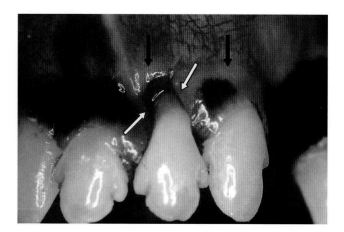

FIGURE 6.18. Gingival cleft: white arrows, mucogingival junction; black arrows.

GINGIVAL HYPERPLASIA

Abnormal proliferation of the gingiva is termed *gingival hyperplasia*. The boxer breed is more prone than others to be affected by gingival hyperplasia. Gingival hyperplasia results in increased pocket depths, caused by *increased* gingival height, *not* attachment loss. The resultant pseudopocket can accumulate plaque, which, if untreated, may progress to attachment loss. Gingival hyperplasia is treated by gingivoplasty and strict home care to help slow recurrence (Figure 6.17).

TOOTH MOBILITY

Normally there is physiological tooth movement of less than 1 mm. Teeth may become pathologically mobile in response to increased occlusal forces, outside trauma, or normal forces exerted on a reduced periodontium. Mobility per se is not diagnostic of periodontal disease, but it reflects a pathologic adaptation to stresses placed on the periodontium.

With progression of periodontal disease, tooth support erodes. Eventually, if enough support is lost, the tooth will be lost.

The mobility (M) index uses the following divisions:

* 0 is normal
* M1 occurs when the tooth moves a distance slightly less than 1 mm.
* M2 mobility exists when the tooth moves about 1 mm.
* M3 mobility is present when the tooth moves a distance greater than 1 mm, and/or may be depressed into the alveolus.

MUCOGINGIVAL DEFECTS

Type I mucogingival defects are characterized as pockets that extend apically to or beyond the mucogingival junction. Treatment for type I mucogingival defects includes pocket reduction by performing apically repositioned flap surgery.

Type II mucogingival defects are present when the alveolar mucosa acts as the marginal gingiva without a zone of attached gingiva (fissures or clefts). Such lesions are called *nonpocket deformities*. The sulcular (pocket) depth may be less than 2–3 mm (Figure 6.18).

The goal of mucogingival surgery for Type II mucogingival lesions is to obtain more resistent tissue to withstand masticatory stress. Lateral pedicle and free autogenous gingival grafts are two examples of mucogingival surgery to accomplish this goal. These advanced procedures carry a guarded prognosis and will fail without excellent home care.

Gingival recession is the exposure of the root surface by an apical migration of the gingival margin. Gingival recession can be measured from CEJ to the free gingival margin.

Gingival recession classification breaks into the following categories:

* *Class I* occurs when recession is present coronal to mucogingival junction (Figure 6.19).
* *Class II* occurs when recession is present at the mucogingival junction but is not accompanied by bone loss interproximally (Figure 6.20).
* *Class III* recession occurs past the mucogingival junction with soft tissue and bone loss interproximally (Figure 6.21).

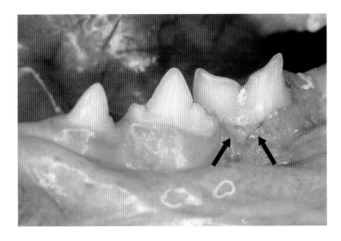

FIGURE 6.19. Class I gingival recession affecting a feline's mandibular molar.

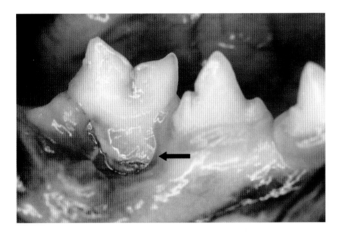

FIGURE 6.20. Class II gingival recession affecting a feline's mandibular molar.

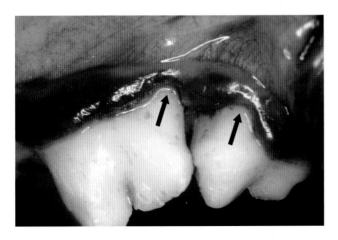

FIGURE 6.21. Class III gingival recession affecting a canine's maxillary fourth premolar and first molar.

FURCATION INVOLVEMENT

The *furcation* is a normal anatomical area at the trunk of a multirooted tooth where the roots begin to diverge. Normally this area is sealed from the oral environment by the periodontium. Furcation involvement, invasion, or exposure occurs secondary to periodontal disease. When the integrity of the periodontium has been lost and junctional epithelium migrates apically, oral microflora can gain access and multiply, resulting in progressive disease. There are three clinical furcation classifications:

- *Class I involvement* is diagnosed when an explorer can just detect an entrance to the furcation. A portion of alveolar bone and periodontal ligament is intact at the furcation. Generally, there will be less than 1 mm exposure (Figure 6.22).
- *Class II involvement* occurs when an explorer can enter the furcation, but does not exit the other side. The undermined furcation is occluded by gingiva or bone on one side (Figures 6.23,6.24).
- *Class III exposure* is diagnosed when the periodontium is destroyed to such a degree that the furcation is open and exposed. An explorer can pass from side to side (Figure 6.25).

Radiographs are helpful in locating furcation involvement. The slightest radiographic change in the furcation area should be investigated clinically. Diminished radiodensity in the furcation suggests furcation exposure (Figure 6.26).

Furcation involvement usually carries a guarded-to-poor prognosis. Treatment for furcation involvement is an advanced procedure, which success depends on the degree of exposure, the skill of the veterinarian, and the ability of the client to provide home care.

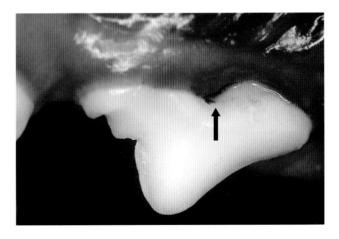

FIGURE 6.22. F1 furcation involvement of a maxillary third premolar in a dog.

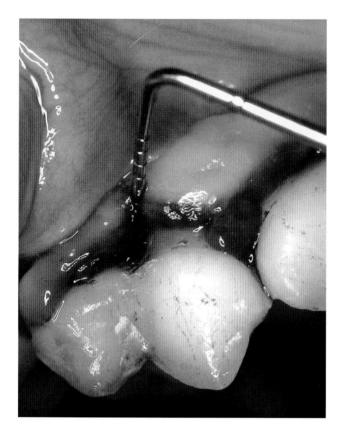

FIGURE 6.23. Class II furcation exposure in the maxillary first molar of a dog.

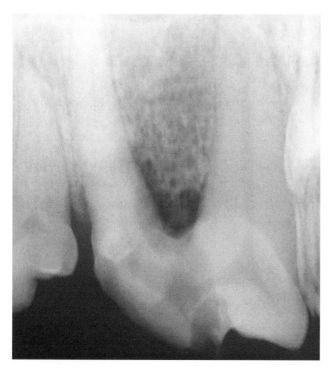

FIGURE 6.24. Radiograph showing anadvanced Class II furcation of the maxillary fourth premolar in a dog.

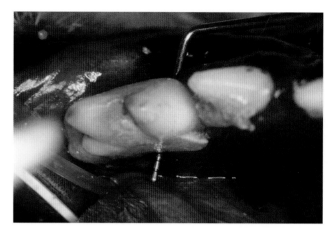

FIGURE 6.25. Class III through-and-through furcation exposure of the mandibular first molar in a dog.

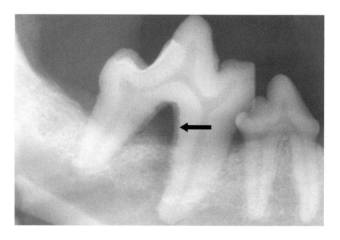

FIGURE 6.26. Radiograph of mandibular first molar showing Class III furcation exposure.

CHRONIC ULCERATIVE PARADENTAL STOMATITIS (CUPS)

Chronic ulcerative paradental stomatitis (CUPS), also referred to as contact ulcers or kissing lesions, appears as marked ulceration of the buccal mucosa adjacent to calculus and plaque-laden teeth. Affected animals (often Maltese, and other small breeds) may have a hyperimmune response to plaque (Figure 6.27).

CUPS patients should be evaluated medically, including organ function profiles, thyroid function, autoimmune disease evaluation, urinalysis, and lesion biopsy to rule out other causes of stomatitis. In patients where elevated alkaline phosphatase values are reported, tests to rule out Cushing's disease should also be performed.

Initial care involves teeth cleaning, both above and

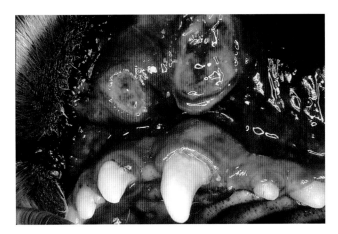

FIGURE 6.27. Chronic ulcerative paradental stomatitis (kissing lesions).

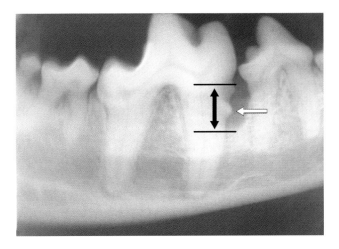

FIGURE 6.28. Less than 50% bone loss affecting the mesial root of the mandibular first molar. White arrow points to calculus attached to the root.

below the gum line, and polishing followed by intraoral radiographs. Those teeth affected by grades 3 and 4 periodontal disease should be extracted. Antibiotics are indicated to help control infection. Pain medication is also indicated. Use of the CO_2 laser to photovaporize the lesions has also been used to treat the ulcers, with mixed results. The use of steroids in control of CUPS is controversial. Home care, including daily teeth brushing; application of a gel and/or oral rinse containing zinc might be helpful in controlling plaque and for ulcer care. If initial therapy and weeks of home care are not effective, extraction of the rubbing teeth is usually curative.

RADIOGRAPHIC APPEARANCE OF PERIODONTAL DISEASE

Intraoral radiography provides critical information when making periodontal therapy decisions by imaging the supportive bone mesial (rostral) and distal to the affected teeth. Unfortunately, due to superimposition, it is difficult to radiographically evaluate the lingual-buccal plane.

If clinically and radiographically greater than 50% of the bone and tooth support remains, periodontal procedures together with a healthy patient and stringent home care will often result in a saved tooth. A guarded prognosis is given when 50–75% bone loss exists. If greater than 75% support is lost, the prognosis for saving the tooth is poor (Figures 6.28–6.30).

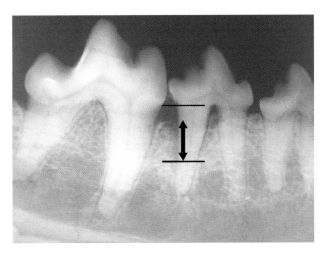

FIGURE 6.29. Between 50–75% bone loss affecting the distal root of the mandibular fourth premolar.

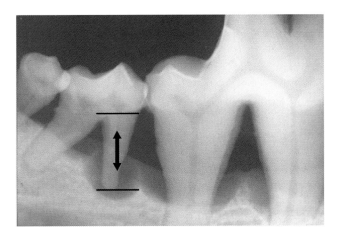

FIGURE 6.30. Between 75–100% bone loss affecting all of the mandibular molars.

When evaluating periodontal disease, radiographs are checked for:

- Alveolar bone changes
- Trabecular patterns
- Interdental bone height
- Presence of the lamina dura completely around the root
- Size of periodontal ligament space
- Amount of bone loss

PERIODONTAL THERAPY

Criteria the veterinarian should consider when choosing periodontal therapy includes the following:

- The client's *ability and commitment* to perform aftercare, return for follow-up progress visits, and incur the related expenses. The pet owner who has little success in removing plaque may not be able to provide essential home care for advanced tooth-saving procedures.
- The degree of *patient cooperation* and general health.
- The *importance (function) of the tooth.* The carnassial teeth, maxillary fourth premolar, and mandibular first molars are *important* teeth because they act as scissors to cut food into small pieces. Also important are the molars, which grind food, and the mandibular canines, which provide structure for the rostral mandible. Incisors and first, second, and third premolars perform the least important functions.
- The clinician's *ability* to perform periodontal procedures to minimize attachment loss and maintain at least 2–3 mm of attached gingiva in dogs, and 0.5–1 mm in cats.

PROFESSIONAL ORAL HYGIENE

Prophy is an abbreviation of the word *prophylaxis,* which is defined by the American Academy of Periodontology as the "removal of plaque, calculus, and stains from the exposed and unexposed surfaces of the teeth by scaling and polishing as a *preventative measure* for the control of local irritation factors." The dentist is usually presented with a generally healthy mouth; the hygienist cleans the teeth and reschedules 6 months to 1 year later for another prophylaxis. In human dentistry, prophys are performed to *prevent* dental disease.

When used in the veterinary context, "prophy" is a misnomer for teeth cleaning and periodontal care. To call proper attention to the extent of dental care per-

formed, the level of disease should appropriately identify the type of necessary cleaning procedure. Examples are: "dental cleaning-gingivitis," "dental cleaning-established periodontitis," and "dental cleaning-advanced periodontitis."

THE PROFESSIONAL TEETH-CLEANING VISIT

The dental visit for oral examination and cleaning must be performed in a consistent manner. All procedures are important and interlinked. When one step is not performed, long-term patient benefit may be compromised.

A teeth cleaning packet example includes the following:

- Sickle scaler—H6/7 (Burns 951-9464, Schein 378-0698), S6/7 (Schein 101-9032) (Figure 6.31)
- Curette—Gracey 12/13 (Burns 950-9545), 11/12 (Schein 600-7601), Barnhardt 5/6 (Burns 843-3035, Schein 600-5410, P8 Cislak), Columbia 13/14 (Burns 950-9598, P10 Cislak, Schein 100-4313) (Figures 6.32–6.34)

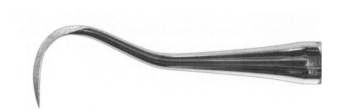

FIGURE 6.31. Sickle scaler.

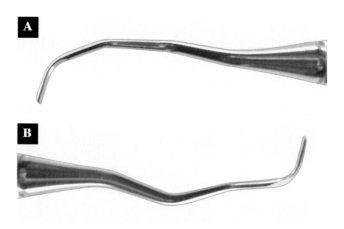

FIGURE 6.32. Gracey 12/13 curette.

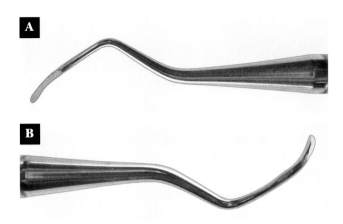

FIGURE 6.33. Barnhardt 5/6 curette.

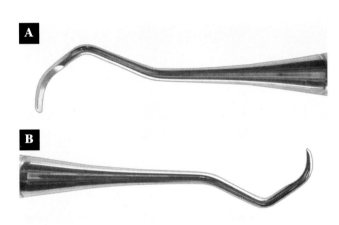

FIGURE 6.34. Columbia 13/14 curette.

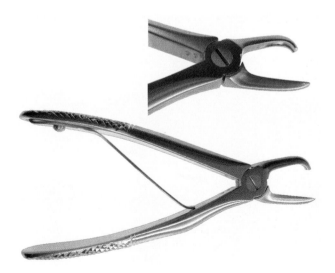

FIGURE 6.35. Calculus-removing forceps.

- Calculus-removing forceps, with one eccentric longer tip, which is placed over the crown, and a smaller tip, which is applied under the ledge of calculus (Burns 271-9120, Schein 102-8318) (Figure 6.35)
- Periodontal probe/explorer, which is a double-ended combination of a thin Michigan (Burns 894-3194, Schein 600-3203) type probe and a No. 23 explorer (Burns 951-2248, Schein 101-2098, Cislak P2) (Figure 6.36) (Burns 271-9105, Schein 100-4807 ST-4)
- Sterile container for the teeth cleaning packet (Figure 6.37)

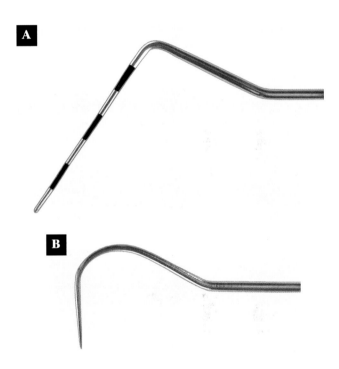

FIGURE 6.36. Periodontal probe (A) and explorer (B).

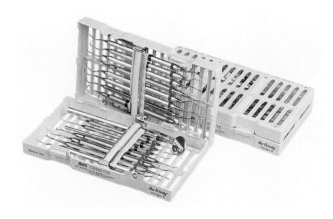

FIGURE 6.37. Hand scaling and examination kit.

Before treatment of the animal, the clinician should obtain general and dental/oral history, review pre-operative diagnostics, and interview the client concerning expectations and abilities to provide aftercare.

STEP 1 *Visual oral examination on the unanesthetized animal.* The face is examined visually for swellings and by palpation for areas of tenderness. The assessable lymph nodes are palpated for pain, texture, and size. The mouth is opened and closed to check the occlusion and pain or crepitus of the temporomandibular joints. The number of teeth is counted in each quadrant. The lips, tongue, palate, pharynx, teeth, and gingiva are examined for lesions. Even a small amount of plaque touching the gingiva is abnormal. Often, fractured teeth have more calculus than the other teeth from chewing on the opposite side due to pain and discomfort (Figure 6.38).

STEP 2 *Visual oral examination under general anesthesia* after the patient is intubated, cuff is secured and inflated, and ophthalmic ointment is applied to the corneal surfaces. The patient is positioned in lateral or dorsal recumbency. The head is supported with a towel to prevent injury. Each tooth is visually examined for fracture, abnormal wear, mobility, and discoloration (Figure 6.39).

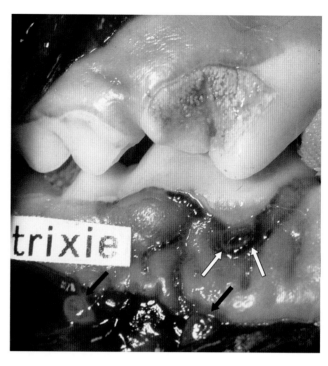

FIGURE 6.39. Gingival swellings and recession caused by endodontic (black arrows) and periodontic (white arrows) disease of the mandibular first molar.

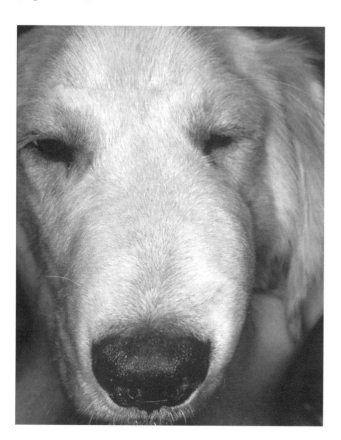

FIGURE 6.38. Swollen muzzle secondary to an abscess caused by a fractured maxillary canine tooth.

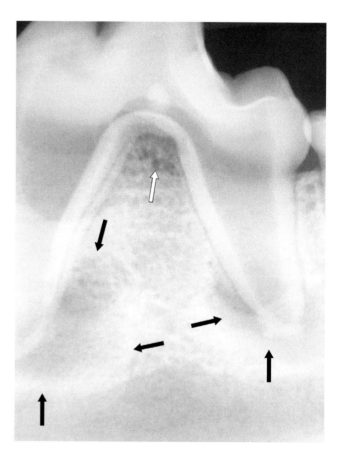

FIGURE 6.40. Radiograph of endodontic (black arrows) and periodontal (white arrow) lesion of the mandibular first molar portrayed in figure 6.39.

STEP 3 *Intraoral radiography* helps the practitioner diagnose periodontal lesions below the gingiva (Figure 6.40).

STEP 4 *Supragingival plaque and calculus removal* is accomplished with the help of hand instruments and/or power scaling equipment. Before the actual teeth cleaning procedure is started, the oral cavity is irrigated with 0.12% chlorhexidine solution. Ultrasonic beavertail or P-10 tips are designed for gross debridement of supragingival calculus (Figures 6.41, 6.42).

Periodontal bactericidal ultrasonic debridement is a term used to describe supra- and subgingival treatment to remove plaque, plaque-retentive calculus, and toxic by-products. The removal of irritants within the gingival sulcus is accomplished using periodontal ultrasonic scalers. Ultrasonic sound waves are made up of alternate compressions and rarefactions. During the low-pressure rarefaction cycle, microscopic bubbles are formed. Through the high-pressure compression cycle, the bubbles collapse

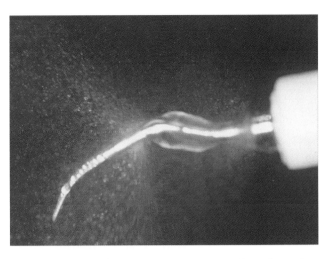

FIGURE 6.42. Ultrasonic instrument used to clean the crown.

or implode. These implosions produce shock waves called *cavitation,* which may disrupt the bacterial cell wall and lead to bacterial cell death.

Acoustic streaming occurs when a continuous torrent of water produces tremendous pressure within the confined space of the periodontal pocket, resulting in a decreased number of bacteria. Gram-negative motile rods in particular are sensitive to acoustic streaming because of their thin cell walls.

STEP 5 *Subgingival periodontal cleaning* and root planing (if indicated). Periodontal disease occurs secondary to the imbalance of subgingival bacteria with the host. The goal of teeth cleaning is to remove irritating plaque and calculus from the gingival sulcus. Calculus, coated with bacteria, left on the root surface contributes to the progression of disease. If subgingival cleaning is not performed, the teeth have not been adequately cleaned. Subgingival root cleaning can be accomplished with curettes or special ultrasonic periodontal subgingival inserts (Hu-friedy) manufactured for subgingival use. The Fineline tips are only for cleaning the root surface. Using them for supragingival calculus removal will often lead to tip breakage (Figures 6.43, 6.44).

Disclosing agents are organic dyes that reveal areas of dental plaque. Disclosing agents are useful both diagnostically and in assessing the efficiency of cleaning procedures. The disclosing solution can be swabbed on the tooth surfaces using cotton pledgets, after the teeth cleaning procedure and before the animal is awakened. Stained calculus and plaque are visualized and removed. The disclosing solution may also be applied in the exam room to monitor client home care. Caution must be used when applying disclosing solution on light-haired breeds. The solution may temporarily stain facial hairs (Burns 951-1218, Schein 100-2491) (Figure 6.45).

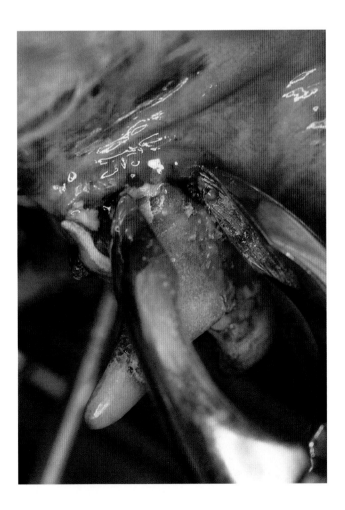

FIGURE 6.41. Small animal extraction forceps used for gross supragingival calculus removal (better choice of instrument would be calculus-rmoving forceps, see figure 6.35).

STEP 6 *Charting* is performed to record the condition of the mouth. A chart contains drawings of teeth and areas to mark pathology and therapy suggested and/or completed. Charted oral pathology includes missing, mobile, fractured, and discolored teeth, as well as feline odontoclastic resorptive lesions, periodontal pocket depths, gingival recession, and other significant lesions. Charting is usually performed before the teeth are cleaned, and may be repeated after supra- and subgingival calculus removal (Burns 342-0691, Schein 100-8927) (Figures 6.46, 6.47).

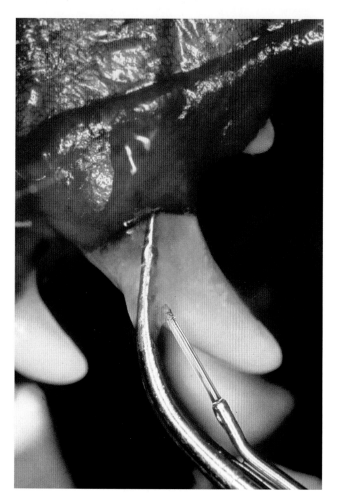

FIGURE 6.43. Subgingival insertion of specialized ultrasonic tip.

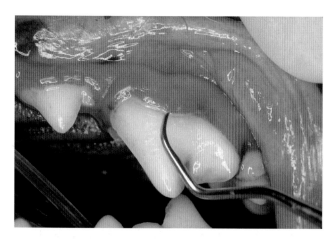

FIGURE 6.44. Use of a curette to remove plaque and calculus from the root subgingivally.

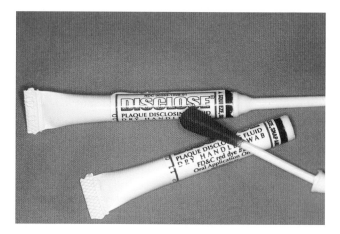

FIGURE 6.45. Disclosing solution (Virbac).

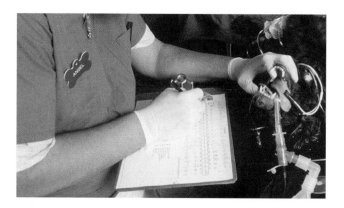

FIGURE 6.46. Technician charting the mouth.

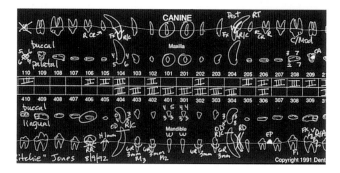

FIGURE 6.47. Completed dental chart.

A periodontal probe is the single most important examination instrument used to evaluate periodontal health. By gently inserting a calibrated periodontal probe just apical to the free gingival margin and tracing the gingival crevice from mesial to distal, a rapid determination of the health of the sulcular tissues can be made. The *clinical sulcus depth* is the distance from free gingival margin to the most apical point that a probe reaches when gently inserted into the gingival crevice (Figure 6.48).

The probe stops where the gingiva attaches to the tooth or at the apex of the alveolus if attachment is lost. Each tooth should be probed on a minimum of six sides. Bleeding on probing is indicative of an inflammatory process in the connective tissue adjacent to the junctional epithelium. If the sulcular lining is intact and healthy, no bleeding will occur. If, however, periodontal disease is present, bleeding will usually take place.

Normal dogs should have less than 3 mm probing depths, and cats less than 1 mm. Abnormal probing depths are noted on the dental record and discussed with the client, and then a treatment plan is mapped out before therapy begins.

Pockets

The periodontal pocket is a pathologically deepened gingival sulcus. *Clinical (absolute) pocket depth* is the distance from the free gingival margin edge to the base of a pocket, measured in millimeters.

Attachment loss (attachment level) is used to evaluate support loss in cases of gingival recession where little or no pocketing exists. The measurement of attachment loss is the backbone of a periodontal examination. The clinical pocket depth plus recession (measured CEJ to free gingival margin) equals the *total periodontal attachment loss* (Figure 6.49).

STEP 7 *Therapy to treat lesions found.* When periodontal disease is not treated, bacteria will continue to reproduce, possibly creating deeper periodontal pockets with more bone destruction, causing pain and eventually tooth loss. Periodontal disease has been shown to be associated with lesions in a patient's kidney, heart, and liver.

The following are goals of periodontal therapy:

* Removing debris from the tooth surface and periodontal pocket(s)
* Minimizing pocket depth
* Minimizing attachment loss
* Maintaining at least two millimeters of attached gingiva
* Producing a gingival contour to promote self-cleaning
* Decreasing future pocket formation

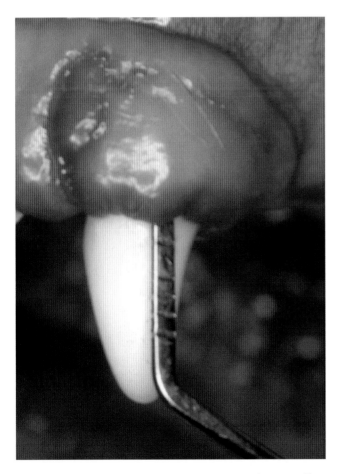

FIGURE 6.48. Periodontal probe inserted subgingivally.

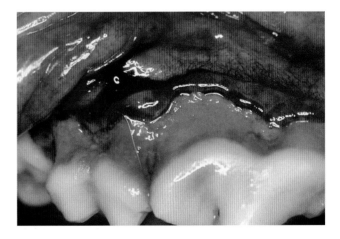

FIGURE 6.49. In areas of gingival recession, measurement of attachment loss is a better gauge of periodontal health compared to probing depth alone.

STEP 8 *Polishing* smoothes minor enamel defects and removes some of the plaque missed during previous steps. Regardless of how careful the scaling/curettage phase of teeth cleaning is performed, minor defects (microetches) of the tooth surface occur. Polishing teeth decreases the surface area of enamel defects, retarding plaque recolonization.

Prophy paste (Burns 951-8652, Schein 100-7869) or flour pumice (Burns 907-6002, Schein 100-5836) is applied to the tooth surface with a prophy cup attached to the prophy angle on a low-speed handpiece. Cross-contamination can be avoided between different animals by using individual paste cups or a tongue depressor to bring paste from the container to the teeth. Metallic prophy angles have screw-on or snap-on fittings. The author prefers plastic disposable polishing angles. Oscillating disposable prophy angles generate less heat on the enamel and do not tangle pet hair (Figures 6.50–6.53).

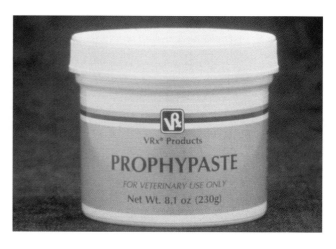

FIGURE 6.51. Large prophy paste container.

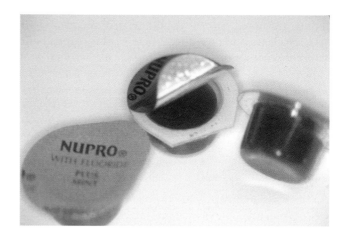

FIGURE 6.52. Individual prophy paste cups.

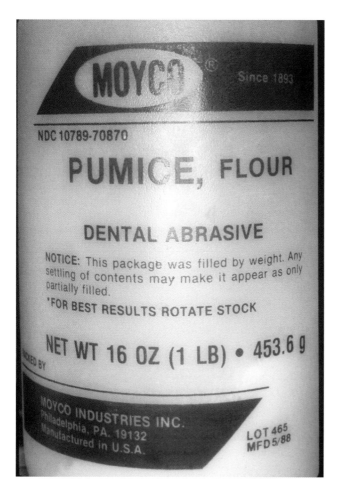

FIGURE 6.50. Flour pumice used for tooth polishing.

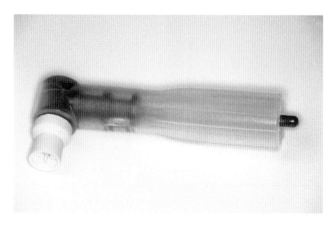

FIGURE 6.53. Disposable prophy angle.

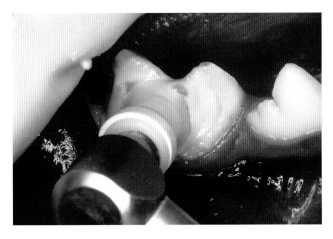

FIGURE 6.54. Polishing technique.

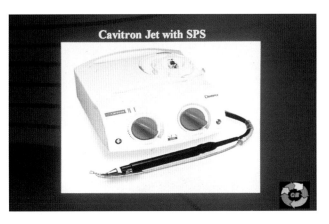

FIGURE 6.55. Prophy Jet air polisher (Cavitron).

The cup is kept in contact with the tooth, using continuous motion. When polishing, light pressure is used until the cup edge flares (Figure 6.54). Care must be taken not to hold the cup on one spot for more than a few seconds to prevent overheating and subsequent damage to the pulp.

Air Polishing

Air polishing uses sodium bicarbonate to "sandblast" the tooth surface smooth in addition or as a replacement to conventional polishing (Figure 6.55).

To use an air polisher, a source of compressed air, CO_2 or nitrogen, plus water is necessary. The air mixes with water and sodium bicarbonate crystals creating an abrasive slurry, which removes minor stains and particulate matter on the tooth surface. Advantages of air polishing include lack of potential iatrogenic pulpal thermal damage and the ability to polish hard-to-reach areas.

Follow these steps when performing air polishing as a prophylaxis technique:

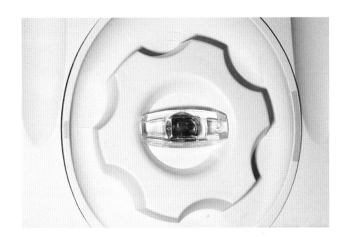

FIGURE 6.56. Sodium bicarbonate port.

- When using the air polisher, place a cuffed endotracheal tube in the patient and gauze sponges in the oropharynx to prevent aspiration.
- For patient protection, apply eye ointment and place a towel over the eyes.
- Avoid striking the unkeritinized tissue. Air polishing should not be used on exposed cementum or dentin (Figures 6.56–6.58).
- Place the tip of the air polishing nozzle 3–4 mm slightly apically on the incisal to the middle 1/3 of the tooth. Using a constant circular motion, sweep around the tooth. Do not direct the tip into the sulcus (Figure 6.59).

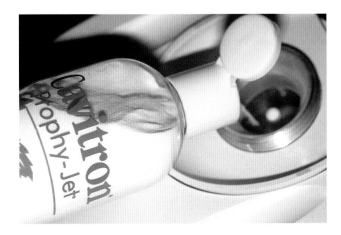

FIGURE 6.57. Filling the bicarbonate port.

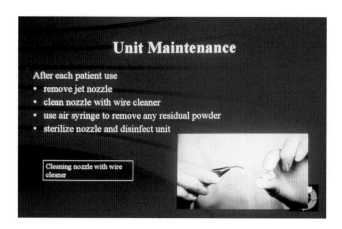

FIGURE 6.58. Air polisher maintenance.

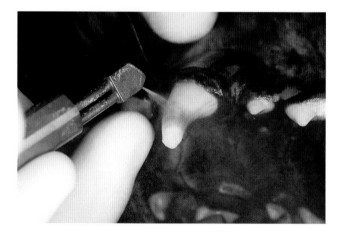

FIGURE 6.59. Proper position for air polishing.

- Use proper angulation of the nozzle tip toward the surface of the tooth, as follows:
  - Distal: 80°
  - Mesial: 60°
  - Occlusal: 90°
- Polish one or two teeth per second. Avoid application to dentin or cementum.

STEP 9 *Irrigation* removes loose debris from the pocket or sulcus. Water spray and/or a 0.05–0.2% chlorhexidine gluconate solution (CHX Oral Lavage Solution, Virbac Products) are commonly used. Chlorhexidine is the most effective chemical agent available for the prevention and retardation of plaque accumulation and gingivitis. Chlorhexidine does not remove established plaque (Figures 6.60, 6.61).

Positive properties of chlorhexidine include:

- Adheres to teeth, pellicle, and soft tissues.
- Gradually releases in therapeutic levels over 6 hours, with residual antibacterial effect for 24 hours.
- Is effective against both gram-negative and gram-positive organisms.
- Inhibits plaque by binding to the pellicle, thereby reducing bacteria on the tooth surface.
- When used before ultrasonic scaling, decreases the volume of aerosolized bacteria to the operator and bacteremia to the patient.
- Does not result in bacterial resistance with long-term usage.

Disadvantages to the use of chlorhexidine in animals include the following:

- Bitter taste, especially for cats

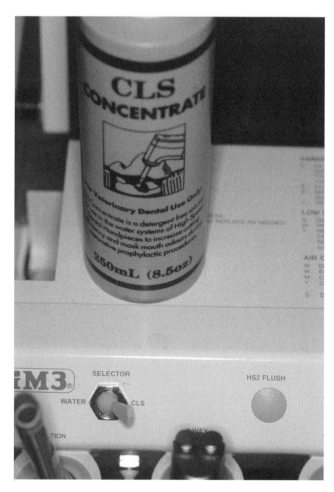

FIGURE 6.60. Chlorhexidine irrigation solution (iM3).

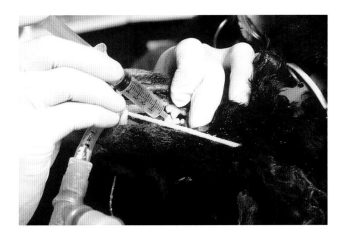

FIGURE 6.61. Application of irrigation solution subgingivally using a syringe.

- Brown or black staining of the pellicle with prolonged use (stain is easily removed through ultrasonic scaling)
- Possible retardation of periodontal healing

The *gluconate form* of chlorhexidine is most commonly used as an irrigating solution delivered with a blunt 23 gauge needle on a 6 ml syringe, or through the air/water syringe on the dental delivery system (CHX Lavage Solution, Virbac Products). Chlorhexidine can also be used as part of the home care process twice daily for 2 weeks followed by daily application for patients affected with periodontal disease (Hexarinse, Virbac Products).

STEP 10 *Fluoride application.* In human dentistry, fluoride is used mainly to prevent caries. In veterinary dentistry, the use of fluoride is controversial. Caries are rare in dogs and virtually unheard of in cats.

Potential fluoride advantages in veterinary dentistry include the following:

- Decreases enamel surface tension
- Reduces tooth sensitivity by sealing exposed dentinal tubules
- Inhibits bacterial metabolism, which might decrease plaque accumulation
- Leaves a cherry-like odor after application (FluraFom Virbac Products)

Fluoride's potential disadvantages include the following:

- Toxicity if used chronically in higher than recommended dosages
- Extension of anesthetic time for application and removal
- Interference with acrylic bonding polymerization

Fluoride-containing preparations include the following:

- Fluoride varnish, which is virtually ineffective in small animals because its effect is short-lived (Burns 950-9131, Schein 100-0045)
- Fluoride gel (Burns 951-7908, Schein 100-8570), Gel-Tin Topical Fluoride Phosphate Anti-caries Gel (Young Dental Manufacturing)
- Fluoride solution (Burns 269-0520, Schein 100-2105)
- Fluoride foam, which can be applied while the animal is anesthetized to clean, dry teeth (FluraFom Virbac Products) (Burns 269-0520, Schein 309-0143) (Figures 6.62–6.64)

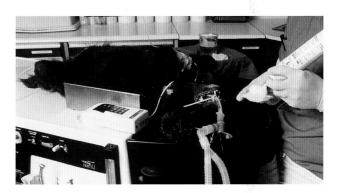

FIGURE 6.62. Application of fluoride foam on a gauze sponge.

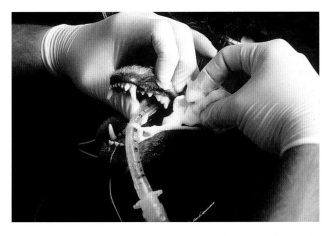

FIGURE 6.63. Application of fluoride foam on the teeth.

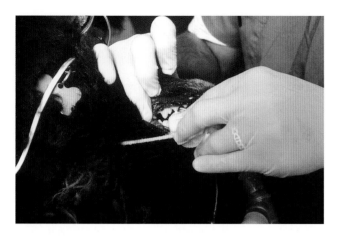

FIGURE 6.64. Removal of excessive fluoride foam with a dry gauze sponge.

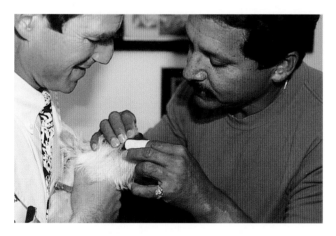

FIGURE 6.65. Allowing pet owner to demonstrate brushing technique.

When using fluoride foam, approximately 1/2 inch of the foam is rubbed over the teeth and allowed to remain for 3 minutes. The foam is removed with suction or with a dry gauze sponge. Irrigation is not used after fluoride application.

STEP 11   After treatment, home care involves daily (twice daily preferred) *tooth brushing,* and/or using oral pads to remove plaque accumulation. Before periodontal treatment is initiated, a discussion with the pet owner concerning commitment and ability to provide aftercare should be conducted (Figure 6.65).

STEP 12   *Follow-up visits* are essential to monitor periodontal healing. The time between oral exams should be based on the degree of disease and the client's ability to provide aftercare. Progress visits are initially scheduled weekly until the owner is comfortable with the home care process. Thereafter, advanced periodontal cases should be rechecked every other week to monthly. Pets that have been treated for stage 1 or 2 disease, and whose teeth are brushed once or twice daily, could be rechecked every 6 months. The reminder interval for recheck can be linked by computer to the degree of periodontal disease (i.e., if the patient is treated for grade 3 periodontal disease, a monthly progress reminder can be automatically generated).

THERAPY OF PERIODONTAL DISEASE

STAGE 1   *Gingivitis* care ideally includes thorough supra- and subgingival teeth cleaning and polishing, followed by daily brushing. Gingivitis will usually resolve within weeks of the oral hygiene visit.

STAGE 2   *Early periodontal disease,* where minimal to moderate pockets are diagnosed associated with gingivitis, can be treated similarly to stage 1 disease +/- root planing, +/- local administration of antibiotic (LAA). Doxirobe Gel (Pfizer) contains a flowable biodegradable solution of 8.5% doxycycline hyclate, which can be applied subgingivally to cleaned periodontal pockets greater than 3 mm in dogs older than 1 year, according to the manufacturer. Upon contact with the gingival crevicular fluid or water, the doxycycline polymer hardens within the periodontal pocket. The biodegradable insertion of doxycycline allows sustained release of therapeutic levels of antibiotic for several weeks at the site of injection. The gel gradually biodegrades to carbon dioxide and water. Doxirobe is not a substitute for scrupulous pocket debridement and other periodontal procedures (Figure 6.66).

Doxycycline insertion:

- Allows direct treatment of localized periodontal disease
- Is bacteriostatic against Porphyromonas gingivalis, Prevoltella intermedia, Camphylobacter rectus, and Fusobacterium nucleatum, which are associated with periodontal disease
- Inhibits collagenase enzymes, which are destructive to the periodontal attachment apparatus
- Directly binds to dentin and cementum for prolonged release, according to the manufacturer.

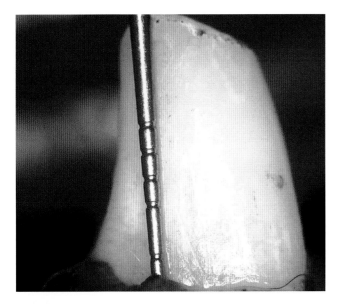

FIGURE 6.66. 4 mm periodontal pocket affecting a mandibular canine in a dog.

- Decreases edema and inflammation, and promotes growth of junctional epithelium resulting in decreased pocket depth, according to the manufacturer.
- Helps rejuvenate tissues of the periodontium, according to the manufacturer (LAA does not regenerate lost tissue)

To insert doxycycline:

1. Hold the two supplied syringes upright to avoid spilling before coupling.
2. Couple the liquid containing syringe A, identified by a red stripe, and syringe B, doxycycline powder.
3. Inject the liquid contents of syringe A into syringe B and then push it back into syringe A, constituting one mixing cycle.
4. Using brisk strokes, complete 100 mixing cycles at a pace of 1 cycle per second, with the final mix into syringe A (red stripe).
5. Hold the coupled syringes vertically with syringe A at the bottom. Pull back the plunger of syringe A, allowing the contents to flow down the barrel for several seconds.
6. Attach the blunt injection cannula to syringe A; the tip is bent to resemble a periodontal probe.
7. Insert the blunt syringe tip into the cleaned pocket, near the base, and inject the gel until it starts to extrude from the top of the pocket (Figures 6.67–6.69).

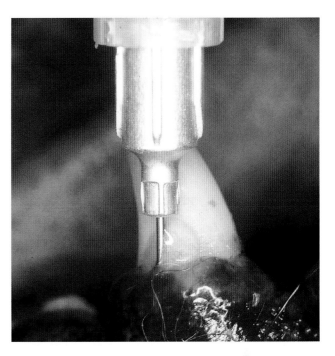

FIGURE 6.67. Doxirobe Gel inserted into the pocket of a manibular canine in a dog.

8. Withdraw the cannula tip from the pocket. To separate Doxirobe from the cannula, turn the tip toward the tooth and press against the tooth surface, pinching a string of the formulation.
9. Apply water drops to the area to hasten gel hardening.
10. Pack the gel into the pocket with a premoistened W-3 plastic beavertail instrument, cord packer, or #7 wax spatula. If necessary, apply more Doxirobe in the pocket until full.

Advise the client not to brush the dog's teeth where the gel was applied for two weeks following local antibiotic gel application.

STAGE 3 AND STAGE 4 *Established and advanced periodontal disease* therapies are based on dental findings after the patient and radiographs are evaluated.

Therapy decisions are based on the following:

- *Percentage of support loss.* Greater than 50% support loss carries a guarded-to-poor prognosis; greater than 75% support loss carries a poor prognosis for long-term success.
- *Type and extent of attachment loss.* Pockets form secondary to the apical migration of the epithelial

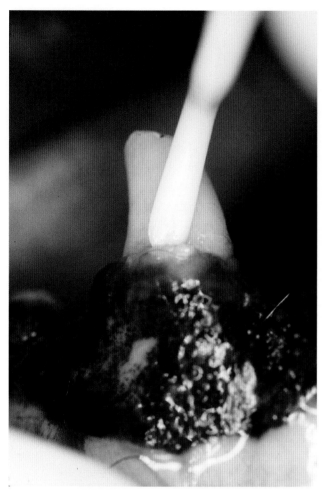

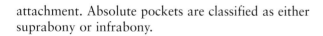

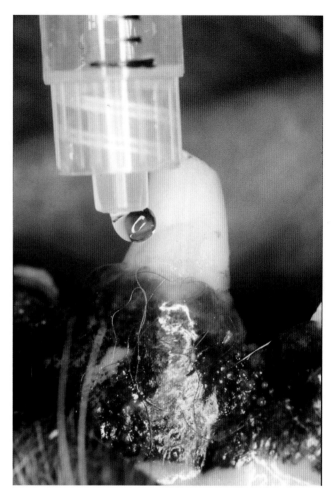

FIGURE 6.68. Plastic applicator used to press Doxirobe Gel into the pocket.

FIGURE 6.69. Water used to harden the Doxirobe Gel.

attachment. Absolute pockets are classified as either suprabony or infrabony.

Suprabony pockets are *above* the margin of alveolar bone. Suprabony pocket bone loss commonly occurs horizontally at similar rates on the mesial and distal surfaces of the teeth (Figures 6.70, 6.71).

When the suprabony pocket is less than 5 mm, treatment includes removal of supra- and subgingival plaque and calculus, root planing, and—in the dog—installation of local antibiotics (Doxirobe). This initial care usually provides tissue shrinkage, connective tissue remodeling, and gain of soft tissue attachment reducing pocket depth. Home care is essential for maintenance.

If greater than 50% of the gingiva and alveolar bone

has receded along the root, or if furcation exposures cannot be cleaned at home, extraction is the treatment of choice unless the owner accepts a guarded to poor prognosis.

For suprabony pockets >5 mm without gingival recession, apical repositioned flap surgery can be performed to visualize and clean the roots so that adequate treatment can be accomplished to help eliminate the pocket.

Infrabony (infra-alveolar vertical bone loss) pockets occur when the pocket floor (epithelial attachment) is apical to the alveolar bone. The infrabony pocket extends into a space between the tooth and the alveolar socket. Often gingival recession will accompany the infrabony pocket. Radiographically, infrabony pockets appear as vertical loss of bone along the root surface.

Infrabony defects are classified, and treatment deci-

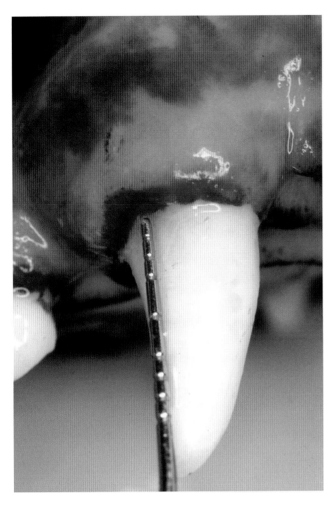

FIGURE 6.70. Periodontal probe before insertion.

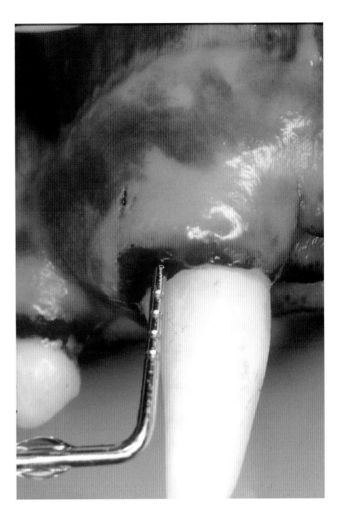

FIGURE 6.71. Periodontal probe extending 5 mm into a suprabony pocket.

sions are structured, by the number of walls remaining around the tooth. An infrabony defect is shaped like a box that has no top. The floor of the box is the base of the pocket. One side of the box or pocket is next to the root surface that has undergone attachment loss. The missing box top corresponds to the entrance to the pocket. The three remaining sides of the box are the potential walls of the defect.

Three-wall (intrabony) defects occur when the soft tissue that lines the pocket is surrounded with three sides of bone and one tooth surface (example: canine palatal defect). Three-walled pockets carry the best prognosis for eventual bone fill after periodontal therapy (Figure 6.72).

Two-wall bony defects are bordered by two osseous walls and two tooth surfaces (Figure 6.73).

One-wall defects occur when only one wall of bone remains around two tooth surfaces. The facial or

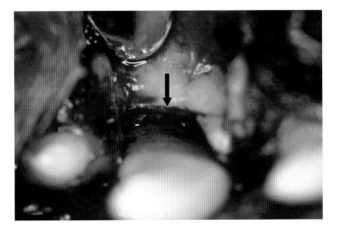

FIGURE 6.72. Three-walled infrabony defect palatal to the left maxillary canine.

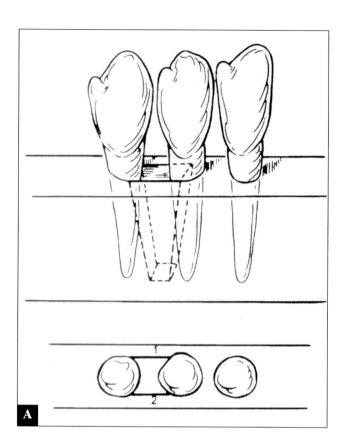

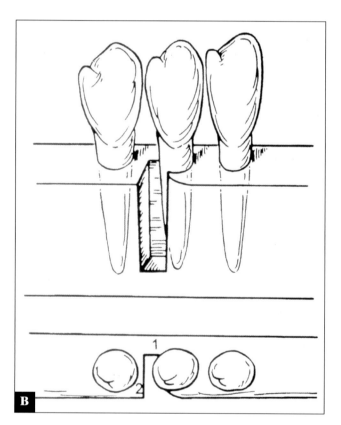

FIGURE 6.73. Two-walled defect.

palatal/lingual portion of the alveolar crest has been destroyed by disease in one-wall defects (Figure 6.74).

Combined (cup) bony defects occur when the tooth sits without any surrounding bony surfaces. Combined bony defects carry the worst prognosis.

PERIODONTAL INSTRUMENTS

Periodontal surgical tray contents include the following:

- *Probe and explorer.* A double-ended combination of a thin Michigan type probe, No. 23 explorer (Burns 951-8624, Schein 100-0805), and a double-ended cow horn explorer for examination of furcation areas (P2 probe/explorer Cislak, Cow horn EXP 3 CH).
- *Disposable number 15 or 15C scalpel blade and number 3 handle.*
- *Periodontal knife* (examples include Goldman-Fox No. 11, (Figure 6.75) (Burns 951-7840, Schein 100-1288), Orban 1-2 (Figure 6.76) (Burns 951-7792, ORB 1/2 Cislak, Schein 600-8598), Bucks 5/6 (Figure 6.77) (Burns 951-7781, Schein 600-3623) or #15 scalpel blade (Burns 808-0175, Schein 953-

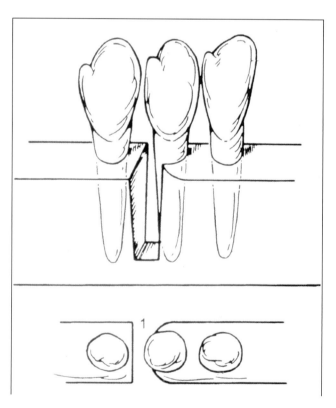

FIGURE 6.74. One-wall defect.

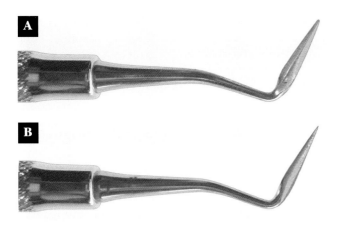

FIGURE 6.75. Goldman-Fox No. 11 periodontal knife.

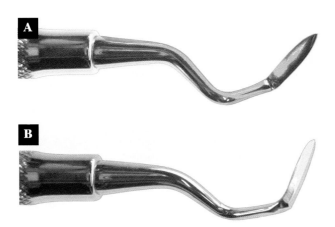

FIGURE 6.76. Orban periodontal knife.

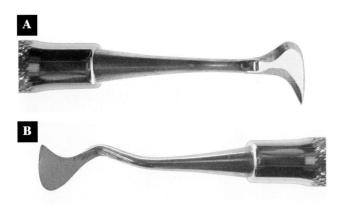

FIGURE 6.77. Bucks periodontal knife.

7101). Orban knives are shaped like spears that have cutting edges on both sides of the blade. Kirkland knives are double-ended with kidney-shaped blades.

- *Periosteal elevators* reflect and retract periosteum from the surface of the bone. Molt (Figure 6.78)

(Burns 951-7875, Schein 100-4888, Cislak EX-1) and Freer (Figure 6.79) (Burns 843-2422, Schein 953-0025, Cislak) are human dental elevators commonly used in veterinary dentistry. The EX 7 and EX 9 (Cislak; Burns 271-9050, 699-2598) are periosteal elevators manufactured specifically for small dogs and felines (Figure 6.80).

- *Curettes* come in a wide selection. Popular examples are the McCall 17/18 (Burns 950-9536, Schein 100-6283, P9 Cislak), Gracey 11/12 (Burns 950-9605, Schein 100-1982, P20 Cislak), and Gracey 13/14, (Burns 950-9605, P21 Cislak, Schein 100-4313).
- *Osseous and gingival reduction contouring instruments* include bone chisels and files for hand use, as well as a selection of diamond burs for the high-speed handpiece.

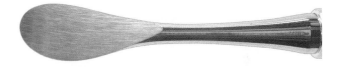

FIGURE 6.78. Molt periosteal elevator.

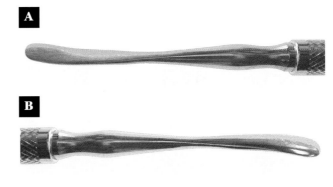

FIGURE 6.79. Freer periosteal elevator.

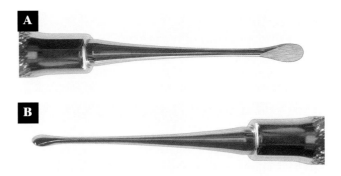

FIGURE 6.80. EX 9 periosteal elevator.

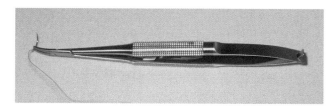

FIGURE 6.81. Castroviejo needle holder.

- *Fine curved cilia scissors.*
- The *Castroviejo needle holder* allows controlled suturing of delicate flaps (Figure 6.81) (Burns 950-6105, Schein 100-2146, 4388 Cislak).
- The *No. 6 India sharpening stone* is used to sharpen periodontal instruments. The sharpening stone can be autoclaved for use during surgical procedures (Burns 843-3204, Schein 600-2191).

FLAP SURGERY

Tissue that is raised from its bed and left attached on at least one side is called a *flap*. The base through which the attachment and circulation is maintained is called the *pedicle*.

Flaps provide an ideal method to allow exposure of the root surface, preserve attached gingiva, and allow the gingiva to be sutured in a fashion that reduces the periodontal pocket and promotes reattachment to the root surface.

During the surgical preparation phase, if chlorhexidine is used as an irrigant, it must be irrigated thoroughly. High concentrations of chlorhexidine may devitalize periodontal ligament cells and interfere with attachment. A strength of 0.05% chlorhexidine is considered safe.

Flap design should meet the following criteria:

- Flaps should be planned for maximum utilization and retention of keratinized gingival tissue to maintain a functional zone of attached keratinized gingiva.
- Flap design should allow adequate access and visibility. Flaps should have ample length to fully evaluate the root surface not covered with bone.
- Involvement of adjacent areas should be avoided.
- Primary closure is preferred to secondary intention healing.
- The base of a flap should be 1 1/2 times as wide as the coronal aspect to allow adequate vascularity.
- Tissue tags should be removed to allow rapid healing and prevent granulation tissue.

- Adequate flap stabilization is necessary to prevent displacement, bleeding, hematoma formation, bone exposure, and infection.

Flap closure should meet these criteria:

- Sutures should be placed from movable to nonmovable tissue when possible. The sutured flap should be tension-free.
- Knots should be tied three to five times (depending on suture type) to prevent loosening. Surgical knots should not lie on the incision line.
- The suture needle should be held anterior to the curvature but not at the tip.
- Rapidly absorbable 3-0 to 5-0 suture material attached to curved P1 or P3 Ethicon needles are preferred by the author. A reverse cutting edge is used to minimize inadvertent tissue tears. In human periodontal surgery, many procedures finish with only tissue approximation, and few—if any—sutures. Sutures impose an additional insult on the tissue, which can slow wound healing, and are plaque-retentive. Additionally, suture tracts provide a site for bacterial invasion.
- A continuous suture pattern should be used if possible, because it reduces the number of knots.
- Inverted knots are preferred, minimizing plaque retention.

Flap Classification

The *full-thickness flap* is used to gain visibility and access for osseous surgery, root planing, and pocket elimination. A full-thickness flap, which includes the periosteum, can be elevated by blunt dissection using a periosteal elevator in a rocking motion until the periosteum is peeled away from the underlying bone (Figure 6.82)

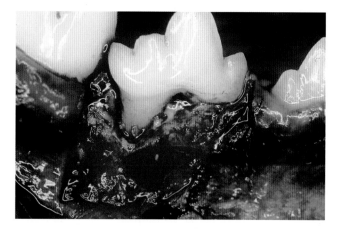

FIGURE 6.82. Full-thickness mucoperiosteal flap around the mandibular fourth premolar in a dog.

The *partial- or split-thickness (mucosal) flap* leaves the periosteum at the donor site, avoids larger blood vessels, and allows suture placement in the periosteum (Figure 6.83). Partial-thickness flaps are indicated:

- Where there are thin bony plates.
- In areas of dehiscence or fenestration where bone must be protected.
- In areas where bone loss is permanent.

Envelope flaps

Envelope flaps are conservative full-thickness elevations coronal to the mucogingival line, used to expose gingival pockets through intrasulcular incisions. The horizontal incision is made along the alveolar margin at least one tooth distal to two teeth mesial to the site of operation. In the unmodified envelope flap, there are no vertical releasing incisions. After the root surface is cleaned and irrigated, sutures are placed to close the flap (Figure 6.84).

Modifications of a basic envelope flap include the following:

- An envelope flap can also be made with one vertical releasing incision. The papilla is included in the mesial extent of the incision to make repositioning and suturing easier (Figure 6.85).

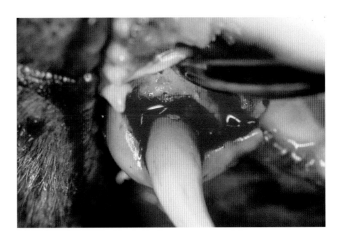

FIGURE 6.84. Envelope flap for the maxillary canine tooth in a cat.

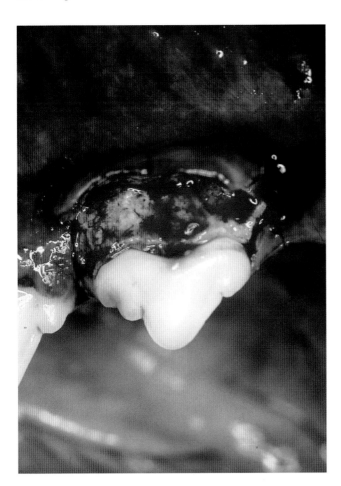

FIGURE 6.83. Partial-thickness flap over the maxillary second premolar in a dog.

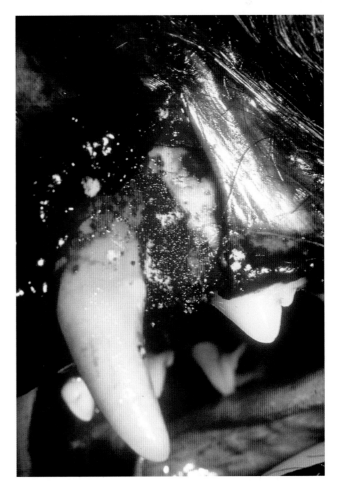

FIGURE 6.85. Triangular flap over the maxillary canine in a dog.

- An envelope flap made with two vertical relaxing incisions (pedicle flap).
- Curved or semilunar flaps do not involve the gingival sulcus. They are placed in attached or unattached gingiva for periapical endodontic surgical access or retrieval of small root tips (Figure 6.86).
- Access flaps expose the involved root surface(s) and alveolar margins for visualization and instrumentation. The access flap, which is not reflected past the crestal bone, gives the clinician entrance to infrabony defects and root surfaces. Under direct vision, defects can be carefully curetted and root surfaces planed. Access flaps are replaced and sutured at their original height.

Access flap

Use the following technique to perform access flap surgery:

1. Make mesial and distal vertical interdental incisions 2 mm apical to the deepest level of the pocket. Placing the incision totally in attached gingiva preserves the rich blood supply during and after surgery and takes advantage of the rapid epithelial migration encountered in this area during wound healing (Figures 6.87, 6.88). If the flap is to be replaced in its original location, it need not be elevated past the mucogingival line.
2. Angling the blade tip toward the root, make a 360° incision in the pocket (Figure 6.89).
3. Use a periosteal elevator (Molt or Freer) to expose the tooth's root surface for cleaning and root planing (Figures 6.90, 6.91).
4. Perform minor alveoloplasty (removing sharp bony spicules), if needed, using either bone-cutting forceps, hand chisels, or a diamond bur in a water-cooled high-speed handpiece.

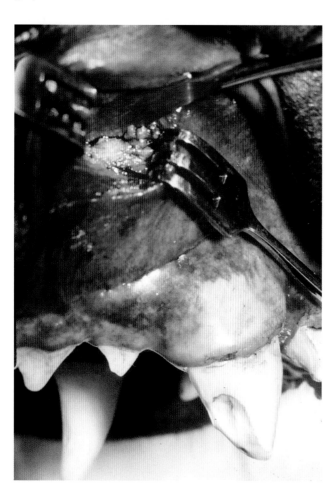

FIGURE 6.86. Semilunar flap for apicoectomy exposure of the maxillary canine tooth in a dog.

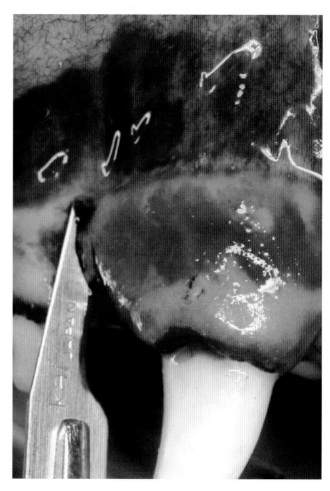

FIGURE 6.87. Distal interdental incision of the gingiva of a maxillary canine tooth in a dog.

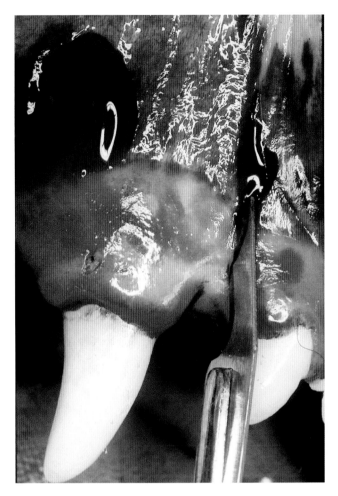

FIGURE 6.88. Mesial interdental incision past the mucogingival junction for greater exposure of the maxillary canine in a dog.

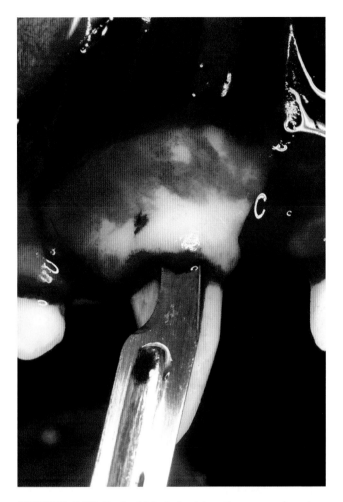

FIGURE 6.89. Scalpel blade incising the coronal periodontal attachment of a maxillary canine in a dog.

5. Plane the root surface and remove granulation tissue with a curette.
6. Place interdental 4-0 absorbable, simple, interrupted sutures to replace the flap.

Apically Repositioned Flap

An apically (re)positioned flap is created to decrease the depth of pockets in areas of alveolar bone loss without sacrificing the attached gingiva. The objective is to reposition the gingiva so it overlies the remaining alveolar bone with the margin extending 2 mm coronally.

The following are indications that an apically positioned flap is needed:

- Suprabony pockets (Figure 6.92)
- Moderate one- and two-walled infrabony pockets

- Crown lengthening
- Furcation involvement to get the furcation exposed for the pet owner to provide home care

The following are contraindications for such a flap:

- Marked bone loss leaving minimal tooth support
- Grade 3 tooth mobility
- Inadequate (less than 2 mm) attached gingiva present pre-operatively
- Non-pocket mucogingival deformity (dehiscence or fenestration)

To create an apically positioned flap:

1. Insert a number 15 blade 360° around the tooth to incise the epithelial attachment.

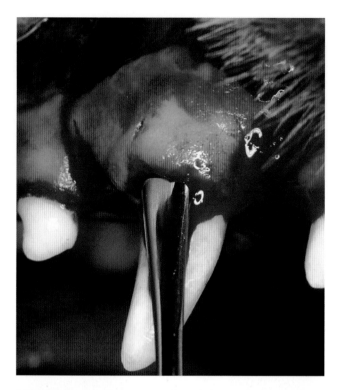

FIGURE 6.90. Elevator used to dislodge the attached gingiva from the buccal alveolar plate of the maxillary canine in a dog.

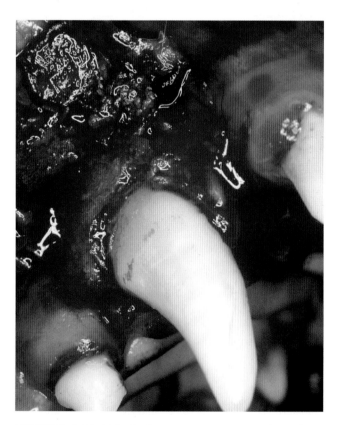

FIGURE 6.91. Full-thickness mucoperiosteal flap of the maxillary canine in a dog..

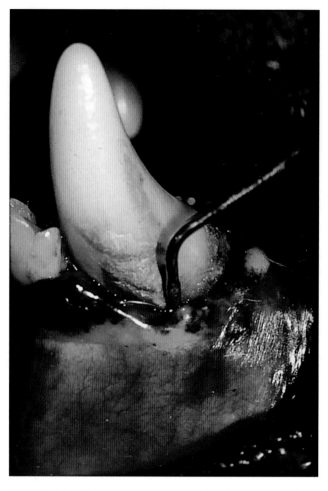

FIGURE 6.92. Suprabony pocket affecting the attached gingiva in a mandibular canine in a dog.

2. Make vertical releasing line angle incisions from the gingival margin and carry them apically past the mucogingival line (Figure 6.93).
3. With a curette, remove loose alveolar connective tissue, muscle, and granulation tissue at the alveolar margin. Debride bone defects to remove residual soft tissue. Use irrigation and compressed oil-free air to disclose missed plaque and calculus (Figure 6.94).
4. After cleaning the exposed root, suture the flap with 4-0 or 5-0 absorbable suture material to a position at the alveolar margin, reducing pocket depth. Leave the redundant tissue to fibrose naturally (Figure 6.95).
5. Apply gentle but firm digital pressure on the gingiva for 60 seconds. The pressure thins the fibrin clot, stimulates initial adhesion between wound edges, and reduces bleeding and hematoma formation.

Reverse Bevel Flap

In the reverse bevel flap (excision new attachment pro-

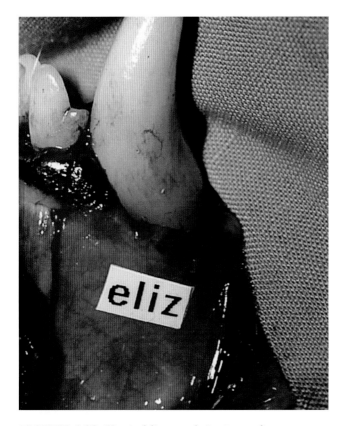

FIGURE 6.93. Vertical line angle incison of a mandibular canine in a dog.

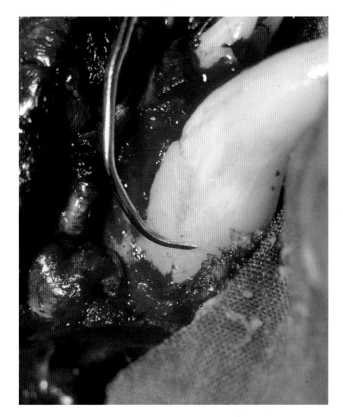

FIGURE 6.94. Curette used to remove subgingival calculus exposed by a flap over a mandibular canine in a dog.

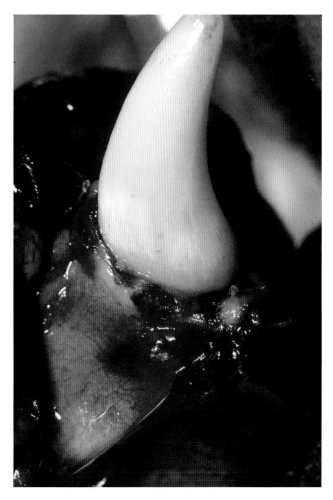

FIGURE 6.95. Sutured apically repositioned flap over a mandibular canine in a dog.

cedure, ENAP), a portion of the diseased pocket epithelium is removed to gain access for root treatment.

Indications for a reverse bevel flap include the following:

- Inflamed and necrotic free gingival margins
- Access to three-walled infrabony defects treated with bone grafts
- Mild-to-moderate cases of gingival hyperplasia
- Suprabony pockets extending apically to the mucogingival junction without osseous deformities

Use the following technique to create a reverse bevel flap:

1. Make the initial reverse beveled incision 1 mm apical to the gingival margin, 10° toward the long axis of the tooth between the diseased and healthy-appearing attached gingiva. The incision leaves a collar of diseased tissue attached to the tooth, which can be removed with a curette (Figures 6.96, 6.97).

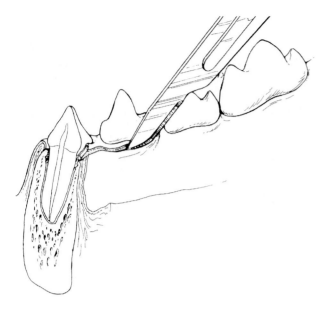

FIGURE 6.96. Reverse beveled incision (illustration by Michael Leonard, provided by courtesy of Nutramax Laboratories, Inc.).

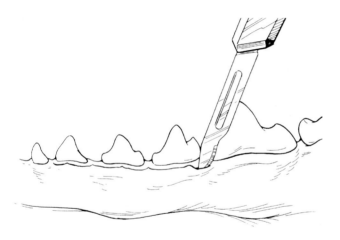

FIGURE 6.97. Reverse beveled incision carried distally.

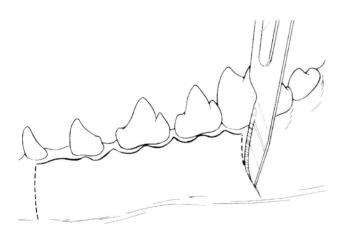

FIGURE 6.98. Vertical releasing incisions (illustration by Michael Leonard, provided by courtesy of Nutramax Laboratories, Inc.).

2. Make interdental releasing incisions mesial (and, if needed, distal) to adjacent healthy teeth (Figure 6.98).

3. When there are no bony defects, use a periosteal elevator to elevate the flap to the alveolar margin. If infrabony defects are found, make a full-thickness mucoperiosteal flap to gain exposure to the diseased bone (Figures 6.99, 6.100).

4. Perform root planing.

5. Perform alveoloplasty, using a hand chisel or a small round bur to create a smooth parabolic flow of the alveolar margin.

6. Place 4-0 or 5-0 absorbable sutures to appose "healthy" attached gingival incised edges (Figure 6.101).

7. With moistened gauze sponges, apply several minutes of digital pressure to help adaptation of the tissues.

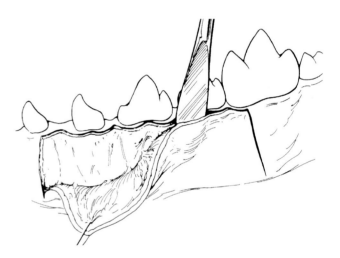

FIGURE 6.99. Flap elevation (illustration by Michael Leonard, provided by courtesy of Nutramax Laboratories, Inc.).

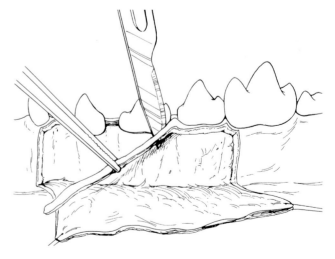

FIGURE 6.100. Removal of diseased gingival collar. Note: gingival exposure is extreme.

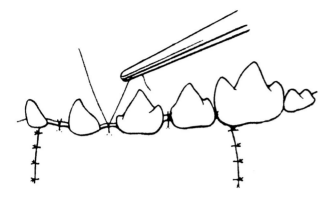

FIGURE 6.101. Sutured "healthy" attached gingiva reverse beveled incision.

Laterally Positioned (Pedicle) Flap

A laterally positioned pedicle flap is an advanced surgical procedure that is indicated where a localized gingival cleft exposes the tooth's root. The apical portion of the cleft defect is usually bound by alveolar mucosa and frequently found in an inflamed state. If the mesial and distal interadicular bone bordering such a defect has normal bone height, the laterally positioned pedicle graft can partially cover the denuded root when healed.

The laterally positioned flap surgery should not be attempted in teeth that are mobile due to periodontal disease, when furcation exposure exists, or in a patient whose caregiver cannot provide adequate aftercare.

Use the following technique to create a lateral positioned flap:

1. Make a vertical incision 2–3 mm on each side of the defect. The vertical incisions on either side of the defect are designed differently. The incision on the side away from the donor site is beveled toward the defect to create a broad recipient connective tissue surface for suturing. The vertical incision on the same side as the donor tissue is beveled away from the defect. The pedicles are elevated further than the mucogingival line because periosteum of the attached gingiva does not allow stretching. The beveled incisions should be generous enough to allow about 3 mm beyond the denuded root for placement and suturing of the donor flap (Figures 6.102,6.103).
2. Remove granulation tissue with a curette after the incisions are made and donor tissue is removed (Figure 6.104).
3. Delineate the distal extent of the split-thickness donor pedicle flap by making a vertical incision apically into the alveolar mucosa. The split-thickness

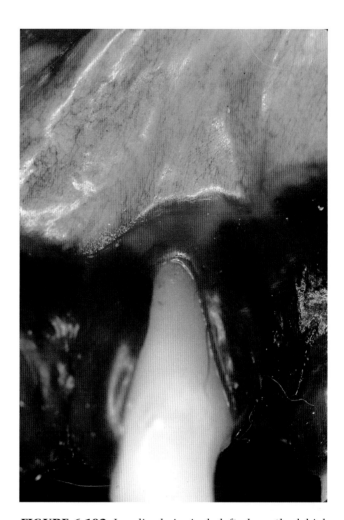

FIGURE 6.102. Localized gingival cleft along the labial surface of the maxillary corner incisor in a dog.

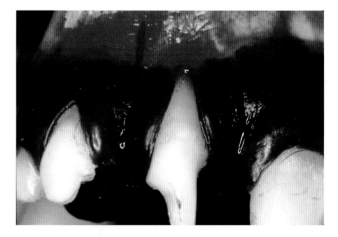

FIGURE 6.103. Incisions on either side of the defect.

flap (which leaves no denuded bone at the donor site) is harvested attached at its base. There must be sufficient dissection apical to the mucogingival junction or the flap will not have adequate mobility.

4. Move the flap laterally over the recipient area with a tissue forceps.
5. Suture the flap in place using 4-0 or 5-0 absorbable suture. The graft should be completely immobilized (Figure 6.105).

Free Gingival Graft

A *free gingival graft* can be used to establish or increase areas of attached gingiva where there is inadequate width, and where neighboring areas are unable to provide adequate donor tissue (lateral sliding flap). This advanced dental procedure is not indicated where there is moderate-to-marked tooth mobility (Figure 6.106).

To prepare the recipient area:

1. Use an apically positioned partial-thickness flap as a recipient bed of periosteum. Establish the lateral borders of the bed with vertical incisions carried close to the bone surface. Join the vertical incisions with a horizontal incision.
2. Separate the flap from the underlying connective tissue by sharp dissection. Position the flap apically and suture to provide a host bed of the desired size (Figure 6.107).

To secure donor tissue:

1. Harvest donor tissue for the free gingival graft from the wide attached gingival area apical to the maxillary canine on the same side of the defect (Figure 6.108).
2. Determine the size of the graft needed by measuring the length and width of the recipient bed with a periodontal probe. The graft should be approximately 20% larger than the recipient site to allow shrinkage and tension-free suturing.

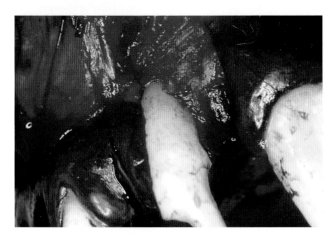

FIGURE 6.104. Cleaned root surface.

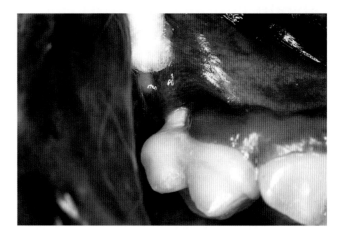

FIGURE 6.106. Marked gingival recession affecting the distal root of the maxillary first molar in a dog.

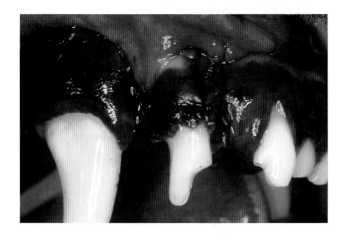

FIGURE 6.105. Resutured flap covering the original defect.

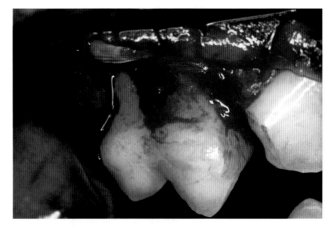

FIGURE 6.107. Flap exposure for cleaning the calculus and plaque from the root surface.

A No. 15 or preferably 10A blade on a scalpel handle is used to incise the graft tissue. The round shape of the No. 10A blade permits apical, mesial, and distal movement of the blade and facilitates removal of a 1 mm split-thickness donor graft (Figure 6.109).

To apply the graft:

1. Suture (using 5-0 or 6-0 absorbable suture with an atraumatic needle) and/or affix the graft with tissue adhesive. Adhesive must not run below the graft or the flap will fail because it won't be able to revascularize (Figure 6.110).
2. Hold a warm, wet gauze sponge against the surface of the graft for several minutes to express excess blood from between the graft and the bed, initiate hemostasis, and allow a thin fibrin layer to provide good adaptation of the graft to the periosteal bed.

Alveoloplasty

Bone defects revealed after flap exposure should be treated before resuturing. Treatment involves recontouring unsupported bone with diamond burs and/or chisels, as well as leveling interproximal craters to allow optimal flap adaptation.

Aftercare for Flap and Graft Surgery

Initial home care instructions include a soft diet, removal of chew toys, and hard treats for 3 weeks. The owner is cautioned not to brush the teeth around the graft site during this period. Chlorhexidine oral rinse is applied to the surgical site twice daily. Oral antibiotics and pain relief medication are also administered (Figure 6.111).

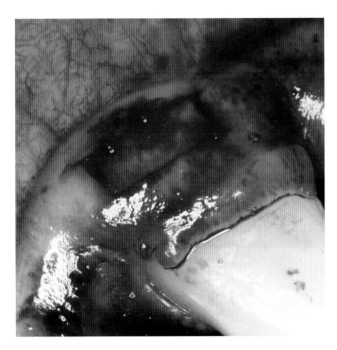

FIGURE 6.108. Template outlined in the attached gingiva overlying the maxillary canine in a dog.

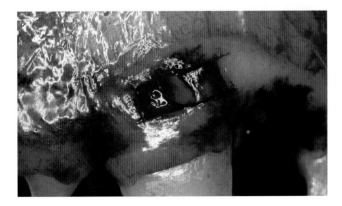

FIGURE 6.109. Harvesting spit-thickness donor tissue.

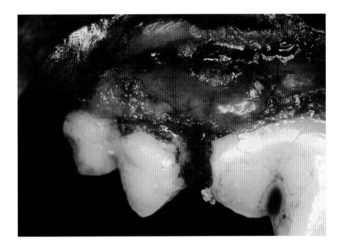

FIGURE 6.110. Graft sutured on recipient periosteal bed.

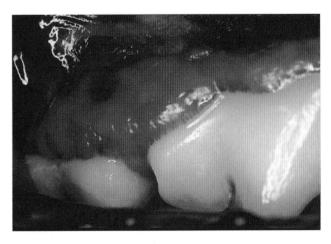

FIGURE 6.111. Area healed 2 months post-operatively.

PERIODONTAL SPLINTING

Periodontal splinting stabilizes mobile teeth by attaching them to nonmobile adjacent teeth. This advanced procedure has a low percentage of long-term success and should only be used in selected cases.

Periodontal splinting can be used:

- To accompany the healing phase of periodontal therapy
- For stabilization after trauma

- For stabilization before and during periodontal surgery
- As a method of temporarily saving teeth that would have been extracted because of advanced support loss. The client should be made aware that periodontal splinting is a controversial procedure that might not be in the patient's best interest because of continuing periodontitis beneath the splint (Figures 6.112–6.116).

After a splint is placed, home care is vital. The area under the splint is difficult to keep clean. If the owner will not agree to home care or if the patient will not allow aftercare, splinting should not be attempted. The splint may be left in place permanently or until the

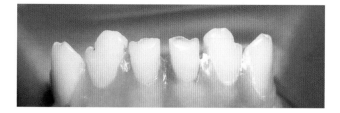

FIGURE 6.112. Mobile mandibular incisors in a dog before splinting.

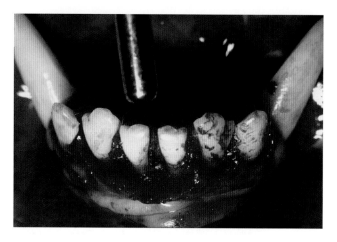

FIGURE 6.114. Flap exposure for cleaning subgingival plaque and calculus from the root surface of the mandibular incisors in a dog.

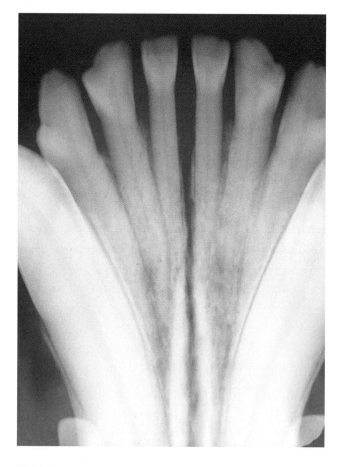

FIGURE 6.113. Radiograph showing marked bone loss around the mandibular incisors in a dog.

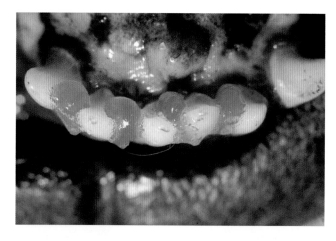

FIGURE 6.115. Phosphoric acid gel to etch the teeth before splinting.

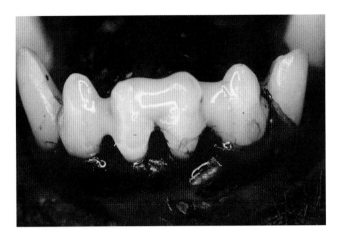

FIGURE 6.116. Bonded (splinted) mandibular incisors.

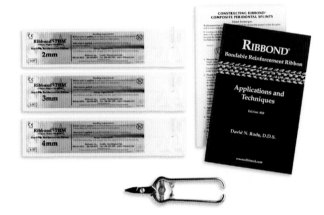

FIGURE 6.117. Ribbond.

underlying healing periodontium provides stability.

Materials used in periodontal splinting include the following:

- Dental acrylic (Triad) or composite (Protemp Garant)
- Composite filling material (Burns 950-9043, Schein 100-1673)
- Bondable reinforcement ribbon (Ribbond) (Figure 6.117).

To fabricate a composite resin splint using Ribbond bondable reinforcement ribbon:

1. Place a narrow strip of tin foil along the labial surface of maxillary or mandibular incisors to determine the length of Ribbond needed.
2. Cut the Ribbond to the predetermined length and place on a clean glass slab. Do not handle the Ribbond with bare hands.

3. Apply and light cure two layers of composite to the labial surfaces of the affected teeth, which are clean and pumice-polished.
4. Place composite on top of the splint without light curing.
5. Place adhesive on the Ribbond.
6. Place Ribbond over the bonded teeth and light cure. Place an additional layer of composite over the splint; then light cure, shape, and polish.
7. Check occlusion after the animal is extubated. Make adjustments if indicated.

PROCEDURES FOR PERIODONTAL REGENERATION

Regeneration procedures include a variety of surgical techniques that attempt to restore the periodontal tissues (alveolar bone, cementum, periodontal ligament) lost through disease. The goal of periodontal regeneration is to replace the bone and lost attachment. Regenerative procedures consist of flap exposure, root planing, and placement of bone, bone induction products, or a membrane over the treated area before resuturing.

BONE GRAFTING

Ideally, bone grafting restores normal bony architecture, rebuilds the periodontal ligament and soft tissue, and prevents further periodontal pocket formation.

The following are areas where bone grafts are indicated:

- Deep extraction sites, in order to preserve the alveolar ridge
- Deep, narrow, three-walled infrabony pockets, such as palatal defects, that do not extend into the nasal cavity (infrabony (below the bone) defects are more amenable to bone regeneration compared to suprabony pockets)
- Endodontic-periodontic defects

Bone grafts should not be used on the following:

- Patients receiving chronic anticoagulant therapy
- Patients receiving immunosuppressant medication
- Patients receiving, or that have received, radiation treatment at the surgical site
- Poorly controlled insulin-dependent diabetics.
- Patients that have an active infection at recipient site

The following is a partial list of materials used for bone grafting:

- Synthetic bioactive ceramic, Consil (Nutramax Laboratories) develops a direct bond to tissue and becomes osseoconductive when implanted into an osseous defect. The ceramic is resorbed within 14 months, leaving bone and periodontal ligament behind. Consil, due to its high pH, can also be used in minimally infected sites to help inhibit bacterial growth (Figure 6.118).
- Autogenous (the patient's) bone harvested from the alveolar margin from an unrelated area or from one of the long bones (humerus or tibia).
- Frozen cadaver bone.
- H.T.R. (hydroxyapatite-coated resin polymer).

A bone grafting instrument setup should include the following:

- No. 3 scalpel handle (Burns 950-2150, Schein 100-7520, Cislak 4208) with No. 15c scalpel blade (Burns 950-2175, Schein 953-7101)
- Molt No. 2 (Burns 699-3504, EX 20 Cislak, Schein 600-6125)), No. 4 (EX 21 Cislak, Schein 600-9526, Burns 699-3504, Schein 100-4888), or Molt double-ended 2/4 (Burns 271-9008, Cislak EX 20/21 DE, Schein 586-9560) periosteal elevators
- Curette (EX 2—#10 Miller Cislak, Burns 843-0572, Schein 600-7080)
- Citric acid for root therapy
- Thumb forceps (Burns 605-1020, Schein 100-5162)
- Needle holder (Burns 700-8650, Schein 100-1125) and 5-0 absorbable suture material with a needle
- Curved iris scissors (Burns 958-1276, Schein 100-5880)
- Consil (Nutramax Laboratories) (Burns 277-0350)
- Dappen dish (Burns 950-9662, Schein 100-9211)

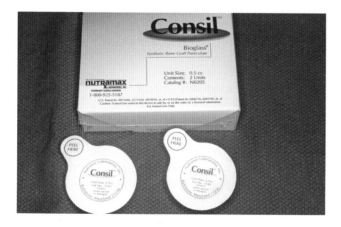

FIGURE 6.118. Consil.

ALVEOLAR MARGIN MAINTENANCE

Use the following technique for alveolar margin maintenance using Consil material (Figure 6.119):

1. If chlorhexidine is used as an irrigant during surgery, rinse it thoroughly. Chlorhexidine can devitalize periodontal ligament cells and interfere with attachment.
2. Create an access flap with interdental and sulcular incisions (Figure 6.119A).
3. Plane the root smooth with a curette and remove excess granulation tissue.
4. Apply several drops of citric acid gel on the root. After 30 seconds, irrigate the area with saline to remove the citric acid.
5. Add four to six drops of the patient's blood, sterile water, or saline to 0.5 ml of Consil material in a dappen dish (Figure 6.119B).

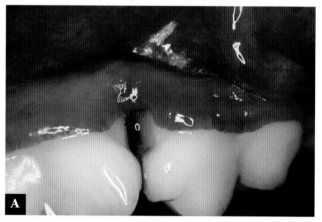

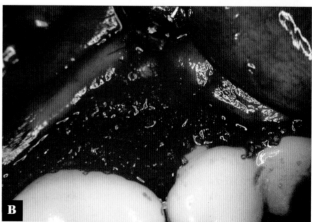

FIGURE 6.119. (A) Gingival recession and bone loss between the maxillary fourth premolar and first molar; (B) mixture of the patient's blood and Consil crystals.

6. Mix the liquid and granules in the dappen dish with a spatula for 10 seconds to achieve the consistency of firm wet sand and apply it into the defect area. Alternatively, carry the Consil granules to the defect and mix with the patient's blood. In 2–3 minutes, a chemical change occurs within Consil that initiates the process of bone regeneration.
7. Suture the access flap.

Post-operative care includes the following:

- Pain and antimicrobial medication are dispensed.
- The patient is fed a soft diet for several weeks.
- Gentle brushing can begin 1 week after surgery.
- The surgical site is reexamined every 2–3 weeks.
- The area is probed and radiographed in 4 months to follow healing.

PALATAL DEFECT SURGERY

Canine palatal defect therapy is indicated in cases where there is >25% attachment loss on the palatal aspect of one or both maxillary canine teeth, and the periodontal probe does not enter the nasal cavity. When deep pockets are diagnosed, pocket therapy should be performed or the tooth extracted and the defect closed. If untreated, the pocket will usually progress until it penetrates the nasal cavity (Figure 6.120).

Use this technique for palatal pocket therapy:

1. Make 4–8 mm mesial and distal incisions to the bone at 20° angles palatally from the affected tooth (Figure 6.121).
2. Use a Molt or Freer periosteal elevator to gently raise a full-thickness flap (Figure 6.122).

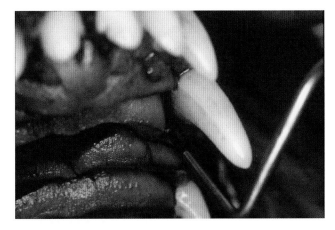

FIGURE 6.120. 10 mm palatal probing depth of the maxillary canine tooth in a dog.

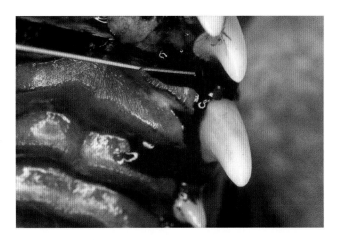

FIGURE 6.121. Interdental incisions.

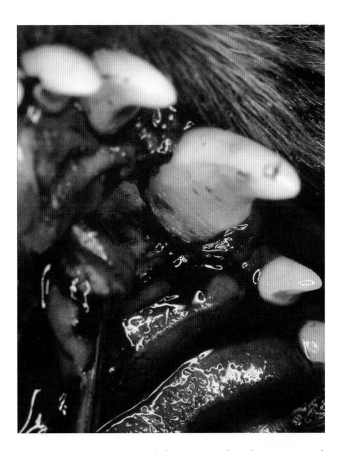

FIGURE 6.122. Palatal defect exposed with a periosteal elevator.

3. Use a thin curette to clean accessible granulation tissue, calculus, and plaque between the root and alveolus (Figure 6.123).
4. Optionally, place several drops of citric acid gel into the defect. After 30 seconds, irrigate the area with saline to remove the citric acid.

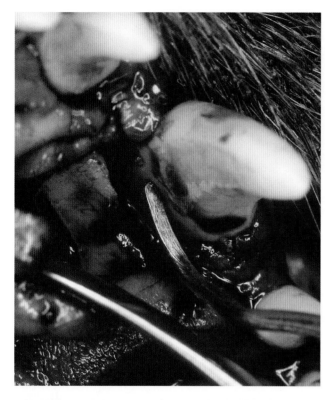

FIGURE 6.123. Curette used to debride the palatal surface of the pocket.

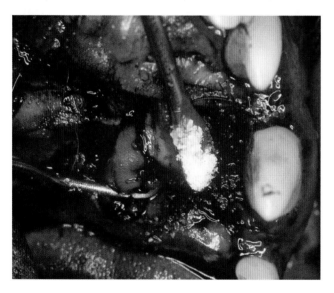

FIGURE 6.124. Consil material placed in the freshly debrided palatal pocket.

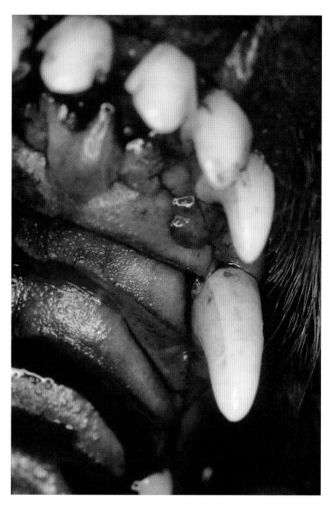

FIGURE 6.125. Sutured flap.

GUIDED TISSUE REGENERATION (GTR)

Granulation tissue growing from the periodontal ligament and bone marrow spaces carries the potential for regeneration. The goal of guided tissue regeneration (GTR) is to repopulate the affected area with periodontal cells that have the capability of redeveloping cementum on the root surface to generate healthy attachment. Barriers are used to avoid the proliferation of the gingival epithelial and connective tissues along the exposed root surface and to selectively guide the growth of bone and periodontal ligament cells into an area where they have been lost. This is considered an advanced periodontal surgical procedure used mostly in Class II furcation defects and two- and three-walled infrabony pockets.

GTR membranes are thin sheets of pliable material placed subgingivally following full-thickness flap expo-

5. Carry bone-grafting particles into the cleaned defect (Figure 6.124).
6. Appose the flap snugly against the tooth and suture with 4-0 absorbable suture on an atraumatic needle (Figure 6.125).

sure. The material is custom-fitted or seated to the specific defect area to allow optimal flap apposition under the periosteum. Nonabsorbable membranes are removed according to manufacturer's directions 1–9 months post-operatively. Absorbable membranes dissolve within 2 months.

ORONASAL FISTULAS

Oronasal fistulas result from periodontal disease of the maxillary teeth, creating communication between the oral and nasal cavities. Oronasal fistulas allow fluid and food to enter the turbinates of the nose, perpetuating nasal discharge and chronic infection. One or both maxillary canines may be affected. Clinical signs include sneezing and/or nasal discharge that is sometimes blood-tinged (Figure 6.126).

If the periodontal probe enters the nasal cavity during exploration of the palatal surface, extraction followed by single- or double-layered flap surgical closure is indicated. If the probe does not extend into the nasal cavity, palatal therapy (described earlier) can be used to decrease pocket depth and increase maxillary canine support.

Single-Layer Flap Oronasal Fistula Repair

A *buccal, single-layer sliding flap* is usually used for small and acute fistulas that occur after the canine is extracted or exfoliated.

Use the following technique to create a buccal single-layer sliding flap:

1. Circumferentially remove a thin mucosal epithelial margin around the opening left after the tooth removal, using a No. 15 blade.

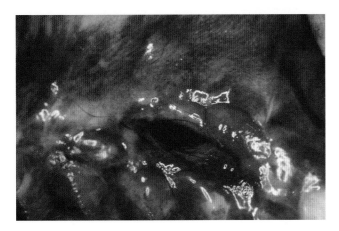

FIGURE 6.126. Oronasal fistula.

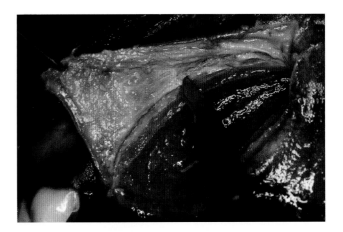

FIGURE 6.127. Scalpel used to incise the periosteal layer to increase its length.

2. Harvest a buccal mucoperiosteum gingival flap by making divergent incisions mesially and distally through the mucogingival line, extending into the buccal mucosa.
3. Gently elevate the flap using a No. 2 and/or 4 Molt or EX 21 (Cislak) periosteal elevator, exposing the periosteum.
4. To improve flap mobility, incise the periosteal layer of the flap in the apical region. If this surgical maneuver is not performed, the flap might fail because of insufficient length to cover the defect without tension (Figure 6.127).
5. Position the flap over the opening to ensure there is no tension before closure.
6. Suture the flap to the edge of the defect using 4-0 to 5-0 absorbable suture material on a reverse cutting needle in a simple interrupted pattern.
7. Confirm that the mandibular canine does not traumatize the flap. If it does, perform a crown reduction and restoration procedure.

Double-Layer Oronasal Fistula Repair

The *double-flap* technique to repair oronasal fistulas is used where the fistula is chronic, large, or when a more predictable outcome is needed than that with the single-layer closure. In the double-flap technique, part of the palatal soft tissue is used to cover the defect; the resulting palate defect area is then covered with buccal mucosa to ensure a double seal:

1. Excise the buccal mucosal edge of the fistula to provide a fresh clean surface for primary healing. Leave the soft tissue lining the palatal edge of the defect intact (Figure 6.128).

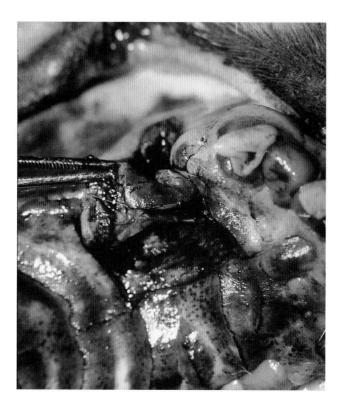

FIGURE 6.128. Palatal flap harvested for double flap technique.

2. Make perpendicular incisions extending palatally from the mesial and distal aspects of the defect. The two incisions are connected on the palate extending several millimeters past the midline. Elevate a full-thickness flap using a periosteal elevator. Control bleeding by prolonged compression with gauze sponges.

3. Rotate the palatal flap on its basilar attachment onto the fistula and suture in place with 4-0 absorbable suture material in a simple interrupted pattern. Turn the oral epithelium to face the turbinates (Figure 6.129).

4. Harvest the second layer as a partial-thickness pedicle flap from the buccal mucosa. Take care to design a mucosal flap large enough to cover the inverted palatal flap and denuded area over the junction between the incisive and maxillary bone. Form the pedicle flap by making two incisions perpendicular to the mucogingival line, extending from the buccal aspect of the defect (Figure 6.130). The space between the two incisions should be at least 1 1/2 times the width of the defect. To gain additional non-tension coverage, partially incise the non-epithelial side in a perpendicular fashion at the base. Suture the second flap (Figure 6.131).

Post-operative instructions after oronasal fistula repair should include the following:

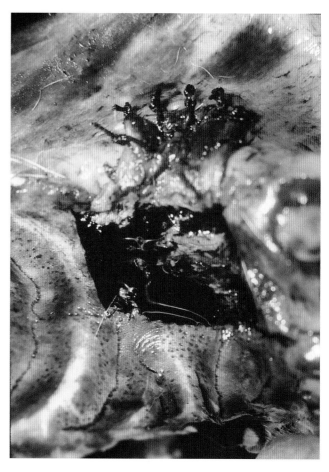

FIGURE 6.129. Palatal flap sutured over the oronasal defect.

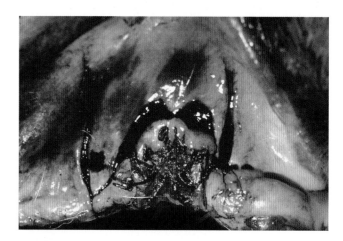

FIGURE 6.130. Buccal flap releasing incisions.

- Administer broad-spectrum antibiotics orally postoperatively for 10 days.
- Dispense pain relief medication for 7 days.
- Pre-wet food to soften for 10 days after surgery.
- Examine the surgical site 3 and 10 days post-operatively to evaluate primary intention healing.

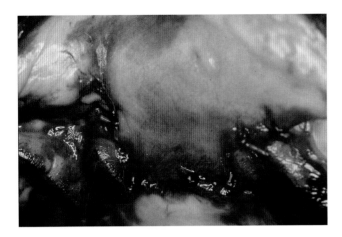

FIGURE 6.131. Completed double flap.

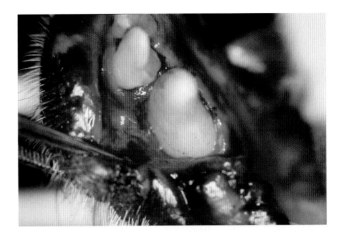

FIGURE 6.132. Tight frenulum around the mandibular canine tooth in a dog, predisposing it to periodontal disease.

MANDIBULAR FRENECTOMY

Frenula are tough bands of tissue connecting the inside surfaces of the lip to the mandibular gingiva behind canine teeth and between the lip and maxillary central incisors. In the presence of marked periodontal disease, the frenulum attachment may trap food and debris against inflamed labial gingiva (Figure 6.132).

Mandibular frenectomy is indicated in patients with gingival recession or pocket formation on the distal labial side of mandibular canine teeth or when periodontal disease around the maxillary central incisors is caused or aggravated by a tight frenulum. By excising the attachment, food will not accumulate as readily in the affected areas.

Frenectomy is performed with the following technique:

1. Local anesthesia.
2. Dissect the frenulum close to the gingival margins with a scalpel blade, iris scissors, radiosurgery, or laser (Figures 6.133, 6.134).
3. Suture the detached labial mucosa close to the periosteum.
4. Root plane the exposed abnormal cemental surface.

GINGIVAL HYPERPLASIA (GH)

Relative, pseudo-, or false pockets exist when there is gingival enlargement (hyperplasia) without destruction of periodontal tissues. If gingival hyperplasia is greater than 2–3 mm when probed, the treatment of choice to reduce pocket depth is a gingivectomy (Figure 6.135).

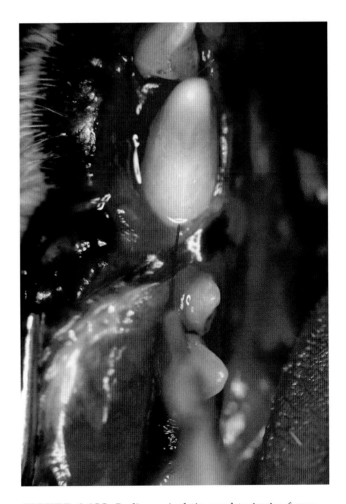

FIGURE 6.133. Radiosurgical tip used to incise frenulum.

attached gingiva must be present both pre-operatively and post-operatively to protect the tooth.

At one time, gingivectomy was the treatment of choice to eliminate pocket depth and to allow exposure of the root surface for cleaning. Although gingivectomy may eliminate a suprabony pocket, healing time of exposed tissue is longer than a repositioned flap procedure. Gingivectomies should be used only in cases of gingival hyperplasia where there is an overgrowth of tissue and at least 2 mm of attached gingiva remains after surgery.

Use the following steps for gingivectomy afer local anesthesia is injected:

1. Place a periodontal probe onto the pseudo-pocket floor, then outside to the measured depth, making slight indentions or bleeding points on the gingiva at the level of attachment.

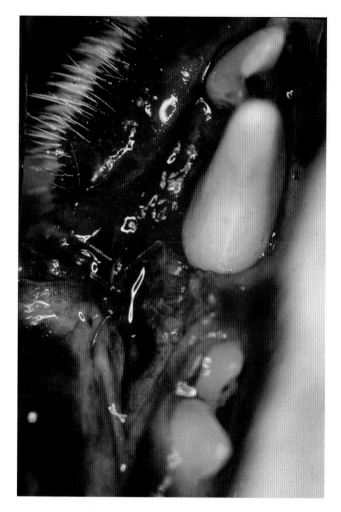

FIGURE 6.134. Incised frenulum before suturing.

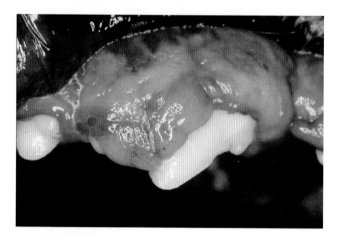

FIGURE 6.135. Gingival hyperplasia.

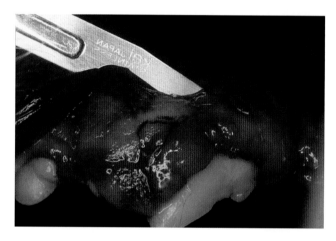

FIGURE 6.136. Scalpel blade angle used for gingivectomy.

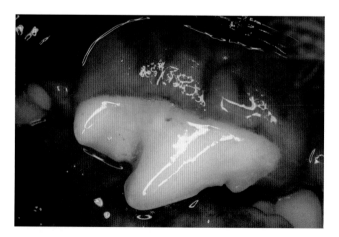

FIGURE 6.137. Gingivectomy site 1 month post-operatively.

Gingivectomy is a coronally directed, externally beveled incision, used primarily for the removal of excess gingiva when no underlying osseous lesions are noted. An adequate band (greater than 2 mm) of

2. Using a scalpel with 15 or 15c blade attached or an electrosurgical or radiosurgical blade, incise a beveled edge to approximate the normal gingiva (Figures 6.136, 6.137).
3. Administer post-operative anti-inflammatory and pain medication; recommend that the patient be fed a soft diet for several days.

HEMISECTION TO SAVE PART OF THE TOOTH

Furcation exposure occurs secondary to periodontal disease. In Class I and Class II disease, periodontal therapy together with a patient able to accept aftercare may result in a saved tooth. Goals of furcation exposure therapy are to decrease pocket depth, eliminate bony lesions, and create a cleanable tooth that is easier to clean to decrease further invasion.

In patients with marked furcation involvement, where one root has at least 50% bone support and the other root(s) have less, the tooth can be sectioned and root canal therapy or vital pulp therapy performed, resulting in preserving a portion of the tooth (Figures 6.138–6.142).

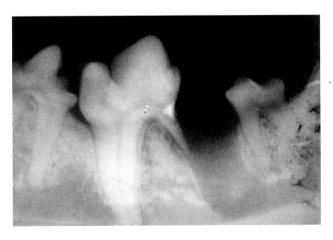

FIGURE 6.140. Hemisection of the distal root and partial coronal pulpectomy (note overhang remaining after hemisection).

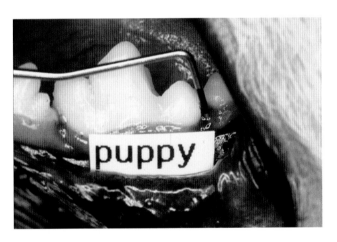

FIGURE 6.138. 9 mm pocket affecting the distal root of the mandibular first molar in a dog.

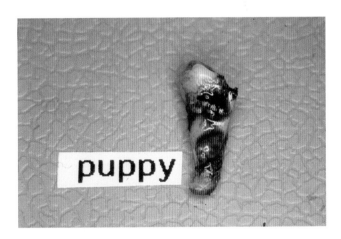

FIGURE 6.141. Hemisected root.

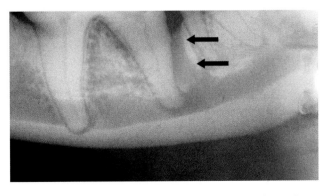

FIGURE 6.139. Radiograph showing vertical bone loss around distal root.

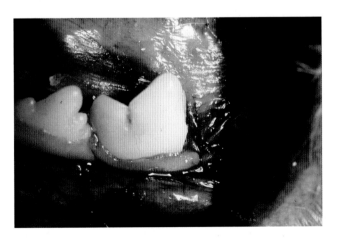

FIGURE 6.142. Remaining vital hemisected mandibular first molar.

USE OF SYSTEMIC ANTIBIOTICS IN PERIODONTAL DISEASE

Antibiotics by themselves will not cure periodontal disease. Antibiotics may be prescribed in patient management, together with scaling, root planing, polishing, or extraction.

Antibiotics may be used in the following circumstances:

- In pretreatment to help decrease bacteremia and operator bacterial exposure in stages 3 and 4 periodontal disease
- The week following treatment in stages 3 and 4 periodontal disease
- In a pulse therapy fashion wherein periodic (first 5 days of each month) doses of an antibiotic approved for small animal dental care is administered on a long-term basis as an adjunct to home care. Pulse therapy is for those cases of treated stage 3 and 4 periodontal disease. This extra-label use of pulse dosing is used extensively in veterinary dermatologic care, and may provide benefits in the periodontally affected patient by;
  - Reducing the bacteria load once monthly, decreasing logarithmic replication
  - Weakening the biofilm glycocalyx, which keeps plaque and calculus together
- Temporarily decreasing halitosis

Pulse therapy should *not* be considered a substitute for proper surgical treatment and home care; even in the patient, that is an anesthetic risk. Further research needs to be performed to substantiate the use and investigate long-term benefits and risks of pulse antibiotic use in the therapy of periodontal disease.

HOME CARE

Regardless of what dental procedures are performed, clinical success is diminished if not combined with an ongoing program of home care. The goal of dental home care is to remove plaque from tooth surfaces and gingival sulci before it mineralizes into calculus, a process that occurs within days of a teeth cleaning. Success depends on the owner's ability to brush teeth daily, as well as the dog or cat's acceptance of the process. True oral cleanliness can be achieved only through the mechanical action of toothbrush bristles above and below the gingiva.

Home care is best started at a young age before the adult teeth erupt. An ideal time to introduce tooth brushing is at the first puppy or kitten visit. The client-animal bond as well as the client-veterinarian bond is enhanced when daily brushing is performed following instructions given at the animal hospital.

Brushing instruction involves more than telling a pet owner it would be a good idea for them to brush their pet's teeth and dispensing a toothbrush. The client needs to be shown how to properly use a pet toothbrush and paste followed by observing the client perform tooth brushing and follow-up examinations to monitor progress.

The small animal client needs to:

- *Start with a healthy comfortable mouth.* Untreated oral lesions can cause a painful mouth and a noncompliant patient. Dental pathology must be treated before the client is instructed to begin brushing teeth.
- *Start early.* At 8–12 weeks of age, brushing once or twice weekly helps familiarize the pet with the tooth brushing routine. At 5–7 months, while the secondary (adult) teeth are erupting, teeth brushing should be performed daily.
- *Choose a proper toothbrush and toothpaste (dentifrice).* Plaque accumulates in the sulcus or periodontal pocket. Toothbrushes have bristles that reach under the gingival margin and clean the space that surrounds each tooth. Devices such as gauze pads, rubber finger toothbrushes, sponges, or cotton swabs remove plaque above the gum line, but cannot adequately clean the sulcus.

Virbac and other companies manufacture toothbrushes specifically for use in small animals. Each dog or cat should have its own brush. Sharing brushes might result in cross-contamination of bacteria from one pet to another. Toothbrushes should be thoroughly cleaned after each use, stored in a clean location, and replaced at least monthly.

- The *fingerbrush* (Virbac Products) is popular for beginners. It fits on the end of the owner's index finger, which reduces resistance of both the pet and owner. Unfortunately, the finger brush's bristles are rubber and do not extend subgingivally to remove plaque. The fingerbrush should be used as the first step to get a pet comfortable with brushing so a pet owner can introduce a bristled brush into daily home care later. The finger toothbrush can be cleaned in a dishwasher (Figure 6.143).

- The *mini-toothbrush* (Virbac Products) has nylon bristles that can extend subgingivally to remove plaque (Figure 6.144).
- The *dual-ended toothbrush* has head sizes to adapt to both small and large tooth surfaces (Figure 6.145).
- The *pet toothbrush* has a single reverse-angle head and extra soft bristles, which makes it ideal for cats and small to medium-sized dogs (Figure 6.146).

- The *cat toothbrush* allows a stroking or swabbing motion in a small cat's mouth. Bristles are soft to ensure a gentle application (Figure 6.147).
- The *two-brush system* brushes both sides of the teeth at the same time (Petosan, Norway) (Figure 6.148).

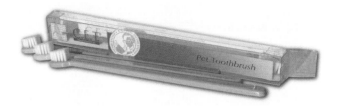

FIGURE 6.146. The pet toothbrush (Virbac).

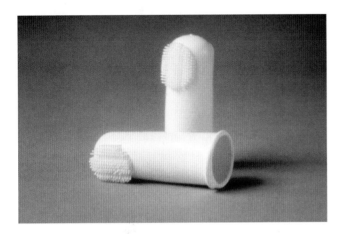

FIGURE 6.143. Rubber finger toothbrush (Virbac).

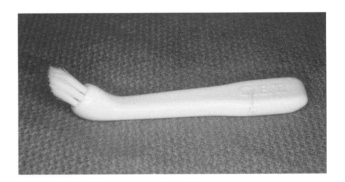

FIGURE 6.147. Cat toothbrush (Virbac).

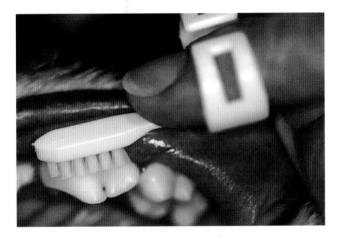

FIGURE 6.144. Mini-toothbrush (Virbac).

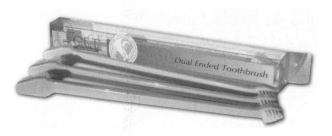

FIGURE 6.145. Dual-ended toothbrush (Virbac).

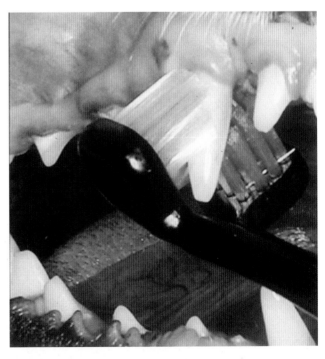

FIGURE 6.148. Two-brush toothbrush (Petosan).

Tooth Brushing Technique

Tooth brushing should be at the same time each day. Before dinner works well using the meal as a reward for cooperating. Follow these steps:

1. Place the pet's head at a 45° angle.
2. With the same hand used to hold the head up, pull the commisure of the lips backward, exposing the cheek teeth, while keeping the mouth closed (Figure 6.149).
3. Rub the toothbrush bristles in small circular motions under the gum line at a 45° angle to the gingiva. Generally, only the outside (facial) surfaces of the maxillary teeth are brushed. Plaque accumulates faster on the buccal surfaces of the maxillary canines and cheek teeth. The incisors, mandibular canines and cheek teeth accumulate less plaque (Figure 6.150). For cats, cotton-tipped applicators can also be used to remove plaque from the gum line (Figure 6.151).

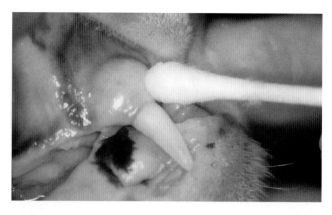

FIGURE 6.151. Q-tip used to remove plaque in cat's teeth.

4. Repeat and reward.
5. If the pet is anxious with the brushing procedure, give reassurance through gentle praise. Expect progress, not perfection. Reward progress immediately with a treat or a play period after each cleaning session.

Each pet is different. Some will be trained in 1 week, and others will take a month or more.

In the author's opinion, scalers and/or curettes should not be used by clients. Hand scaling without proper chemical immobilization and training can injure the gingiva or tooth.

Toothpaste (dentifrice) is used to help clean and polish the tooth surfaces. Human toothpaste should not be used on dogs and cats because it contains detergents and fluoride, which may be irritating to the stomach when swallowed.

> The Veterinary Oral Health Council (VOHC) evaluates the effectiveness of dental products, confirming manufacturer's claims. The VOHC is similar to the American Dental Association's (ADA) seal of approval for human dental products.

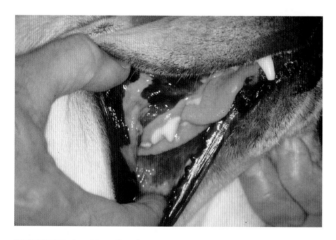

FIGURE 6.149. Cheek teeth exposed for brushing.

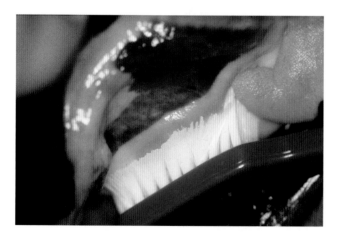

FIGURE 6.150. Proper toothbrush position.

Plaque Retardants

Salivary peroxidase enzyme-enhanced products (C.E.T., Virbac Products) bind to plaque. Peroxidases are found in a number of biologic fluids and in saliva. The antibacterial action of salivary peroxidase takes place because of the peroxidase-catalyzed oxidation of thiocyanate. The mode of action for salivary peroxidase appears to include inhibition of bacterial enzymes containing essential thiol groups:

- Virbac's C.E.T. "dual-enzyme" system consists of glucose oxidase and lactoperoxidase. When saliva and oxygen are added, hypothiocyanite is formed, which produces an antibacterial (antiplaque) effect.
- C.E.T. Tartar Control Toothpaste is marketed for dog and cat owners that do not brush teeth daily.
- DentAcetic Wipes (Dermapet) contains sodium HMP to help chemically decrease calculus while the wipes mechanically remove plaque accumulation (Figures 6.152, 6.153).

For dogs and cats with periodontal disease, chlorhexidine is an effective product to inhibit plaque formation. Chlorhexidine has bactericidal and virocidal

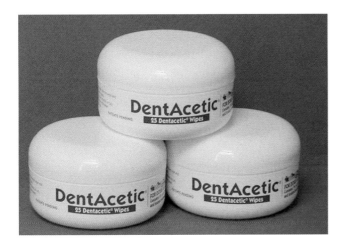

FIGURE 6.152. DenAcetic Wipes.

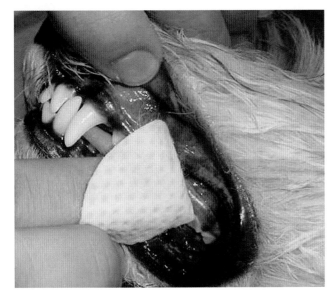

FIGURE 6.153. Dental wipes to remove plaque from the maxillary fourth premolar.

effects against most oral bacteria and some viruses. Chlorhexidine binds to the dental pellicle for 24 hours after application, reducing plaque-forming bacteria. Additionally, chlorhexidine renders existing plaque less pathogenic.

Potential disadvantages using chlorhexidine include staining of the pellicle, unpleasant taste, and desensitized taste buds. Additionally, chlorhexidine can enhance the precipitation of salivary minerals to speed the development of calculus.

Human dental patients are advised to use chlorhexidine as a rinse swished in the oral cavity for approximately 2 minutes. The contact time of application is important for chlorhexidine to bind to the tooth and gingival sulcus. In animals, 2-minute oral rinsing is not practical. Oral contact time in animals is facilitated through incorporation in a gel or chew.

For animals, chlorhexidine is available as:

- *C.E.T. Oral Hygiene Rinse* (Virbac Products) is composed of chlorhexidine gluconate 0.12% plus zinc gluconate to promote healing of ulcerated tissue. The rinse also includes Cetylpyridinium chloride to decrease malodor.
- *C.E.T. 0.12% Chlorhexidine Rinse* (Virbac Products) is used in the clinic as an oral irrigant before dental procedures.
- *C.E.T. Oral Hygiene Gel* (Virbac Products) is composed of chlorhexidine gluconate plus 0.12% zinc gluconate. The gel allows greater binding time with a pleasant taste.
- *Nolvadent* (Fort Dodge Laboratories) is composed of chlorhexidine diacetate 0.1% (Figure 6.154), chlorhexidine solution (Burns 606-3620, Schein 309-3732).
- *C.E.T. HEXtra* Chews are chlorhexidine-impregnated rawhide chews (Figure 6.155).

Chlorhexidine should not be used with fluoride products at the same time. The binding of both products may inactivate each other. A 30-minute to 1-hour wait between use of a dentifrice containing fluoride, and a chlorhexidine rinse or gel is recommended.

Zinc ions disrupt bacterial enzyme systems by displacing magnesium ions. Zinc reduces halitosis by inhibiting the production and release of volatile sulfur compounds. Zinc ascorbate stimulates collagen production to help repair diseased tissue.

Zinc also enhances the antiplaque activity of chlorhexidine. Zinc and chlorhexidine are combined in C.E.T. oral hygiene rinse and C.E.T. oral hygiene gel (Virbac Products).

Zinc and vitamin C are combined in MAXI/GUARD Oral Cleansing Gel (Addison Biological Laboratories).

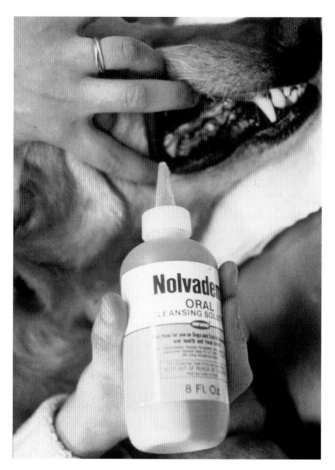

FIGURE 6.154. Nolvadent.

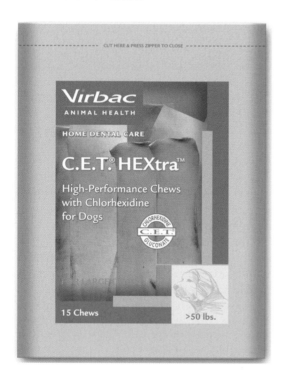

FIGURE 6.155. C.E.T. HEXtra Chews.

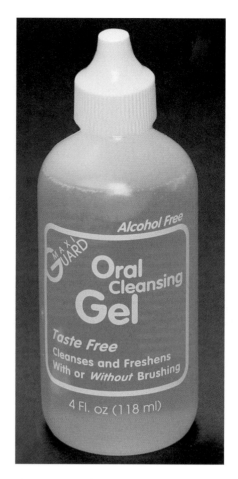

FIGURE 6.156. MAXI/GUARD Gel.

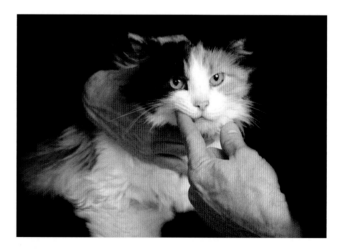

FIGURE 6.157. Application of MAXI/GUARD Gel to a cat's gingiva.

MAXI/GUARD should be mixed (vitamin C added) before it is dispensed to the client. This ensures proper combination and gives the veterinarian or technician an opportunity to discuss application, shelf life, and the product's unique color change feature. The mixture has a shelf life of 6 months in a cool, dark cabinet, or 1 year in the refrigerator. The product is still effective as long as the color remains blue or green. A brown or yellow color indicates the product should be replaced. MAXI/GUARD is also positioned for use in animals that will not tolerate tooth brushing and has been shown to decrease plaque and gingivitis compared to controls (Figures 6.156, 6.157).

Fluoride decreases plaque, desensitizes dentin, and strengthens enamel. Fluoride binds to enamel and dentin (not soft tissues). Fluoride should not be used in conjunction with chlorhexidine preparations. In patients with stages 3 and 4 periodontal disease, 0.4% stannous flouride strength can be used daily. Fluoride preparations include Omni Gel (Dunhill Pharmaceuticals), Gel-Kam (Colgate Oral Pharmaceuticals), and Qygel 0.4% Gel (Veterinary Product Labs).

FluraFom (Virbac Products) contains 1.23% acidulated phosphate fluoride. The foam is supplied for in-clinic application after teeth cleaning. Fluoride foam should not be used as part of a home care program because of the danger of ingestion toxicity. Fluoride

should not be directly placed into a periodontal pocket. Fluoride may delay healing and gingival reattachment (Figure 6.158).

OraVet (Merial) is a waxy polymer applied on teeth after the oral hygiene procedure. The product provides an inert, invisible barrier that, according to the manufacturer, decreases bacteria adhering to the teeth. In theory, the polymer remains on the tooth for up to 8 days following application-repelling plaque. After the 8 days, the client is instructed to apply a thinner polymer weekly. OraVet does not adhere to fluoride-treated teeth. The use of non-fluoride prophy polish and toothpaste are recommended in conjunction with OraVet.

Chew Toys, Dental Devices, and Dental Diets

The main benefit of dental devices and toys is chewing stimulation. Chewing removes some of the plaque and provides exercise to the periodontal ligament. Food and toy manufacturers have tried to create products to replace the need for tooth brushing. Some dental chew devices and foods are effective in decreasing plaque and gingivitis. All chew toys and devices must be monitored. Any pet can abuse a dental device. If the product is too soft, an aggressive dog can break it apart and swallow pieces. If the product is too hard, tooth fractures may occur (Figure 6.159).

The following are potentially dangerous chew products:

- Cow hooves
- Nylon bones
- Ice cubes
- Hard plastic toys

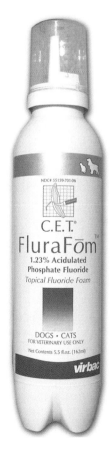

FIGURE 6.158. C.E.T. FluraFom.

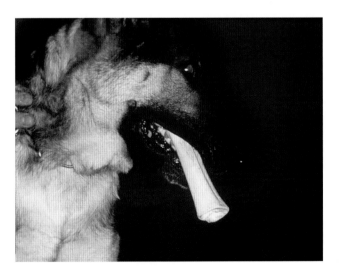

FIGURE 6.159. Dog chewing on bone.

- Tennis balls (chronic chewing will cause attrition and may cause pulpal exposure through enamel and dentin loss)
- Any object that is harder than the tooth
- Knotted rawhide chews (can cause intestinal obstruction)
- Bones

The following are some of the products currently available:

- *Rawhide strips,* which are helpful in controlling plaque—especially when combined with tooth brushing. Rawhide chews are generally safely chewed and digestible if swallowed. Unfortunately, some dogs are "gulpers" who swallow the rawhide

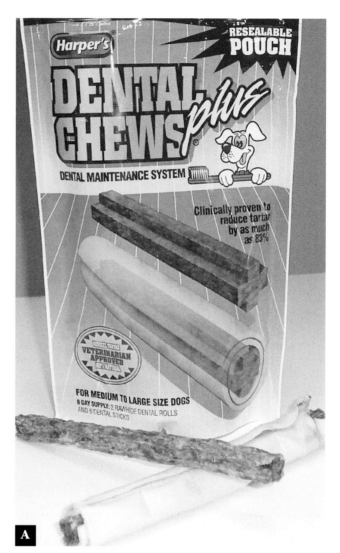

A

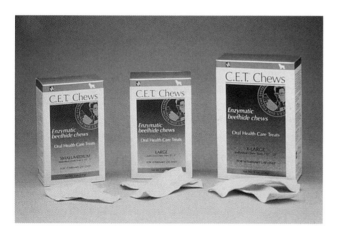

FIGURE 6.160. C.E.T. Chews for dogs.

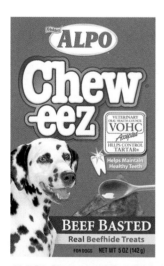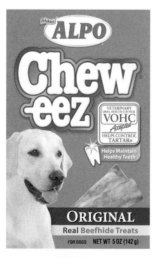

ALPO® Chew-eez® Beefhide Treats are VOHC® accepted as a product that helps control the buildup of calculus

FIGURE 6.161. Chew-eez.

without chewing, potentially causing gastrointestinal problems. Examples include *C.E.T. Chews for dogs* (Figure 6.160) and *C.E.T. Hextra* (fortified with chlorhexadine) (Virbac Products), *Chew-eez Beefhide Treats* (Friskies Petcare) (Figure 6.161), *H.M.P. Rawhide Dental Maintenance System* (Harpers Leather Goods, Inc.) (Figures 6.162A–6.162C). Each H.M.P System box contains a 15-day supply of chews—12 Dental Strips (flat, dark brown strips) and 3 Dental Rolls (Dental Strips wrapped in rawhide). The manufacturer recommends a 5-day cycle: on days 1–4, the dog is given a Dental Strip; on day 5, the dog is given a Dental Roll.

- *Kong Toys,* also sold under the *Tuffy* label, help satisfy a dog's need for exciting object play. The toy bounces in an unpredictable fashion, simulating fleeing prey. As the dog chews the Kong, teeth impinge on the resilient rubber. Kongs come in three chewer-friendly hardness styles: red, black, and blue. *Kong Blue* toys are autoclavable, radiopaque, and avail-

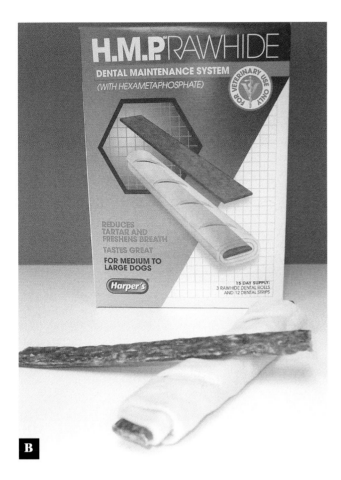

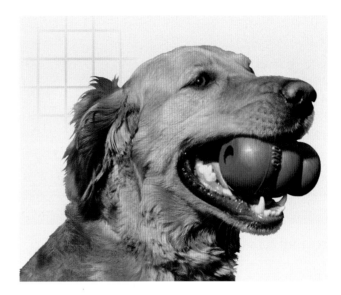

FIGURE 6.163. Kong Blue toys.

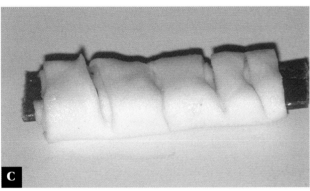

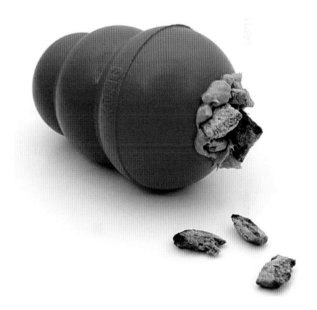

FIGURE 6.164. Dental Kongs stuffed with treats.

FIGURE 6.162. HMP rawhide dental products: (A) Dental Chews *plus* with plus core, (B) HMP Rawhide with HMP strips, and (C) HMP strip combined with rawhide rolls (Harpers).

able only through veterinarians. Kong Blue's rubber has 20% greater tensile strength than the black toys (Schein: King 259-6683, Kitty 259-1891, Original 259-9086, Ultra 259-1789) (Kong Company) (Figure 6.163, 6.164).

- *Dental Kongs* contain "chew-clean" grooves where toothpaste may be applied. The small and medium

sizes have floss rope attached. According to the manufacturer, the rope helps clean the back teeth. Caution should be observed, because the ropes might lacerate gingiva.

- *Pedigree RASK/DENTABONE* (Waltham) is an oral hygiene chew made from rice and milk protein. When fed as a daily supplement, according to the manufacturer, RASK/DENTABONE reduced gingivitis, calculus, and malodor (Figure 6.165).
- *Dental Chew* (Nylabone Products) is made from a plastic material softer than nylon. Dental Chew is positioned for nonaggressive chewers. Fortunately, if

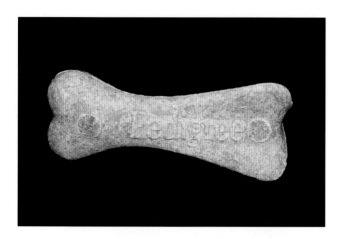

FIGURE 6.165. RASK/DENTABONE (Waltham).

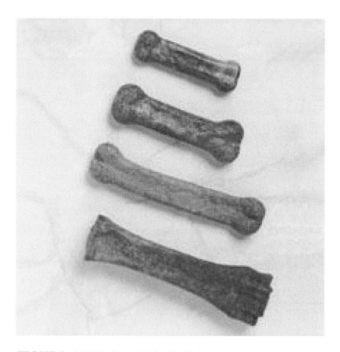

FIGURE 6.166. Roar-Hide (Nylabone).

- *Rhino* (Nylabone Products) is a rubber dog dental device with special dental "pyramids to maximize chewing enjoyment while cleaning the teeth and exercising the jaws," according to the manufacturer.
- *C.E.T. Chews for cats* are made from freeze-dried fish, treated with an antibacterial enzyme system to provide abrasive cleansing action. According to the manufacturer, the coarse texture of the processed fish cleans teeth by helping remove plaque and food debris (Figure 6.167).

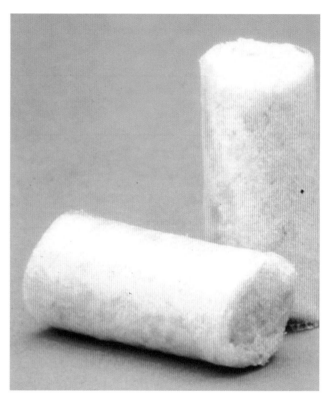

FIGURE 6.167. C.E.T. cat chews.

swallowed, Dental Chews are detectable radiographically.
- *Roar-Hide* (Nylabone Products) is designed to avoid problems sometimes associated with large rawhide chews. The rawhide in Roar-Hide is ground into small digestible rice-sized pieces, heated, and then injected into a mold (Figure 6.166).
- Nylon chewing devices (*Dental Dinosaur, Hercules, Galileo,* and *Plaque Attacker*) (Nylabone Products) have "dental tips," which the company claims aid teeth cleaning and gum massage.
- *Gumabone* (Nylabone Products) is more pliable than the nylon bones.

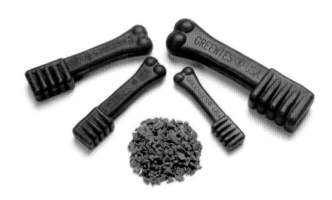

FIGURE 6.168. Greenies.

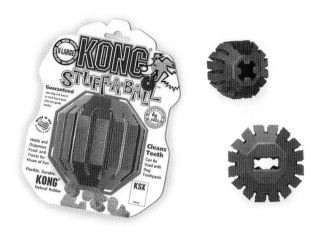

FIGURE 6.169. Kong Stuff-A-Ball dental device.

- *Greenies* are digestible chews, which when fed daily, according to the manufacturer, decrease calculus accumulation (Figure 6.168).
- *Kong Stuff-A-Ball* is a nontoxic natural rubber fetch toy marketed to hold toothpaste and clean teeth above and below the gum line. Kong Stuff-A-Ball is sold in three sizes and two hardnesses (Figure 6.169).

Diets/Treats

Dry foods decrease plaque while the pet is chewing. "Dental" diets claim to control plaque and gingivitis by chemical and/or mechanical methods. *Feeding a specialized calculus-control diet does not take the place of daily tooth brushing.* Dental diets are not treats; they are a complete food and should be fed as the pet's only food, rather than as an occasional treat. For clients that feed specialized dental diets and brush their pet's teeth, the interval between professional teeth cleaning visits is usually months longer than with clients that do not feed a dental diet.

The following dental diets are available:

- *Canine and Feline t/d* (Hills Pet Nutrition) is a kibble formulation with transverse fibers that "squeegee" plaque and calculus from the tooth surface. The unique fiber structure resists crumbling as the tooth penetrates. When fed as a sole diet, t/d decreases supragingival plaque better than regular kibble. Canine and Feline t/d has been approved by the VOHC to help control plaque and calculus (Figure 6.170–6.174).
- *Science Diet Oral Care* is positioned for pets that have healthy mouths and has been VOHC-approved to help control plaque and tartar.

- *Tartar Check* (Heinz Pet Products) is a snack biscuit containing sodium hexametaphosphate (HMP) to help control calculus. Sodium hexametaphosphate sequesters calcium, forming soluble complexes that diffuse into the saliva and are subsequently swallowed. The hexametaphosphate and pyrophosphate

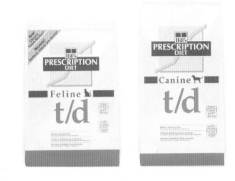

FIGURE 6.170. Canine and feline t/d.

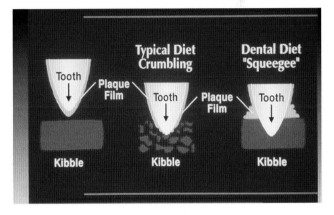

FIGURE 6.171. Diet mechanical placque removal.

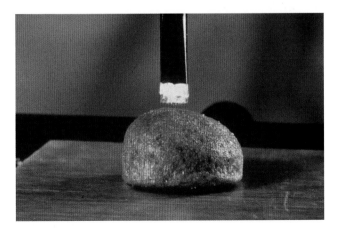

FIGURE 6.172. Screwdriver coated with paint before insertion into t/d food.

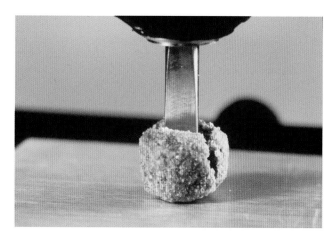

FIGURE 6.173. Food stays intact during insertion.

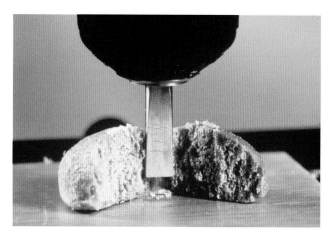

FIGURE 6.174. Paint removed from tip.

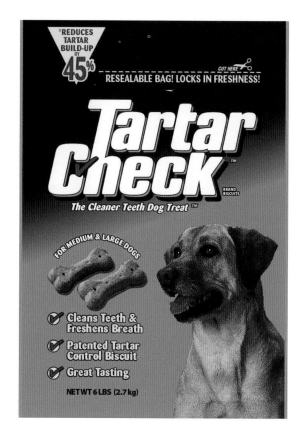

FIGURE 6.175. Tartar Check.

act as calcium chelators, binding calcium and decreasing mineralization of plaque into calculus. Tartar Check has been approved by the VOHC to help control tartar (Figure 6.175).

- *Friskies Dental Diet* for cats has larger kibbles and a unique texture that has been approved by the VOHC to help control plaque and tartar.
- *Eukanuba Dental Defense* incorporates sodium hexametaphosphate on the outside of the kibble in the canine diet and pyrophosphates in the feline diet. In addition to the chemical binding to the substances in plaque for easier elimination, these additives also make the kibble tougher to puncture, providing mechanical cleansing action. The Iams Chunk Dental Defense Diet for Dogs and the Eukanuba Adult Maintenance Diet for Dogs have been approved by the VOHC to help control tartar. (Figure 6.176).

Table 6.3 summarizes periodontal care.

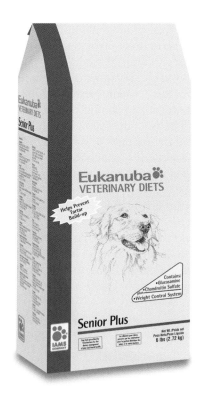

FIGURE 6.176. Eukanuba dental defense diet.

Table 6.3. Periodontal care at a glance.

Pathology	Present	Treatment
Stage 1 gingivitis	Minimal calculus and inflammation progressing to gingival edema	Teeth cleaning, subgingival hand instrumentation, polishing, irrigation, home care.
Stage 2 early periodontitis	Bleeding on probing, less than 25% attachment (support) loss	As above plus root planing, closed curettage (if indicated), instillation of Doxirobe into cleaned pockets.
Stage 3 established periodontitis	As above, plus andattachment loss between 25%–50%, Class I and early II furcations; M1 mobility may be observed in single-rooted teeth	Case-by-case and tooth-by tooth determination similar to stage 4 disease based on the tooth's importance, client's ability to provide home care, mobility, and absolute pocket depth. Stringent home care.
Stage 4 advanced periodontitis	As above, plus possible tooth mobility and/or attachment loss >50%	As above plus flap surgery and or extraction.
	Pockets >5 mm with suprabony ledges, infrabony (1- or 2-walled)	Apical reposition flap and osteoplasty replacing the flap margins at the new height of bone.
	3-walled infrabony pockets	Flap exposure and placement of bone graft materials.
	Class III furcation exposure	Extraction if support loss is >50%.

7
Endodontic Equipment, Materials, and Techniques

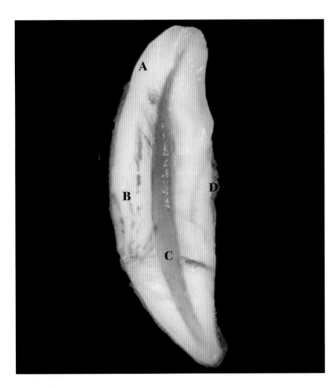

FIGURE 7.1. Anatomy of a canine tooth and surronding tissues: A = *enamel* B = *dentin*, C = *pulp*, D = *cementum*.

Endodontics is the dental discipline that deals with disease, diagnosis, and treatment of the pulp and associated structures. The steps outlined in this chapter indicate the author's current techniques, which are constantly evolving based on new materials, instruments, and research. Other equally valid technique variations are currently in use.

ANATOMY AND PHYSIOLOGY

The *dental pulp* consists of richly vascularized and high-

ly innervated connective tissue. When traumatized, the pulp reacts to irritants through inflammation. If untreated, inflammation spreads up and/or down the pulp, eventually becoming irreversible. Toxic products from damaged tissue and microorganisms in the tissue sustain inflammation (Figures 7.1, 7.2, 7.3).

The *pulp cavity* consists of a *pulp chamber* located in the crown and *root canal* in the root. An *apical delta* containing minute openings is present at the root apex.

Soft tissues in the pulp cavity include blood vessels, sensory nerves, connective tissue, and undifferentiated cells. Odontoblasts, which form dentin throughout the tooth's life, line the pulp cavity wall. Before eruption, the odontoblasts produce *primary* dentin. Once the root formation has neared completion, the odontoblasts produce *secondary* dentin causing the dentinal walls to thicken and decreasing the pulp cavity size. Reparative or *tertiary* dentin is produced in response to thermal, mechanical, occlusal, or chemical trauma to the odontoblasts.

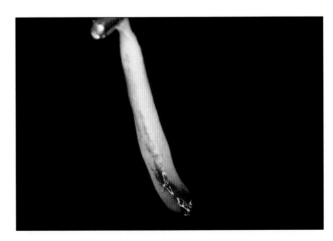

FIGURE 7.2. The pulp removed during conventional root canal therapy in an acutely fractured tooth.

z

175

Glossary

Access site is an entry into the tooth for root canal therapy.

Anachoresis is the hematogenous exposure to bacteria.

Apex is a terminal tip or end of a root.

Apexification is the process of apical closure of the root by hard tissue deposition in a non-vital tooth by the action of cementoblasts and odontoblasts.

Apexogenesis is the normal development of the apex of a tooth root.

Apical delta are multiple foramina at the tooth's apex where the blood vessels and nerves pass through the apex typified by canine and feline teeth.

Apical foramen is a single opening in the apex typical of human teeth, through which nerves, blood vessels, and lymphatics pass.

Apicoectomy is the surgical removal of the apex of the tooth.

Barbed broach is an instrument with numerous protruding barbs from a metal shaft used to engage the dental pulp for extirpation.

Complicated fracture involves pulp in the fracture line.

Conventional (standard) endodontics is standard root canal therapy with access through the crown.

Coronal pulp is located in the crown portion of the pulp cavity.

Crown-root fracture involves enamel, dentin, and cementum in the fracture line.

Direct pulp capping is application of a pulp dressing directly to the exposed pulp.

Gates Glidden drills are endodontic instruments used to widen the coronal access.

Gutta percha is a rubber-like material used to fill prepared root canals.

Hedstrom file is an endodontic instrument used to remove dentin from the sides of the pulp cavity.

Lentulo spiral fillers are wire instruments used in a low-speed handpiece to mechanically move paste-filling materials into the root canals.

Obturation is part of endodontic treatment wherein the root canal is filled.

Periapical is the area that surrounds the root tip (apex).

Periradicular is the area that surrounds the root.

Pulp is the tissue made up of blood vessels, nerves, cellular elements, odontoblasts, lymphatic vessels, and connective tissue.

Pulp (root) canal is the part of the pulp cavity within the root.

Pulp cavity is the space in a tooth bounded by the dentin, consisting of the pulp chamber and root canal.

Pulp chamber is the part of the pulp cavity within the coronal portion of the tooth.

Pulpectomy is the complete removal of the pulp from the pulp chamber and root canal (pulp cavity).

Pulpitis is the inflammation of the pulpal tissue.

Root canal is that portion of the pulp cavity within the root.

Root canal therapy (standard root canal therapy, conventional root canal therapy) is the process of removing the pulp of a tooth and filling it with an inert material.

Step back technique is a debridement procedure, which uses smaller files at the apex progressing up the canal with larger files.

Step up technique (crown down method) starts at the coronal portion of the root canal with larger files progressing toward the apex with smaller instruments.

Stops are small, round, pieces of rubber or plastic that are placed on endodontic instruments to mark the working length.

Surgical endodontics is the removal of the root apex (apicoectomy) to enable placement of a retrograde filling. Surgical endodontics is performed when conventional root canal therapy cannot provide an adequate apical seal.

Tertiary dentin also called reparative dentin forms in response to irritation of the pulp through chronic crown trauma.

Vital pulpotomy (partial vital pulpectomy) is the surgical removal of a portion of the dental pulp.

Working length (distance) is the distance between the access opening to the apical extent of the root canal, which is typically 1–3 mm coronal to the root apex.

Dentin is porous. Each square millimeter contains between 30,000 and 40,000 dentinal tubules that communicate between the pulp and dentin-enamel (DEJ) or dentin-cementum (DCJ) junctions. If there is near pulp exposure from deep carious lesions, fractures, abrasion, or attrition, bacteria can travel through the exposed dentin tubules to the pulp. Bacteria also can invade the pulp through the bloodstream (anachoresis). Near pulp exposure will also transmit painful stimuli (heat, cold, pressure) from the oral environment to the pulp.

All teeth are susceptible to fracture. In the mature dog, the maxillary canines and maxillary fourth premolars are most commonly fractured, followed by the mandibular canines and incisors. In the cat, the maxillary and mandibular canines are most commonly fractured followed by the incisors.

Companion animals fracture their teeth by forceful contact with substances harder than the natural tooth:

- Cage doors
- Airplane crates
- Chain-link fences

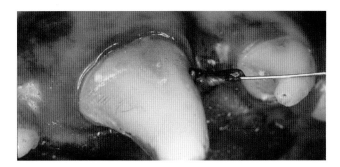

FIGURE 7.3. A necrotic pulp removed from a tooth with chronic pulpal exposure.

- Hard chew toys or dental devices
- Ice cubes
- Bones
- Cow hooves
- Auto accidents
- Steel reinforced training devices
- Dog fights

MATERIALS USED FOR ENDODONTIC CARE OF FRACTURED TEETH

Paper (absorbent) points are rolled sterile papers used to absorb irrigation solutions in the prepared canal. Paper points are long, narrow, and tapered to fit into the root canal. Like gutta percha, paper points are available in multiple sizes and lengths (55 mm fine: Schein 100-2683, medium: 100-8242, coarse: 100-9339; 25 mm #15–40: Schein 100-0672, #45–80: 100-2142, #90–140 100-1776; 60 mm #15–25: Burns 721-7240, #30–40: 271-7241, #45–55: 271-7242, #60–80: 271-4243) (Figure 7.4).

Gutta Percha is a combination of zinc oxide (66%), gutta percha rubber (23%), and radiopaque barium sulfate (11%). Gutta percha is used as a core-filling material in endodontics. Gutta percha advantages include being an inert material, radiopaque, nonirritating, and removable for re-treatment if root canal therapy fails. Gutta percha points are slender, tapered, and pointed, to fit contours of the root canal. The various widths and lengths correspond to file sizes (60 mm #15–20 Burns 271-7215, #30–40 Burns 271-7216, #45–55 Burns 721-7217, #60–80 Burns 721-7218, #15–40 assorted Schein 100-8393) (Figure 7.5).

Zinc oxide-eugenol (ZOE) is a sealer cement used to seal the apex and act as caulking between the canal wall and solid gutta percha (Burns 952-3250, 951-2081;

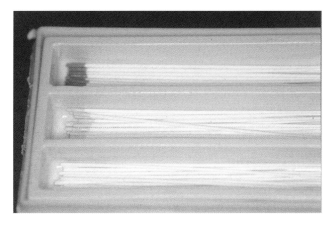

FIGURE 7.4. 55 mm fine, medium, and coarse paper points.

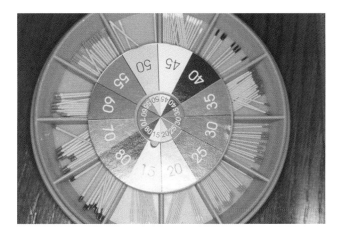

FIGURE 7.5. Various widths of gutta percha in a tray.

Schein 100-4540, 100-1757) (Figure 7.6). Apical sealer cement is also available without eugenol:

- AH 26: Dentsply International Inc. (Burns 804-1050, Schein 117-8362) (Figure 7.7)
- ThermaSeal Plus (Figure 7.8)
- Sealapex-Kerr (Schein 123-2799) (Figure 7.9)
- Kerr Pulpsealer
- Ketac Endo

Calcium hydroxide cement (base) has many uses for endodontic care. Calcium hydroxide offers the following features:

- Acts as an insulating material compatible with composite restoratives
- Can be sandwiched under a restoration between the bonding material and gutta percha

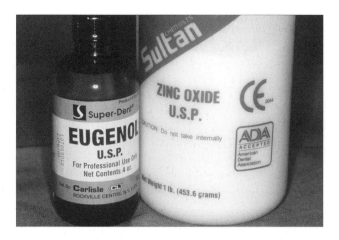

FIGURE 7.6. Zinc-oxide/eugenol sealer cement.

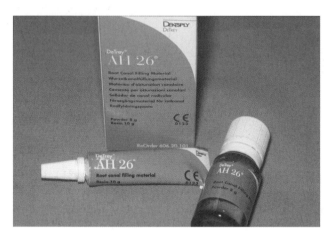

FIGURE 7.7. AH 26 sealer cement.

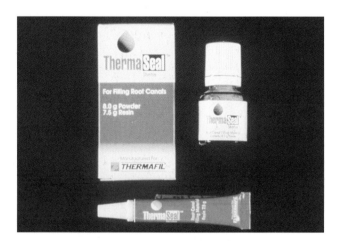

FIGURE 7.8. ThermaSeal Plus.

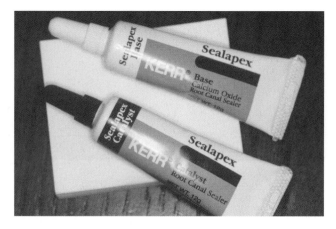

FIGURE 7.9. Sealapex.

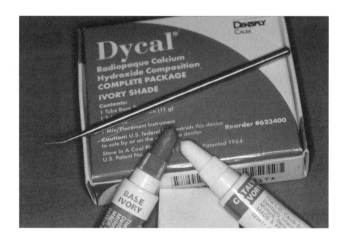

FIGURE 7.10. Dycal calcium hydroxide paste.

- Can be used during the apexification process to stimulate hard tissue closure, and on top of the pulp to help create a dentinal bridge by irritating the pulp-triggering formation of tertiary dentin.

The powder should be stored in a leakproof bottle. Calcium hydroxide has a limited shelf life, reacting with carbon dioxide in the air. The surface layer of powder should be discarded before each use.

Calcium hydroxide is supplied as the following:

- *Self-cured paste* where a base and liquid catalyst are mixed for approximately ten seconds on a paper pad. Mixing is complete after a uniform color is obtained. The calcium hydroxide is delivered to the tooth with a moistened paper point or ball-pointed instrument (Figures 7.10,7.11). Calcium hydroxide paste also comes premixed in a syringe. The syringed paste is introduced into the tooth by placing pressure on a plunger or by turning a screw-type device

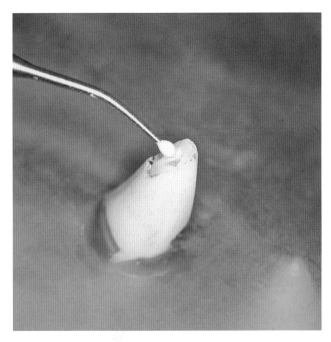

FIGURE 7.11. Application of calcium hydroxide paste with ball applicator.

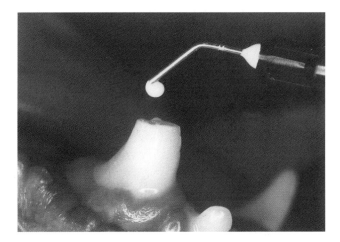

FIGURE 7.12. CaOH paste applied on vital pulp through a blunt needle.

(Hypocal: Burns 834-0850, Schein 100-0036). As the material is introduced into the canal, the needle tip is slowly withdrawn. Unfortunately, this method of placement may lead to incomplete filling or trapping of bubbles within the pulp (Dycal: Burns 813-1200).

- *Light cured flowable paste* (Ultrablend Plus: Ultradent Products, Inc. (Figure 7.12).
- *Powder* packaged in plastic containers available in 11.5 gm, 500 gm, and 2.5 kg units (Burns 834-0850). The powder is scooped onto a glass slab (Schein 100-4432) and packed into a retrograde amalgam carrier (Burns 950-0910, Schein 100-1293) for delivery (Union Broach: Burns 953-4225, Schein 317-1676) (Figures 7.13–7.15).
- *Points* or rigid sticks of calcium hydroxide used for insertion into prepared pulp chambers.

Sodium hypochlorite (common household bleach) acts as a solvent for necrotic tissue, a lubricant, and disinfectant for irrigation of the root canal. Sodium hypochlorite may be diluted with one to two parts distilled water or as it comes from the bottle (Figure 7.16).

To apply sodium hypochlorite, a sterile 2–5 cc disposable plastic syringe with a blunt 20–23 gauge endodontic needle is used. The needle may be bent at an angle to facilitate access to the canal. Damage to the periapical structures and severe pain may occur if sodium hypochlorite solution leaks out of the apex.

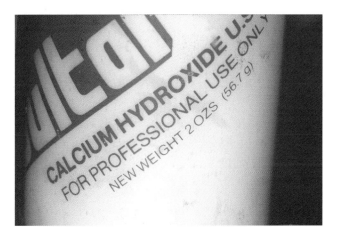

FIGURE 7.13. Calcium hydroxide powder container.

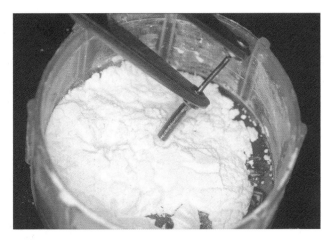

FIGURE 7.14. Calcium hydroxide powder placed in a sterile syringe cap for loading into a retrograde carrier.

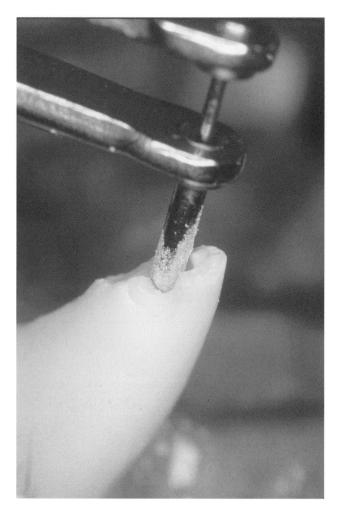

FIGURE 7.15. Calcium hydroxide powder placed on top of vital pulp tissue.

Ethylenediaminetetracetic acid (EDTA) is available in both liquid and gel forms. EDTA is a file lubricant, a dentin softening agent, and an effervescent that helps lift debris from the canal. Liquid EDTA is delivered via syringe (LightSpeed), GlyGel, Gel EDTA (RC-Prep; Premier Dental Products Co.: Burns 878-1820, Schein 378-4499) (Figures 7.17, 7.18).

Mineral tri-oxide aggregate (MTA) is composed of calcium and silicate compounds. It is supplied as a powder which, when hydrated, sets in 2–4 hours. When set, MTA is biologically compatible with adjacent tissues. MTA is gaining wide acceptance in small animal dentistry for use in vital pulp therapy (direct pulp capping), surgical endodontics, root perforations, and one-step apexification procedures (Pro-Root Tulsa Dental).

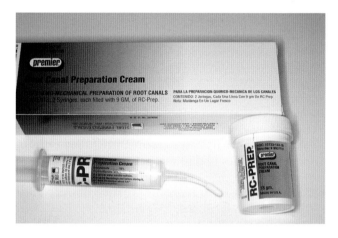

FIGURE 7.17. RC-Prep.

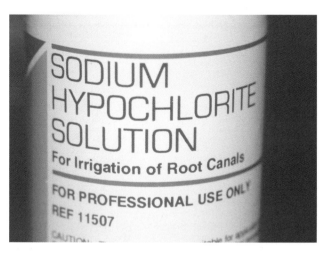

FIGURE 7.16. Sodium hypochlorite used as a solvent, lubricant, and disinfectant.

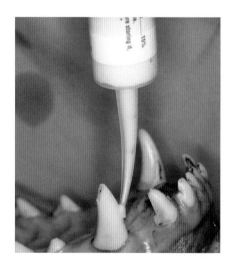

FIGURE 7.18. RC-Prep application during the debriding process.

INSTRUMENTS USED TO ENDODONTICALLY CARE FOR FRACTURED TEETH

The goal of conventional endodontics is to remove toxins, microbes, and necrotic debris by thoroughly debriding the pulp cavity and then sealing the space to prevent further infection. Burs, files, broaches, spreaders, and pluggers are used to accomplish this goal. It is essential that endodontic instruments and accessories are sterile before placement into the canal. A sterilized endodontic pack can be prepared with the necessary instruments.

Barbed broaches are short-handled, hand-operated instruments with barbs along the shaft, used for removal of the entire pulp or pulpal fragments in the root canal. Barbed broaches are available in lengths up to 47 mm and sizes fine to coarse. Broaches are also used to remove paper points or separated (broken) lodged endodontic files. They are not used to shape or enlarge the canals and may bind or fracture if the operator uses too large a broach in the canal (Burns 47 mm assorted 264-9480, Schein 47 mm assorted 100-6351) (Figures 7.19–7.21).

Endodontic files are used to enlarge, debride, shape, and smooth the root canal to clean the canal and prepare for obturation (Figure 7.22).

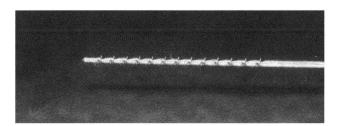

FIGURE 7.19. Barbed broach fine hooks used to grab the pulp for removal.

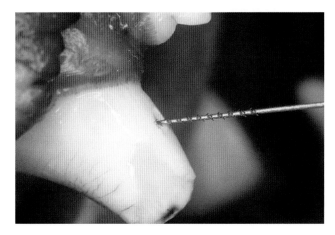

FIGURE 7.20. Barbed broach inserted into access.

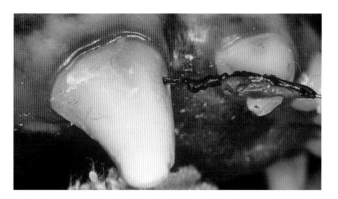

FIGURE 7.21. Removal of necrotic pulp during the debriding process.

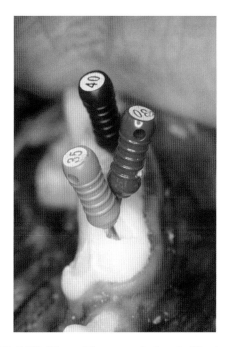

FIGURE 7.22. Three 21 mm endodontic files inserted into a maxillary fourth premolar's root canals.

Kerr (K) files cut or shave the canal on insertion and withdrawal. K files are used in a push-in/pull-out fashion, or with a 1/4 turn after the file is extended to its apical base before withdrawal. K files are stronger and more flexible than Hedstrom files and less prone to breakage. File length chosen depends on the root canal length from tooth access to apex. Files can be purchased in groups of five in one size or assorted sizes.

K files are available in the following lenths:

• 21 mm length (Burns #30 951-2599, #35 951-2601, #40 951-2603; Schein #30 100-9072, #35 100-9254, #40 100-9336)

- 31 mm length (Schein #30 222-1719, #35 222-1978, #40 222-6617)
- 60 mm length (Schein #15–80 264-9478) (Burns 21 mm K #15–40: 951-2617, 21 mm K #45–80 951-2619, 31 mm K #15–40 951-2765, 31 mm K #45–80 951-2767) (Figure 7.23).

Hedstrom (H) files are sharper than K files. Hedstrom files cut on the up (pull) stroke, and K files cut on both clockwise and counterclockwise rotations and on insertion and withdrawal. To prevent a corkscrew apical penetration, Hedstrom files should not be rotated. Hedstrom files cut efficiently and quickly, and they are used when significant removal of dentin is desired. such as flairing the access in the coronal third of the tooth. H files are not intended for use in the apical third. H files commonly used in veterinary medicine include the following:

- 40 mm length (Schein #15–40 widths: 100-8146, #45–80 widths: 100-9141, #90–110 widths: 100-9291)
- 60 mm length (Schein #15–40: 100-7643, #45–80: 100-8303, #90–100: 100-8583; Burns: 60 mm H files #15–80 widths: 264-9458)
- 120 mm long H files (Burns #20–80 widths 264-9466) (Figures 7.24,7.25)

Nickel titanium (NiTi) files have become the preferred file of choice of many human and veterinary dentists. These instruments are used by hand or in a powered handpiece turning 360° at speeds ranging from 150–2000 rpm. NiTi files, available in Hedstrom or Kerr varieties, are more flexible than files made from stainless steel. The LightSpeed file (LightSpeed Technology #20–140 widths in 21, 25, 31, and 50 mm

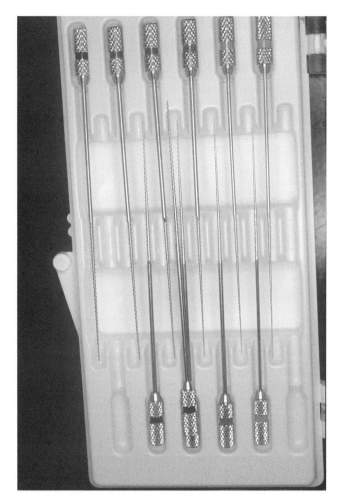

FIGURE 7.25. Package of 60 mm Hedstrom files.

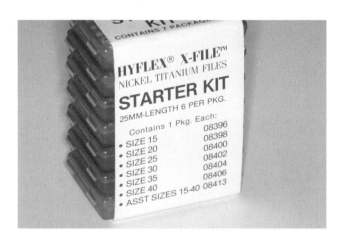

FIGURE 7.26. Packages of Nickel Titanium (NiTi) files.

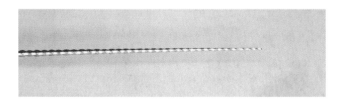

FIGURE 7.23. Kerr (K) file working end.

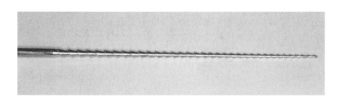

FIGURE 7.24. Hedstrom file working end.

lengths) is designed with the largest part of the instrument at the tip. This file is especially useful for cleaning the apical part of the root canal (Figure 7.26).

File Measurement

WIDTH   The International Standards Organization (ISO) sets standardization from one manufacturer to another regarding lengths and widths of flutes, tapers, relationship between successive sizes, and coloration (Figures 7.27, 7.28). Most files are purchased with color-coded handles, which correlate with various widths. ISO width sizes are numbered 6–140 (0.06–1.4 mm at the tip). File handle color correlates to the diameter at the working end (e.g., all #10 file handles are purple, #15 are white, #20 are yellow, and so on, as noted in Table 7.1).

The most commonly used file sizes for teeth other than large dog canines are the 8–80 widths in 21–25 mm lengths.

Table 7.1. Color-coded file sizes.

Color	File Size
Pink	06
Grey	08
Purple	10
White	15,45,90
Yellow	20,50,100
Red	25,55,110
Blue	30,60,120
Green	35,70,130
Black	40,80,140

Handle colors by convention of the International Standards Organization (ISO) are:

- Standard ISO file widths typically increase in 0.05 mm increments (15, 20, 25, etc).
- LightSpeed instruments are available in .025 mm increments (20, 22.5, 25, 27.5, etc.).
- ProFile Series 29 files (Dentsply Professional) are manufactured with a width change of 29% between successive files. ProFile files do not conform to the standard ISO handle colors (Figure 7.29).

LENGTHS   Files are also measured by *lengths*: Human dental files are sized 21, 25, and 30 mm, sufficient for working on small animal incisors, premolars, and molars. The endodontic system in large dog canine

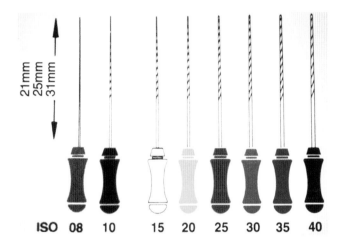

FIGURE 7.27. Color-coded file handles, sizes 8–40.

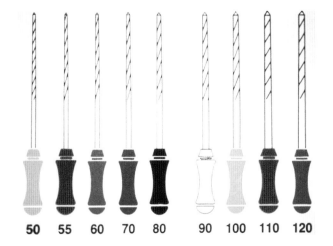

FIGURE 7.28. Color-coded file handles, larger sizes.

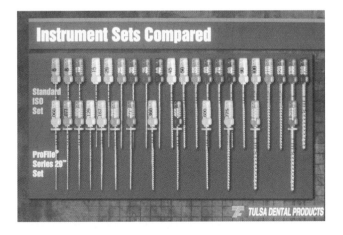

FIGURE 7.29. Comparison of ProFile Series 29 files with standard file widths.

teeth are longer than 31 mm and require 45 mm, 50 mm, or 60 mm files to reach the apex (refer to Figure 7.25).

With repeated use, endodontic files become dull, fatigue, and eventually separate (break). Should the instrument separate within the root canal, retrieval is attempted. In some cases, apical surgery or extraction of the tooth becomes necessary. As instruments are prepared for sterilization, they should be individually checked for signs of wear, weakness, or fracture. Some practitioners color-code the files with endodontic stops relating to the number of times each file is used. The safest practice is to use new files with each patient. To mitigate the expense of using fresh files for each case, a sterile endodontic surgical pack fee can be charged to the client for each case.

Rotary files are attached to a high-torque, slow-speed handpiece of a 10:1 reduction gear contra-angle to mechanically prepare the canal. Rotary file use is technique-sensitive. The risk of file fracture and/or root perforation is increased if rotary files are not used correctly (Figure 7.30).

Endodontic stops are small, round pieces of rubber or plastic that act as visual references to assist the veterinarian in preparing the canal. The stops are placed toward the file handle with the assistance of a confirming radiograph before root canal therapy is initiated, and readjusted when the file is at the internal apex, as confirmed by a working-length radiograph. All succeeding files are fitted with endodontic stops at the working length (Burns 951-9792, Schein 100-5271) (Figures 7.31, 7.32). Some of the newly designed instruments, such as LightSpeed, have length-measuring rings, eliminating the need to set and reset stops during treatment.

Gates Glidden drills are long-shank, flame-shaped, rotary cutting instruments used on slow-speed contra-angle attachments to enlarge the coronal portion of the root canal, allowing easy access for filing. One to six rings are placed on the shaft, indicating the blade's width size. The drills should be matched to the size of

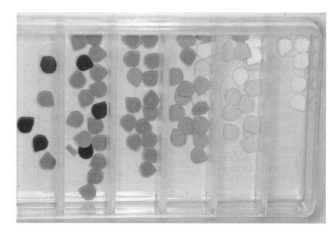

FIGURE 7.31. Endodontic stops.

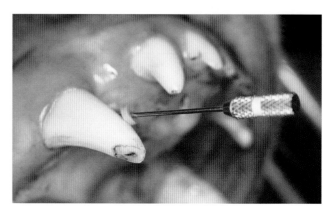

FIGURE 7.32. Endodontic stop attached to a 60 mm Hedstrom file inserted into a dog's maxillary canine pulp cavity.

the endodontic file size desired (#1 = #50 file, #2 = #70 file, #3 = #90 file, #4 = #100 file, #5 = #120 file). The operator should use caution not to take these drills too deeply into the canal, causing ledging or lateral penetration (Burns assorted #1–6: 951-1370, Schein assorted #1–6: 100-9919) (Figures 7.33, 7.34).

Spiral paste fillers, also called *Lentulo spiral fillers*, are used to mechanically carry root canal sealer cement into the prepared root canal before placement of gutta percha. Spiral fillers may be used by hand or at very low speeds in a latch-type 10:1 reduction gear contra-angle. The diameter of the spiral filler used should be slightly smaller than the anticipated gutta percha size. The loaded filler is inserted into the pulp chamber without the spiral filler rotating. After insertion into the canal to its full length, the handpiece is activated. A clockwise pumping motion is used while partially withdrawing the spiral to unload the sealer cement. (40 mm assorted Schein 100-8948; 60 mm assorted Burns 264-9485, Schein 100-4273) (Figure 7.35).

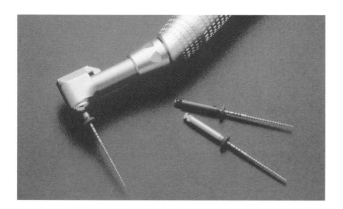

FIGURE 7.30. Tulsa dental rotary file system.

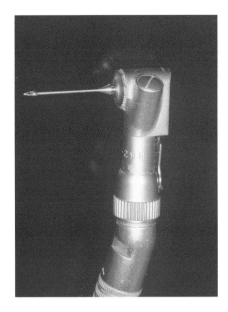

FIGURE 7.33. Gates Glidden drill attached to a 10:1 contra-angle reduction gear.

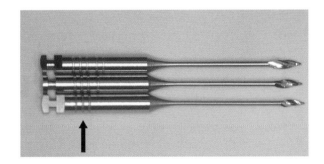

FIGURE 7.34. Gates Glidden drill size ring markings.

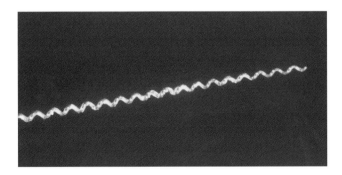

FIGURE 7.35. Lentulo spiral filler.

Spreaders and pluggers are available in multiple diameters and lengths used to compact and adapt gutta percha to the prepared canal. The *spreader* is a hand-operated, smooth-pointed, tapered metal instrument to laterally pack gutta percha into the canal space and

force sealant into dentinal tubules, allowing room for additional gutta percha (Burns 951-8917, Schein 100-0936 #3). The blunt-tipped *plugger* pushes gutta percha toward the apex.

For short teeth (incisors, premolars, and molars), human pluggers and spreaders can be used. For large dog canines, longer Holmstrom (Burns 271-9095, Schein 102-4718, Cislak Holmstrom plugger/spreader kit) plugger and spreader combinations are necessary (Figures 7.36–7.38).

College pliers, also called *cotton pliers* or *endodontic locking pliers*, enable the operator to pick up and hold paper points or gutta percha points in place for

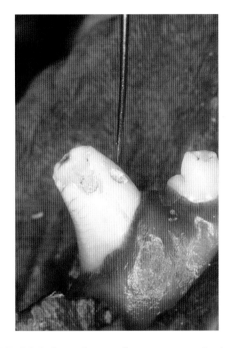

FIGURE 7.36. Spreader to adapt gutta percha into root canal(s).

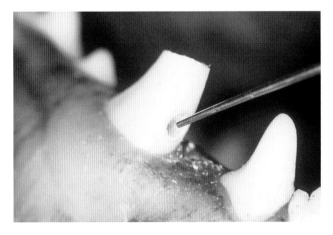

FIGURE 7.37. Blunt-tipped plugger.

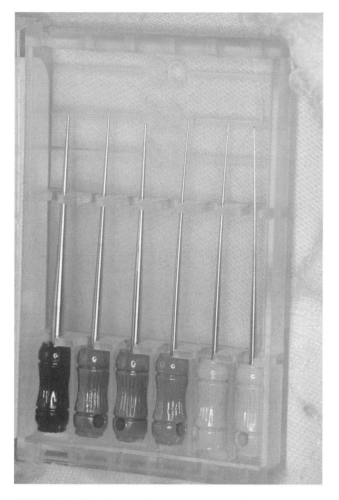

FIGURE 7.38. 21 mm finger spreader pack.

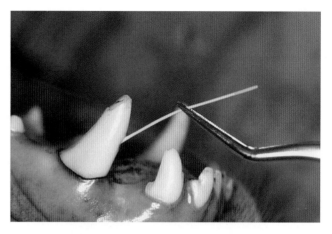

FIGURE 7.39. College pliers to pick up gutta percha and paper points.

FIGURE 7.40. Spatula for mixing sealing cement.

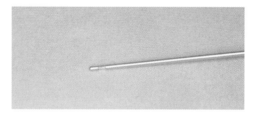

FIGURE 7.41. Endodontic irrigation needle.

insertion into the prepared root canal. College pliers can also be used for holding cotton pledgets for cleaning tooth surfaces. They are available in both locking and nonlocking styles, with plain or serrated tips (Burns 951-8139; Schein 100-3313 nonserrated, 101-1514 self-locking, 101-4026 serrated; Cislak #17 D.P. #4083, #18L Locking #4089) (Figure 7.39).

Spatulas are instruments used to mix dental materials. Cement spatulas are thin and nonflexible (Burns 950-8857, Schein 100-6676) (Figure 7.40).

Irrigation needles and *syringes* are used to flush fluids into the canal and remove dentinal shavings and debris that accumulate during instrumentation. Irrigation needles have a slotted tip or a lateral opening for fluid to exit around the needle and not through the apex, preventing apical damage from overzealous irrigation (23 g x 1 1/4: Burns 950-3610, Schein 194-1410; 27 g x 1 1/4: Burns 950-3612, Schein 194-2242) (Figure 7.41).

PROCEDURES USED TO CARE FOR FRACTURED TEETH

> If the practitioner chooses to do nothing with a tooth affected with pulpal exposure, the exposed pulp will necrose, eventually leading to periapical pathology and patient pain. Extraction or endodontic repair of the fractured tooth are the only sound treatment options. Leaving the tooth untreated to "watch and see what happens" is unjustifiable.

When presented with a fractured tooth with pulpal or near-pulp exposure, the practitioner has two choices:

1. Extract the tooth.

2. Perform endodontic therapy, which allows the tooth to be saved and returned to function. Endodontic therapy is also less invasive than surgical extraction where incision of gingiva, bone, and tooth are involved.

Specific endodontic therapy depends on:

- *Severity of damage to the tooth structure.* The ultimate goal of endodontic care is to preserve the functioning tooth. When pathology renders the tooth nonfunctional, extraction is the treatment of choice.
- *Degree of periapical and periodontal changes.* Tooth support is critical to long-term success of an endodontic treatment. If marked periodontal disease is present before therapy, success may be impossible unless heroic measures are taken and strict home care is provided.
- *Functional significance of the tooth.* Although endodontic care can be performed on any tooth, in the dog, the canines, maxillary fourth premolars, and mandibular first molars are considered the most essential teeth.
- *The owner's expectation and desires.* Before commencing endodontic therapy, the owner must be made aware of the prognosis, aftercare, and fees involved. If the patient is a show dog, the client should be informed that the American Kennel Club does not approve crown restoration of fractured teeth.
- *The clinician's ability to perform endodontics or availability for referral.* If the client refuses, the veterinarian is unable to perform endodontics, or referral is not available, extraction may be the only option for care of the fractured tooth with pulpal exposure.
- *Patient's use and habits.* Dogs with chewing vices—for example, gnawing fences or rocks—might not be candidates for root canal treatment with composite restoration.
- *The part of the tooth affected.* Some fractures are limited to enamel and require little or no therapy. Others involve dentin only, which may require endodontic care. Finally, some fractures expose enamel, dentin, and pulp, and require endodontic therapy or extraction.

PULP TRAUMA

Pulpitis without obvious loss of tooth structure often appears as a discolored tooth. Pulpitis can be caused by direct blunt trauma, hyperthermia from ultrasonic scaling or overly aggressive polishing. The resulting inflammation may be sufficient to cause vascular damage, hemorrhage, and pulpal swelling. Because the pulp is contained within a solid unyielding chamber with limited blood supply and no collateral support, the inflammatory process that is so beneficial in the healing response in other body areas creates swelling leading to pulpal necrosis. Pulp infection can enter through anachoresis (the process of bacteria exposure by a hematogenous route) and progress to apical disease.

Pulpitis discoloration presents as one of four colors:

- *Pink* is consistent with initial trauma, which may be medically treatable.
- *Purple* is the color of hemoglobin in the dentin tubules shortly after the pulp begins to die. Root canal therapy or extraction is indicated. Occasionally these teeth have a *yellow* discoloration.
- *Gray* indicates a nonvital tooth with a necrotic pulp. When the odontoblasts die and their processes into the dentinal tubules regress, blood and/or necrotic pulpal by-products can enter the vacated tubules approaching the dentinal enamel interface. Root canal therapy or extraction is necessary (Figure 7.42).

Treatment of choice for pulpitis is root canal therapy for all presentations except those teeth with a pink discoloration at the coronal tip. Some of these minimally affected teeth may resolve with antibacterial and anti-inflammatory medication. In the medically treated tooth, follow-up radiographs and clinical examinations for several years is indicated.

Worn Teeth

Chronic abrasion from self grooming, tennis ball chewing, and/or misaligned opposing teeth might result in trauma to the pulp. This persistent low-grade trauma

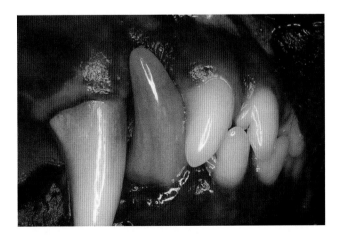

FIGURE 7.42. Discolored mandibular canine affected by pulpitis.

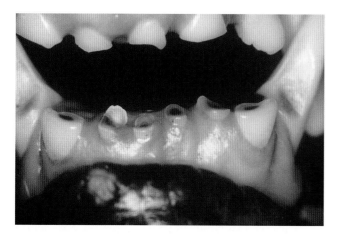

FIGURE 7.43. Worn teeth with tertiary dentin.

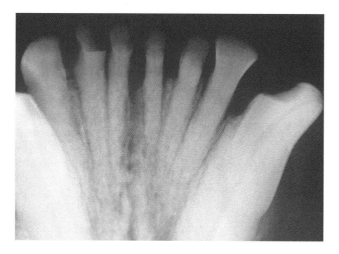

FIGURE 7.44. No radiographic evidence of periapical disease.

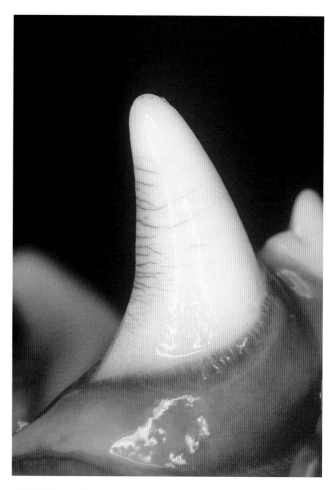

FIGURE 7.45. Craze lines.

causes odontoblasts to produce tertiary (reparative) dentin for repair and protection. Tertiary dentin appears as a reddish-brown or black shiny spot in the center of the worn surface.

As long as the rate of wear is gradual, reparative dentin production will keep up with loss of tooth structure without causing pulpal exposure. If the rate of wear is faster than the rate of tertiary dentin production, the pulp becomes exposed, leading to pulp necrosis. Probing the worn area with an explorer and radiographic examination will help evaluate the endodontic and periodontic involvement of worn teeth to see whether therapy is indicated (Figures 7.43, 7.44).

Crown infraction (crack or craze lines) usually occurs from direct trauma to the enamel and manifests as single or multiple lines in horizontal, vertical, or oblique directions that do not cross the dentoenamel junction. Therapy is usually not indicated (Figure 7.45).

FRACTURE CLASSIFICATION

There are numerous fracture classification systems. The author prefers staging fractures. *Class 1* enamel (uncomplicated) fractures occur from minor trauma. The dentin or pulp is not exposed in stage 1 fractures. Intraoral radiographs should be taken as a baseline and to check for additional root fracture. The tooth should be re-radiographed 6 and 12 months later for evidence of periapical pathology.

Treatment of enamel fractures entails smoothing and recontouring the surface with a white stone or fine diamond bur on a water-cooled high-speed handpiece to remove sharp edges, then applying a bonding agent (Figures 7.46, 7.47).

Class 2 (uncomplicated, near pulpal exposure) fractures extend through enamel into the dentin without pulpal penetration. In stage 2 fractures, bacteria have an indirect pathway to the pulp through the dentinal

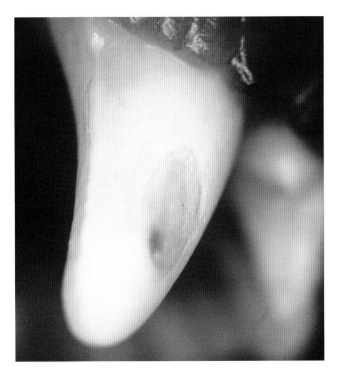

FIGURE 7.46. Class 1 fracture: enamel loss on canine tooth.

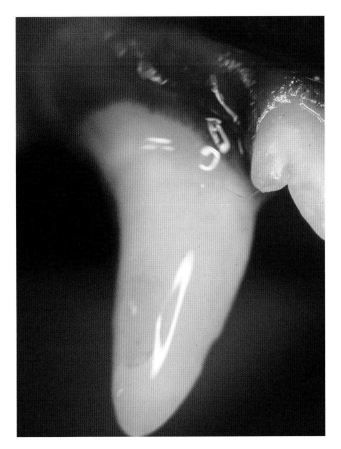

FIGURE 7.47. Restored enamel loss.

tubules. If the injury is recent and a pink spot (pulpal blush) is evident on the fracture site, a near exposure is present. If untreated, the pulp may become necrotic and appear as a dark spot through the thin dentin (Figure 7.48).

Class 2b (near pulp exposure) fracture extends below the gum line. Enamel and dentin are exposed, sparing the pulp.

Treatment for class 2 fractures depends on the age of the animal (younger animals have less distance between dentin and pulp) and the degree of penetration into the dentin:

- If intraoral radiographs show apical closure and do not reveal periapical pathology and the patient is between 9 months and 6 years old, root canal therapy can be performed with predictable results. Alternatively, pulp capping (indirect) with or without crown restoration can be performed with a guarded prognosis:
  - *Indirect pulp capping* covers exposed dentin with a bonded composite or a cast crown.
  - *Direct pulp capping* covers the exposed pulp (exposed with a round bur), with calcium hydroxide followed by restoration. With current dentin bonding systems, calcium hydroxide may be unnecessary or detrimental by actually decreasing the amount of surface area for bonding.

    When pulp-capping procedures are used, follow-up radiographs should be taken at 6-month intervals after injury for several years to examine the pulp cavity for decreased size (indicating a vital tooth) or internal resorption and for periapical pathology.
- If intraoral radiographs do not reveal periapical pathology and the patient is older than 6 years, a "wait and see" approach can be taken. Those that are older than 6 years with fractures that just enter

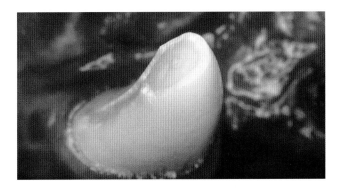

FIGURE 7.48. Class 2 fracture–near pulpal exposure.

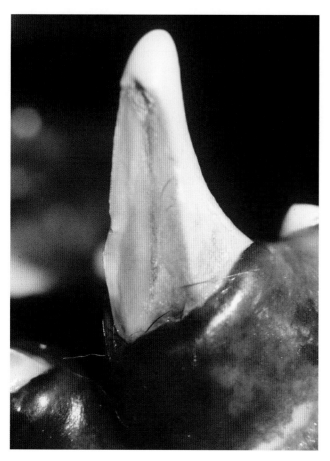

FIGURE 7.49. Class 2b fracture.

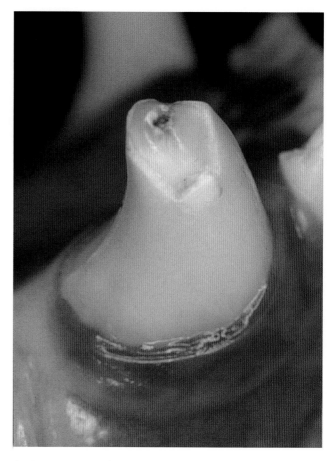

FIGURE 7.50. Class 3 fracture.

the dentin usually have sufficient dentin to protect the pulp for endodontics therapy (Figure 7.49).

- If periapical pathology exists with a radiographically closed apex, root canal therapy and crown restoration is the treatment of choice usually resulting in a saved nonpainful tooth.
- If periapical pathology radiographically exists and there is an open apex (fracture occurred before the patient was 9 months old), either apexogenesis, apexification, or surgical endodontic care is indicated.

Class 3 (complicated) fracture penetrates into the pulp chamber, directly exposing vital pulp tissue. The pulp usually appears as a red or brown spot on the cut surface of the fracture. When exposure exists, endodontic therapy should be performed (vital pulpotomy, conventional root canal, or surgical root canal) or the tooth extracted (Figure 7.50).

When pulp is exposed, there is direct communication between the oral bacterial environment and the vascular system. The initial bacterial exposure eventually leads to pulpal necrosis, apical granuloma formation, periapi-

cal abscessation, pain, and possible compromise of distant organs. The process may occur within a month or may be prolonged, smoldering for 3–5 years.

Animals experience pain similar to humans when a tooth fractures with pulpal exposure. A majority of dogs and cats presented with fractured teeth do not show any signs. When the pulp necroses, the pain decreases until periapical lesions form. The mere fact that an animal does not appear to be in pain is no excuse to avoid treating the fractured tooth.

Dogs and cats can show dental pain in various ways:

- Chewing on one side
- Dropping food from the mouth when eating
- Excessive drooling
- Grinding of teeth
- Pawing at the mouth
- Facial edema/swelling
- Regional lymph node enlargement
- Shying away when the face is petted
- Refusing to eat hard food
- Refusing to chew on hard treats or toys

Class 3b (complicated crown and root) fractures have enamel, dentin, and pulp chamber exposure, with extension below the gum line. Treatment for Class 3b fractures is the same as class 3 fractures, with additional attention to the fracture segment located subgingivally (Figure 7.51).

Slab fractures occur when a slice of the crown separates from the buccal or lingual/palatal surface of a tooth. After the fracture segment is removed, pulpal exposure may be visualized. The fracture often extends subgingivally. Slab fractures most commonly occur on the buccal surface of the maxillary fourth premolar in a dog that has been chewing bones or cow hooves. Treatment options include root canal therapy and restoration with gingival surgery to eliminate the pocket, or extraction (Figure 7.52).

Class 4 (root) fractures extend into the cementum, dentin, and pulp. Root fractures are classified by the anatomic location of the fracture (cervical, middle, or apical third). Cervical root fractures often present with a highly mobile crown.

Treatment consists of either tooth extraction or removal of the fractured coronal segment and root canal therapy. Fractures located in the apical third of the tooth should heal without intervention by deposition of new cementum, with osseous material on the outside and reparative dentin forming internally to heal the fracture. Teeth affected by middle-third root fractures causing minimal crown mobility should be splinted to adjacent teeth for 6 weeks for stability. Follow-up radiographs are recommended. Cervical-third fractures are usually extracted with the root, or the crown is removed and the root treated endodontically (Figure 7.53).

PATIENT/FRACTURE AGE

Age of the patient is also important when choosing endodontic therapy options. Teeth of patients younger than 9 months have open apices. Conventional root canal therapy is not performed on these animals because sealing the apex cannot be assured. Treatment options include partial coronal pulpectomy (vital pulpotomy) to promote apexogenesis or an apexification procedure based on the pulp health. Patients older than 9 months with pulpal exposure and closed apices should be treated with conventional root canal therapy.

Age of the fracture might also influence the endodontic treatment. Shortly after pulpal exposure, inflammation occurs less than 2 mm from the exposure site. Healthy pulpal tissue can be found several millimeters deeper within the pulp, which might respond to

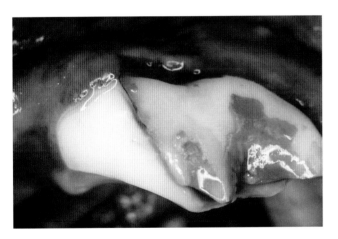

FIGURE 7.51. Class 3b fractured maxillary fourth premolar.

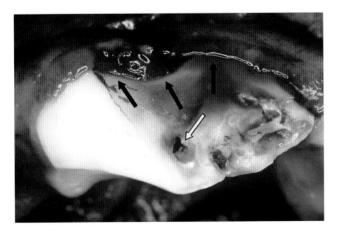

FIGURE 7.52. Slab segment removed revealing pulpal exposure (white arrow) and subgingival involvement (black arrows).

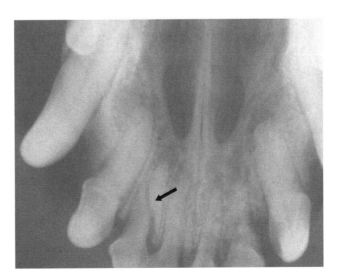

FIGURE 7.53. Root fracture maxillary intermediate incisor.

conservative vital pulp procedures. In acute fractures, the pulp appears pink or red at the fracture surface. The pulp of a long-standing fracture will appear brown or black.

Partial coronal pulpectomy (vital pulpotomy) is an endodontic procedure in which the vitality of the pulp is preserved and tooth maturation is allowed to continue. The procedure involves removal of a portion of the pulp in the chamber of the crown, leaving the pulp in the root undisturbed. Partial coronal pulpectomy can be performed if the fracture is less than 48 hours old in the patient older than 9 months, or less than 2 weeks in the patient younger than 9 months. If the patient is young and the root is not fully formed, the vital pulp therapy might allow root closure to continue.

Partial coronal pulpectomy generally takes less time to perform than conventional endodontics, and when successful, will salvage the tooth's vitality. The intention, when performing a vital pulpotomy, is to stimulate the pulp to form a dentinal bridge to cover the exposed pulpal tissue. Unfortunately, the dentinal bridge does not "seal" the pulp from the oral environment. The long-term prognosis of partial coronal pulpectomy is poor in cases of trauma-induced fractures. Conventional endodontics is the treatment of choice for the traumatically injured tooth that has a closed apex because it carries greater long-term success than vital pulpotomy.

The following are indications for vital pulp therapy (partial coronal pulpectomy, vital pulpotomy):

- To repair an acutely (less than 48 hours) fractured tooth in a young dog or cat whose apex is immature and open. If the patient is less than 9 months of age, conventional endodontic procedures should not be performed because proper debridement and an apical seal cannot be perfected. A successful vital pulpotomy allows *apexogenesis* of the immature tooth to occur with eventual root thickening and apical closure. The best prognosis results when the tooth is treated within 24 hours. In the young animal, if the fracture is present for greater than 2 days, it is considered infected, and *apexification* would be the desired outcome after calcium hydroxide is applied to the apex to stimulate hand tissue deposition. In the mature animal with a closed apex, conventional endodontics result in a more predictable outcome compared to vital pulp therapy after an acute fracture.
- As a part of the crown reduction procedure to potentially decrease biting damage from an aggressive patient (disarming).
- For repair of iatrogenic pulpal exposure.

The following are contraindications for vital pulpotomy:

- Non-vital pulp
- Suppurative pulp
- Pulp that will not stop bleeding (indicating irreversible pulpitis)
- Radiographic evidence of periapical changes secondary to pulpal necrosis

Materials for vital pulpotomy include the following:

- #701, #2, #3, #4 round burs, #330 burs
- Sterile saline
- Cotton dressing forceps
- Paper points
- Retrograde amalgam filler
- Chlorhexidine solution (0.12%)
- Calcium hydroxide powder
- Hypocal (Bellman), Pulpdent paste (Caulk/Densply), Dycal (Caulk/Densply)
- MTA (Densply)
- Restorative material

Use the following steps to perform a partial coronal pulpectomy (Figure 7.54):

1. Administer antibiotics and pain control medication pre-operatively.
2. Infuse a local anesthetic with epinephrine around the tooth or perform a nerve block to desensitize the pulp.
3. Take a dental radiograph to determine root maturity and to evaluate pathology.
4. Clean and polish the teeth ultrasonically.

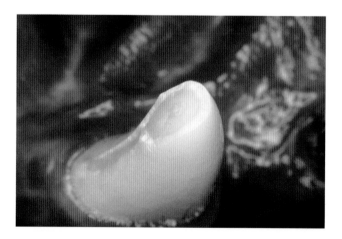

FIGURE 7.54. Near pulpal exposure in an acutely fractured canine.

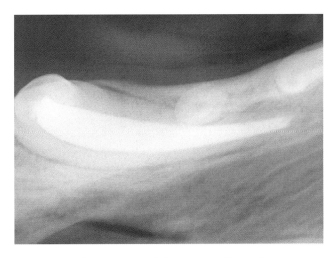

FIGURE 7.63. Root canal therapy performed once apex closed.

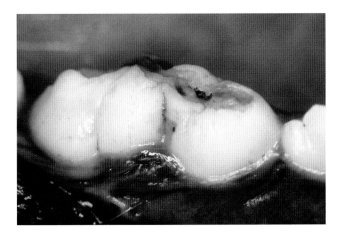

FIGURE 7.64. Crown fracture of a mandibular first molar in a 7-month-old rottweiler.

point where preservation of the pulp is no longer possible. Calcium hydroxide is used to bring a bony closure to the apex. After this has been accomplished, conventional endodontics can be performed. This advanced procedure should not be attempted if the clinician is at a beginning or intermediate level.

Even after apexification in the immature patient, the root and crown will be thin, dry, and weak, which makes it subject to fracture. The long-term prognosis for these teeth in large, orally oriented dogs is guarded even with metallic crown restoration, because the tooth might fracture between the alveolar crest and margin of the prosthetic crown (Figures 7.64, 7.65).

Equipment and materials for calcium hydroxide filling of canal include the following:

- High/low-speed delivery system, burs (round, pear, and inverted)
- Barbed broaches
- Lentulo spiral filler (Burns 25 mm assorted 951-7700, 60 mm assorted 264-9487; Schein 25 mm 100-3791, 60 mm 100-8948)
- Calcium hydroxide (powder, paste, or light cured)
- Retrograde amalgam filler
- Sterile paper points (Burns 25 mm #15–40 951-7614, #45–80 951-7640; Schein 25 mm #15–40 100-0672, #45–80 100-2142, #90–140 100-1776; 60 mm: Burns 271-7240, Schein 100-8242)
- Restorative

The technique for pulp removal and canal filling for apexification to occur includes the following steps:

1. Remove necrotic contents of the immature root canal with barbed broaches to a point just short of the radiographic apex (Figure 7.66). Endodontic stops are used to help prevent over-instrumenting the canal. If periapical lesions are present, surgical exposure and debridement may also be indicated.
2. Frequently irrigate the canal with sterile saline. Avoid using bleach.
3. After instrumentation, dry the canal with premeasured paper points before placement of the calcium hydroxide paste. When using paper points, care must be taken not to disturb the apical tissue, causing additional hemorrhage (Figure 7.67).
4. Fill the canal with calcium hydroxide/sterile saline paste (mixed with barium sulfate 8:1). The calcium hydroxide stimulates cementum to create an apical seal. Lentulo spiral fillers with endodontic stops

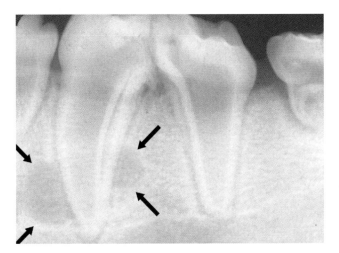

FIGURE 7.65. Radiographs of the fractured tooth in figure 7.64 consistent with pulpal necrosis.

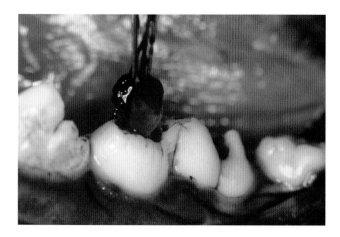

FIGURE 7.66. Removal of necrotic pulp.

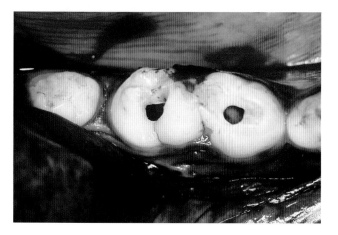

FIGURE 7.67. Appearance of canals after pulp removal.

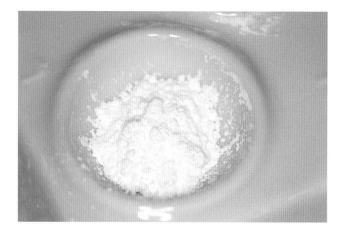

FIGURE 7.68. Calcium hydroxide powder placed in a dappen dish.

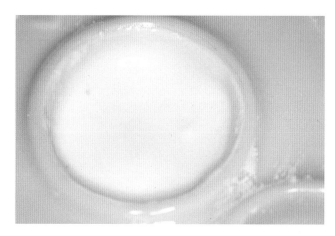

FIGURE 7.69. Calcium hydroxide liquid mixture before placement into root canals.

attached are used to introduce calcium hydroxide paste into the canal. The spiral is placed on a 10:1 contra-angle reduction gear in a low-speed handpiece. Place the turning Lentulo into the canal and apply the calcium hydroxide paste to the spiral, which carries the paste downward. The goal is to completely fill the root canal with calcium hydroxide without introducing trapped air bubbles (Figures 7.68, 7.69).

5. Glass ionomer base cement can be applied coronal to the calcium hydroxide before access restoration.
6. Restore the access, using a composite resin.

The calcium hydroxide dressing should be changed every 3–6 months in dogs and 1–2 months in cats until apexification is complete. When apical calcification is confirmed radiographically, conventional endodontics can be performed (Figures 7.70–7.74).

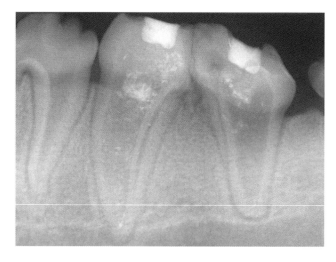

FIGURE 7.70. Radiograph of calcium hydroxide liquid placement into root canals.

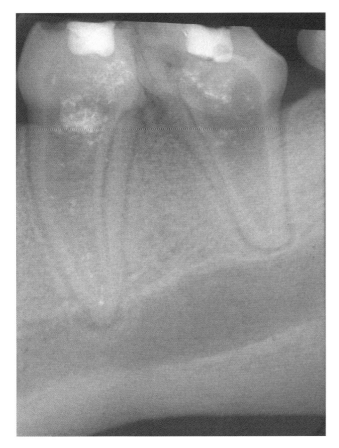

FIGURE 7.71. Radiograph 3 months after calcium hydroxide placement (note resolution of periapical lesion).

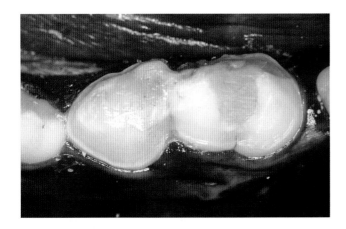

FIGURE 7.72. Restoration of fracture site with acrylic resin.

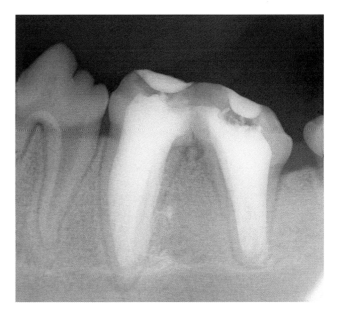

FIGURE 7.73. Radiograph of root canal therapy after apexification.

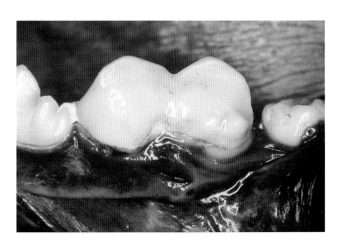

FIGURE 7.74. Crown restoration.

CONVENTIONAL ENDODONTICS (STANDARD ROOT CANAL THERAPY)

Conventional endodontics involves removing the pulp (pulpectomy), disinfecting the pulp chamber, sealing the apex, and restoring the access opening.

Indications for conventional endodontics include:

- Pulpitis from trauma
- Caries or resorptive lesions near or entering pulp in the canine
- Care for an avulsed tooth 3–6 weeks after reimplantation
- Pulp exposure from fracture, attrition, or abrasion

Contraindications for conventional endodontics include:

- Concurrent advanced periodontal disease requiring extraction
- An open apex
- Apical external resorption (Figure 7.75)
- Perforating internal resorption (Figure 7.76)
- Vertical root fracture

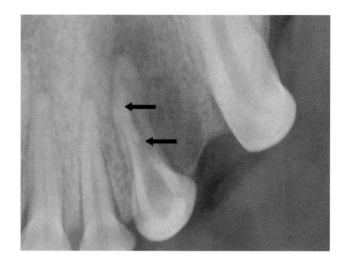

FIGURE 7.76. Radiograph of perforating internal root resorption.

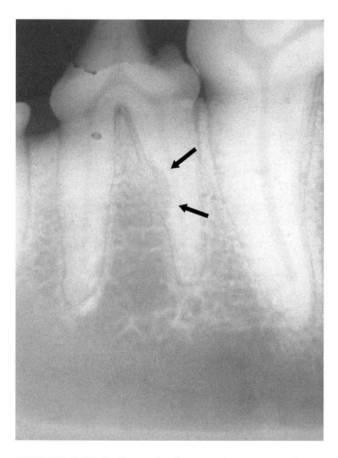

FIGURE 7.75. Radiograph of external root resorption.

Radiographs

At least five radiographs are needed during the endodontic procedure:

1. The *initial* radiograph is taken before therapy to identify peculiarities of the tooth to be treated, location of the pulp chamber orifices and root angulation.
2. The *working length* film is exposed with a file in the canal to full working length in the pulp cavity. The working length film is used to determine the measurement of successive files.
3. The *master file* film is exposed when the master file is at the apex.
4. The *completion* film is exposed when the root canal is finished.
5. *Follow-up* radiographs are taken 4–6 months postprocedure the first year followed by periodic rechecks dictated by the case.

Setup for conventional endodontics includes the following:

- Round or pear-shaped bur for access (Burns 952-5116, Schein 100-0288)
- Barbed broaches (Burns 25 mm asst 950-1790, 47 mm asst 264-9480; Schein 100-6351)
- Gates Glidden burs sizes 2–6 (Burns 951-1370, Schein 100-9919)
- Files 10–40 diameter, 21–60 mm long (Burns H files 60 mm #15–80 264-9458, #15–40 25 mm 951-2487, 25 mm #45–80 951-2489; Schein 100-8146, 100-7643)
- RC Prep (Burns 854-7304, Schein 378-4499)
- Sodium hypochlorite (Burns 952-0052, Schein 100-7562) or 0.12% Chlorhexidine (causes less apical inflammation due to leakage)
- Sterile saline

- Absorbent paper points—various widths and lengths (Burns 951-1802, Schein 100-2683)
- Gutta-percha points (Burns #15–40 31 mm 951-4288, #45–80 31 mm 951-4289, #15–80 60 mm 271-7215-18, 951-4288; Schein assorted 100-8393, 25 mm: #15–40 100-6273, #45–80 100-9997, #90–140 100-1871, 60 mm 100-8226)
- Root canal sealer AH-26 (Burns 804-1050, Schein 117-8362) or zinc oxide (Burns 952-3250, Schein 100-4540), Eugenol (Burns 951-2081, Schein 100-1757)
- Various-sized Holmstrom spreader/plugger combinations (Burns 271-9095, Schein 102-4718, Cislak Holmstrom pluggers/spreaders) plus shorter-sized spreaders and pluggers
- Restorative materials (Burns 867-7296, Schein 777-2647)
- Finishing disks (Burns 868-0690, Schein 294-8195)
- Slow-speed handpiece with latch type contra-angle and 10:1 reduction gear

Accessing the Canal (Coronal Access)

Keep the following general considerations in mind:

- Local anesthetic is injected before the root canal procedure is begun.
- Unsupported or fractured tooth components should be removed, leaving sound structure. This includes discarding the slab portion of the maxillary fourth premolar fracture plus rounding of rough edges.
- Cat and small dog teeth are usually entered from the fracture site. In medium and larger dogs, an additional access is drilled, if needed, to create a straight path through the pulp cavity to the apex. The initial penetration into enamel is made with a No. 2 round carbide or diamond bur in a high-speed drill at a right angle to the crown. (Figure 7.77).
- After the enamel has been pierced, the bur is angled toward the pulp cavity, removing a section of the pulp chamber (Figure 7.78).

Incisors are accessed either palatally/lingually or labially. The first (central) and second (intermediate) incisors are accessed halfway between the gingival margin and incisal edge. The third incisor is entered one-quarter the distance from the gingival margin to the incisal edge (Figure 7.79).

Access to the *canine teeth* is made on the mesial aspect of the tooth just coronal to the gingival margin (Figure 7.80). The maxillary third incisor might interfere with the ideal access to the maxillary canine pulp chamber. In those cases, a longer surgical length bur mounted on a low-speed handpiece is used.

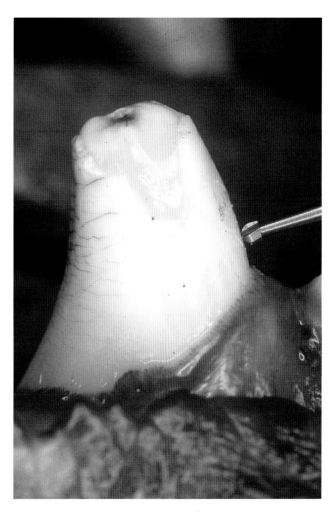

FIGURE 7.77. Perpendicular placement of round bur for access of a mandibular canine tooth.

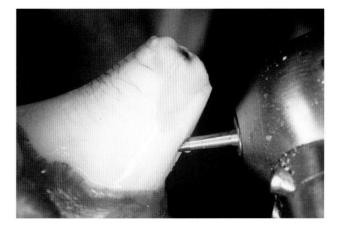

FIGURE 7.78. Redirection of bur to follow the root canal after initial enamel penetration.

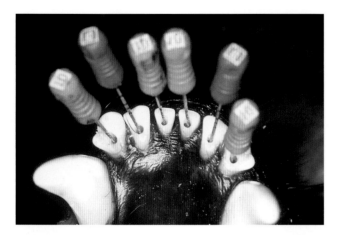

FIGURE 7.79. Lingual mandibular incisor access sites.

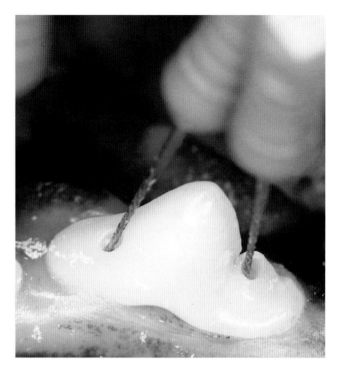

FIGURE 7.81. Mandibular second premolar access site.

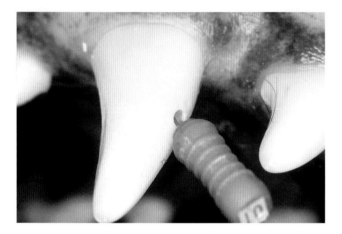

FIGURE 7.80. Maxillary canine access site.

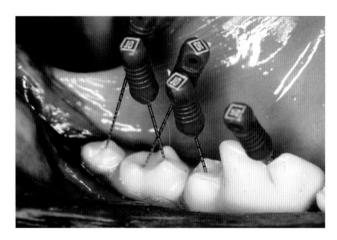

FIGURE 7.82. Mandibular first, second, and third molar access sites.

Access to the *premolars* and *molars* is made over the pulp chambers of these teeth on the buccal or occlusal surfaces. Avoidance of the cusp tip and developmental grooves is preferred because it weakens the tooth. The maxillary first molar may be entered over the center of the mesial developmental groove and the center of the distal cusp (Figures 7.81, 7.82).

The *maxillary* fourth premolar has three roots. At one time, the palatal root was not considered essential to saving the tooth, and it was amputated during the conventional endodontic procedure. Unfortunately, the maxillary fourth premolar with an amputated palatal root is prone to fracture because the tooth cannot withstand shearing forces without the tripod support of the palatal root.

In the maxillary fourth premolar, all three roots may be entered from two buccal access sites. The mesiobuccal and palatal roots are accessed just buccal and slightly distal to the developmental groove of the mesiobuccal cusp. The distobuccal access is at the buccal aspect of the tooth and slightly distal to the development groove on the midsaggital plane. The palatal root is accessed buccally from the transcoronal approach or directly over the root (Figures 7.83–7.87).

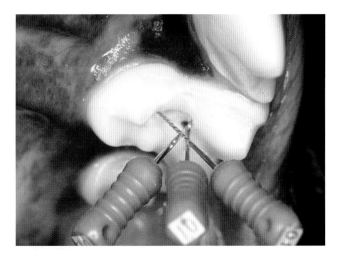

FIGURE 7.83. Maxillary first molar access sites.

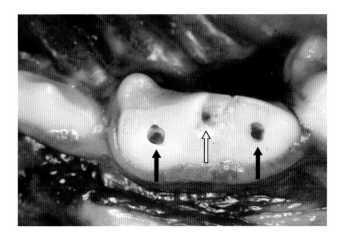

FIGURE 7.84. Access sites on the maxillary fourth premolar (black arrows). Pulpal exposure due to fracture (white arrow).

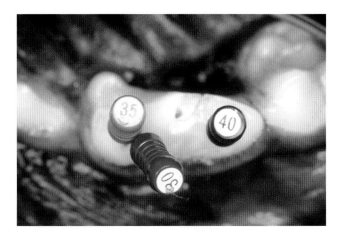

FIGURE 7.85. Placement of endodontic files in the maxillary fourth premolar root canals.

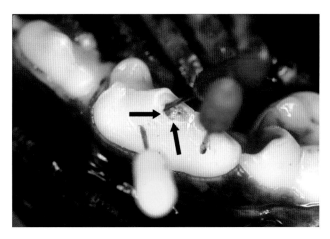

FIGURE 7.86. Access of maxillary fourth premolar mesiobuccal root through the fracture site.

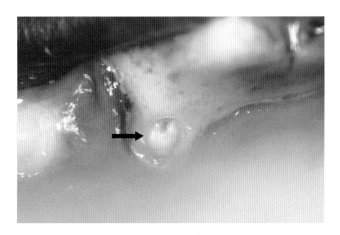

FIGURE 7.87. Palatal root access from a direct coronal palatal approach.

Preparing the Canal—Debridement and Shaping

Cleaning and shaping procedures are designed to remove deleterious debris from the root canal system while producing a smooth funnel shape for complete filling. This process is called *debridement* or *instrumentation*. The thoroughness of debridement facilitates successful dimensional sealing during the obturation (filling) phase.

Pre-operative radiographs are important to evaluate the shape of the root. Most small-animal root canals are slightly curved. Sharply curved canals present a challenge to the veterinary dentist, particularly if flexible NiTi files are not used. If the files used to prepare the canals are not curved (pre-bent) to mimic the canal shape:

- Penetration of the canal lateral to the normal curvature (*ledging*) might occur during the debridement process. If ledging continues, perforation of the root wall may result. When ledging is observed, a smaller file can be prebent to finish debridement, and both the ledged and anatomic canals are obturated.
- The inside of the curve may be shaved excessively (*stripping*).
- The apex may become overly enlarged (*zipping* or *apical transposition*).

For debridement:

1. Use a barbed broach to remove gross pulpal tissue. Barbed broaches work best on intact vital or recently devitalized pulp contents. Carefully introduce the broach into the canal until it makes light contact with the pulpal tissue. Rotate the broach 180° to engage the pulp and gently pull it back. Take care not to break the broach in the pulp cavity. Repeat the process multiple times to remove the entire pulp. If the entire pulp is removed with the broach, minimal additional filing is necessary (Figures 7.88, 7.89).
2. Hedstrom and Kerr files shape and clean the canals. Use the working length radiograph to determine the file length needed to reach the apical terminus. Endodontic stops are small round pieces of rubber or plastic placed on files at the estimated working length (length from the access to apex). Stops are applied to prevent placing the instrument too far into the canal through the apex into the periapical tissues. Establish the working length when the tip of the file rests on the apical floor of the canal.
3. The first file used should just barely engage the canal walls when it is carried to the working length. Hedstrom files can be inserted and partially removed without rotation. The Hedstrom file

works on the pull stroke. Use Hedstrom files to flare the coronal third of the pulp cavity. Use K files to prepare the middle and apical thirds of the root canal in small (<31 mm long) canals. Turn K files

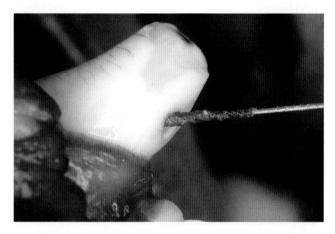

FIGURE 7.89. Necrotic pulpal tissue wrapped around the barbed broach.

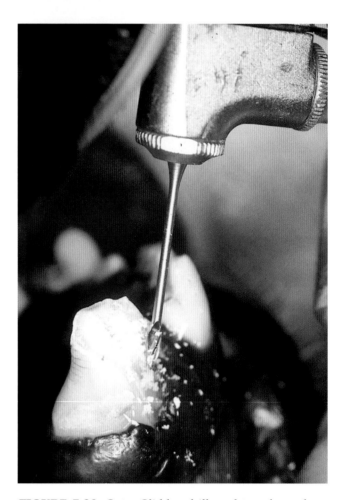

FIGURE 7.90. Gates Glidden drill used to enlarge the coronal third of the pulp chamber.

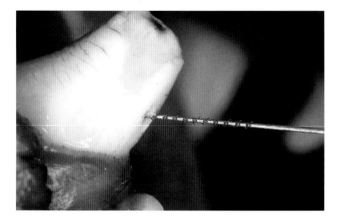

FIGURE 7.88. Barbed broach inserted into the access of a mandibular canine tooth.

clockwise 90°, remove 1–2 mm, and reinsert multiple times. Apply chelating agents on the first two or three files introduced into the canal to soften dentin for easier debridement and for file lubrication. (RC Prep, Premier Dental Products Co.: Burns 878-1820, Schein 378-4499).

4. Use Gates Glidden files to flare the coronal third of the pulp cavity, rapidly removing dentin and allowing unimpeded access to the apical root canal. Gates Glidden drills are susceptible to breakage and should not be forced. Only when straight-line access is possible, should Gates Glidden drills be used to flare the coronal third. Each bur should be used only two or three times. Apply a lubricant (RC Prep), if needed, on the bur tip to decrease friction.

Gates Glidden burs come in six sizes (#1–6): #1 corresponds to a number 50 K file, #2 corresponds to #70 file, and so on. The #1 file should not be used due to its small diameter and its great predisposition to breakage. Instead of the Gates Glidden drills, some veterinarians choose large Hedstrom files to flare the coronal third of the pulp cavity (Figure 7.90).

5. After the coronal third of the pulp cavity is flared, gently direct a Hedstrom file apically in a filing motion until the endodontic stop touches the access area (Figure 7.91).

6. Take a radiograph to verify that the file is within the tooth's apical terminus. If the file tip has not reached the apex, continue filing. The working-length distance may vary from 0.1–5.0 mm from the radiographic apex because of differences in the patient age, size of tooth, and root canal anatomy (Figures 7.92, 7.93).

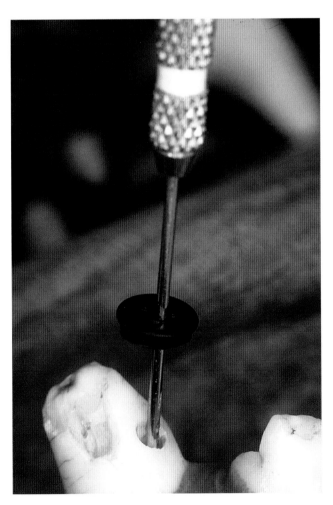

FIGURE 7.91. Number 15 Hedstrom file with endodontic stop inserted in the root canal.

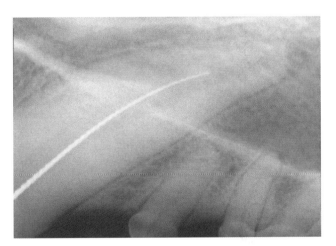

FIGURE 7.92. Radiograph showing the file 5 mm short of apex.

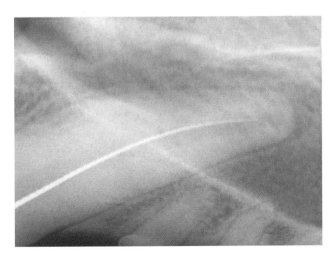

FIGURE 7.93. Radiograph showing the file 3 mm short of apex.

7. After the working length is established, slide an endodontic stop to the tooth level and apply at the same level to all successive files (Figures 7.94, 7.95).

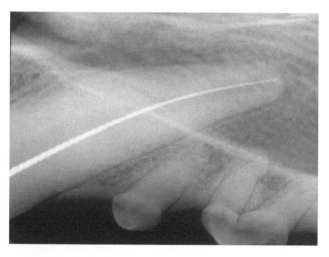

FIGURE 7.94. Working length confirmed with file at the apex.

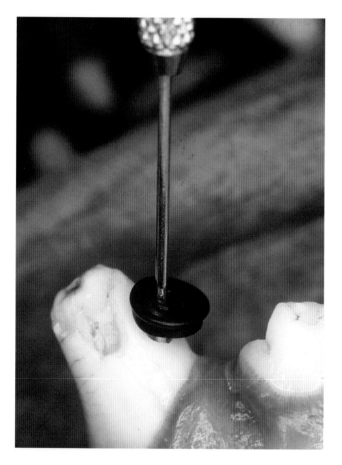

FIGURE 7.95. Endodontic stop slid to the access site to set the working length.

8. Instrumentation of a file is complete when it can be inserted to the full working distance and withdrawn without any resistance. Introduce progressively larger files, enlarging the canal until a size is found that does not easily reach the working length. Then with apical pressure, cut the dentin until the apex is reached. This file is termed the master file.

With the *step back* method, the veterinarian uses smaller diameter files nearest the apex progressing to larger sizes at decreasing distances. Alternatively, the *crown down* method may be employed, where the veterinarian works from the crown of the tooth, shaping the canal as he or she moves toward the apex. The first instruments are the engine-driven Gates Glidden reamers (drills) or manual Hedstrom files for the coronal flaring, Hedstrom or K files follow in the mid-root region followed by smaller K files toward the apex.

9. Between files, irrigate the canals with 5.25% sodium hypochlorite full strength or diluted 50% with sterile saline or 0.12% chlorhexidine to remove dentinal debris, dissolve soft tissue, disinfect, and provide a bleaching effect. Introduce the irrigation solution by using a slot-ended endodontic needle to prevent periapical extrusion of dentin debris and bleach. Bleach should be employed when the practitioner knows the apex is closed. Irrigate the canal with sterile saline between the last three file sizes to remove the hypochlorite irrigation solution (Figures 7.96–7.98). Some practitioners alternate hydrogen peroxide with the bleach and saline.

10. As the procedure progresses, reinsert the last file that reached the apex to the full apical extent, to *recapitulate* the canal, removing dentinal debris that might have accumulated near the apex.

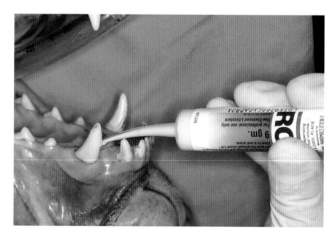

FIGURE 7.96. Application of RC prep for file lubrication.

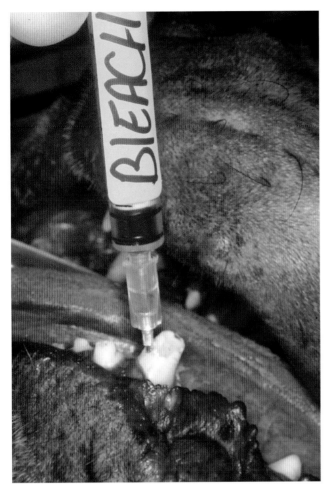

FIGURE 7.97. Application of sodium hypochlorite (bleach) for disinfection.

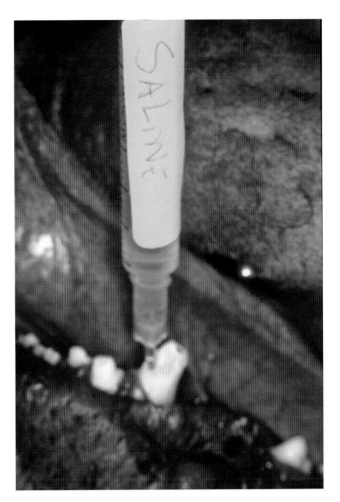

FIGURE 7.98. Application of sterile saline for irrigation.

11. When file flutes reveal clean dentinal shavings (Figure 7.99), irrigate the canal with saline and dry by repeatedly placing sterile paper points into the opening of the tooth to the apex (Figure 7.100). When the points are removed dry, the tooth is ready to be filled (obturated) and sealed. Blood present on the paper points indicates either apical perforation, a lateral canal, or inadequate pulp removal. If bleeding persists, take radiographs to confirm that the apex has not been perforated. If the apex is intact, use additional filing to remove all the pulpal contents and stop the bleeding.

Rotary Debridement

Debridement may also be accomplished with rotary instruments, using a slow-speed (approximately 2000 rpm) handpiece. The LightSpeed technique uses small Gates Glidden-like nickel titanium instruments to enlarge and debride the root canal system. The K3 sys-

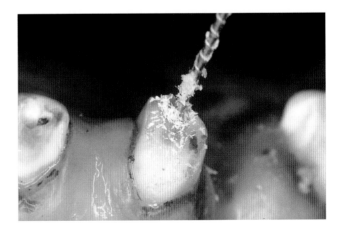

FIGURE 7.99. Clean dentinal shavings.

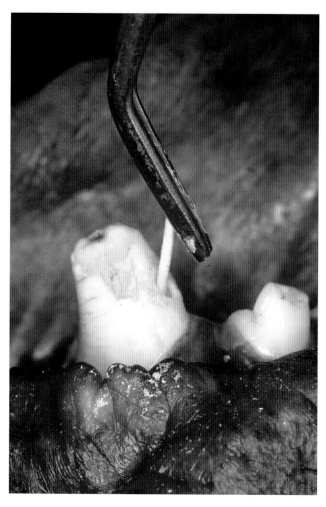

FIGURE 7.100. College-tipped pliers holding a paper point to dry the root canal.

LightSpeed NiTi Rotary Instrument

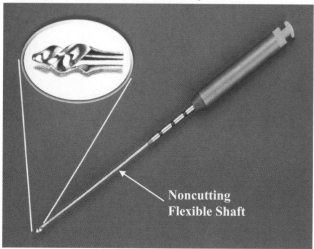

Noncutting Flexible Shaft

FIGURE 7.101. LightSpeed nickel titanium file for rotary debridement.

tem (SybronEndo) uses nickel titanium rotary files to shape and clean the canals. Rotary instrumentation reduces time and increases filing efficiency (Figure 7.101).

In the *modified crown down* technique, the coronal third of the canal is enlarged using Gates Glidden drills, followed by rotary files to prepare the apical and the middle thirds. During debridement of the apical third, endostops are placed at the appropriate working length on each instrument to be used. For the best results, the canal should be filled to the orifice with liquid EDTA (LightSpeed Technology Inc.) during instrumentation. Irrigation with diluted sodium hypochlorite is recommended after every three instruments.

Use the following technique for rotary debridement (using LightSpeed instruments):

1. Use a hand file (#15 K file) to establish canal patency and working length. An endostop is placed at the working length for additional files to enter the canal.
2. Use Gates Glidden drills or large Hedstrom files to enlarge the coronal third of the pulp cavity (Figure 7.102).
3. Begin with a LightSpeed size #35, in hand. If the #35 is easily placed to working length, continue with sequentially larger LightSpeed instruments until reaching a size that binds short of working length (Figure 7.103). Begin rotary debridement with this instrument (in the handpiece). Conversely, if the LightSpeed #35 binds short of working length, continue (by hand) with sequentially smaller LightSpeed instruments until finding a size small enough to reach working length. Begin rotary debridement with the very next larger LightSpeed instrument.
4. Progress to the next larger instrument, continuing this procedure with sequentially larger instruments until the apical third is completely prepared. When it takes at least twelve pecks to advance the next largest file, the apical canal has been properly prepared. The last instrument used to working length is called the master apical rotary (MAR).
5. After the apical third of the canal is instrumented, prepare the middle third. Using the pecking technique, rotate sequentially larger instruments into the canal.
6. Recapitulate the canal to the working length with the master apical rotary (MAR) size.

Make Access and Preflare Coronal 1/3 with Gates-Glidden Drills

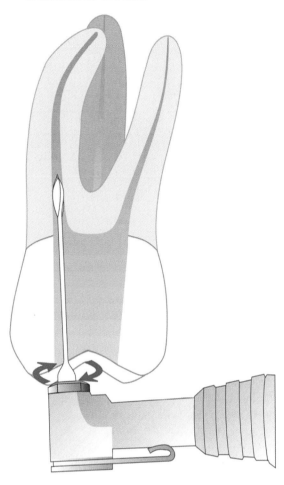

FIGURE 7.102. Rotary coronal canal preparation (human tooth shown).

Use "pecking" motion to advance instrument to working length

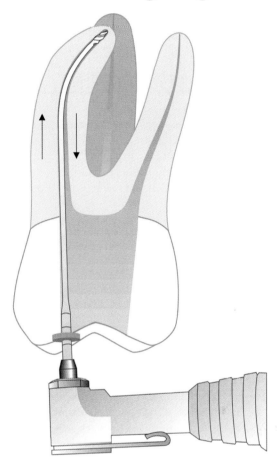

FIGURE 7.103. Rotary apical preparation (human tooth shown).

Obturation

Obturation is the three-dimensional filling and sealing of the entire root canal, preventing leakage and establishing an environment allowing periapical healing. After the tooth has been successfully prepared (cleaned and shaped) and disinfected, the root canal(s) and pulp chamber(s) are obturated with permanent filling material. Healing the periapical tissues occurs when the nutritional supply to the bacteria is stopped by the sealing properties of obturation (Figure 7.104).

Use the following steps for obturation:

1. Place a gutta percha master cone (same size as the master file) into the pulp chamber to the apex and

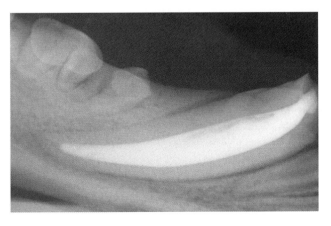

FIGURE 7.104. Properly filled and sealed root canal of the mandibular canine in an 11-month-old dog.

radiograph. Position the cone to a depth that feels snug. Good apical fit is evidenced by receiving a tug-back when the point is at the floor of the canal. Mark the master cone with cotton pliers at the line where it is flush with the opening of the tooth, and remove for application of root canal sealer cement.

2. Use root canal cement to seal the apex, dentinal tubules, and accessory canals and to fill irregularities in the canal. Zinc oxide/eugenol (ZOE) (Burns 952-3250, 951-2081; Schein 100-4540, 100-1757) is a commonly used sealer. Eugenol might interfere with composite restoration. The trend is to use calcium hydroxide–based sealers with little to no eugenol (Sealapex-Kerr) or an intermediate (glass ionomer, calcium hydroxide) filler if composite restoration is planned. To merge zinc oxide and eugenol, mix a dime-sized amount of zinc oxide powder and several drops of eugenol liquid to a creamy consistency with a #5 spatula on a glass slab for approximately 1 minute. Incorporate small amounts of powder into the liquid and wipe over a large area of the mixing pad. Mixing is finished when a half-inch string of the cement can be drawn between slab and spatula (Figures 7.105–7.107).

3. Methods used to apply apical sealing cement include the following:
   • For large canals instrumented with greater than size 40 file, the cement can be loaded on a Lentulo spiral filler powered by a low-speed handpiece with a 10:1 contra-angle reduction gear. The spiral is dipped into the cement mix and inserted approximately halfway into the canal. The spiral is rotated counterclockwise to distribute the cement to the apex and onto the dry walls of the canal. A spreader two sizes smaller than the master cone is used to push the sealer to the internal apex.
   • The endodontic master file can be loaded with apical cement and rotated counterclockwise in the canal releasing the cement into the apex.
   • Gutta percha points can be dipped in sealer cement before insertion into the canal carrying the sealer to the apex (Figures 7.108–7.110).

4. Use a plugger to vertically compact the gutta percha apically. The plugger should be slightly smaller than the root canal width. For canals up to 30 mm, cut the master cone to 10–15 mm in length, place it in the canal, and vertically compact it (Figure 7.111).

5. Use a spreader to laterally compact the master cone and sealer against the root canal walls (Figure 7.112).

6. Cut multiple accessory cones to 10–15 mm lengths. The apical third of the root canal is filled by plac-

ing these accessory gutta percha points in the space made by the root canal spreader alongside the master cone. The accessory cones are vertically and laterally condensed until the operator cannot compress the spreader within 10 mm of the apex.

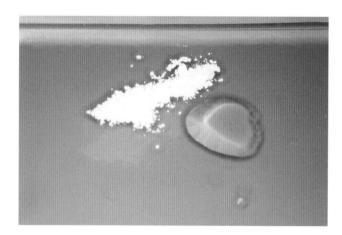

FIGURE 7.105. Zinc oxide/eugenol on glass slab.

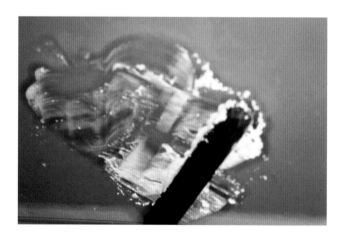

FIGURE 7.106. Mixing zinc oxide/eugenol.

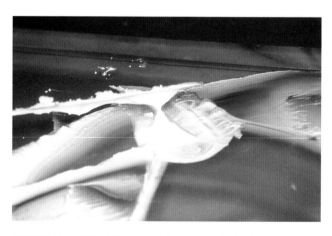

FIGURE 7.107. Mixture strings up 1/2 inch.

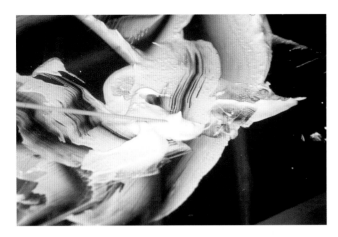

FIGURE 7.108. Application of zinc oxide/eugenol to a gutta percha point.

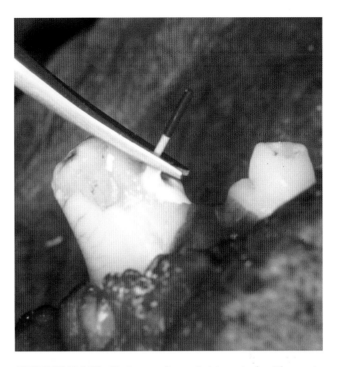

FIGURE 7.110. Gutta percha point inserted with a cotton tip pliers to the apex.

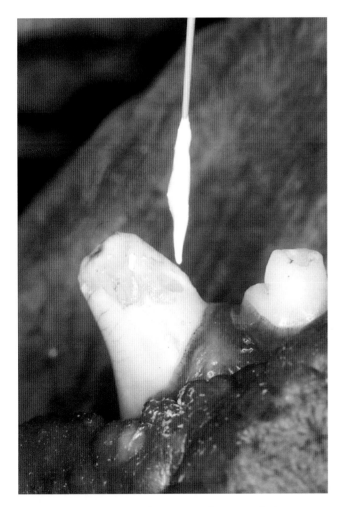

FIGURE 7.109. Coated gutta percha point before insertion into prepared canal.

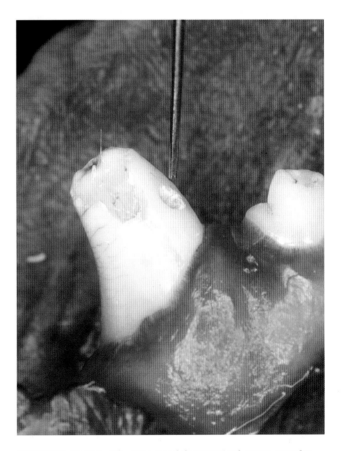

FIGURE 7.111. Plugger used for vertical gutta percha compression.

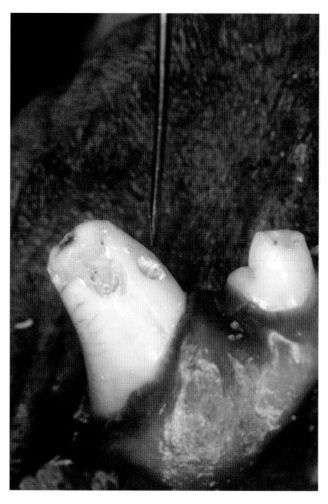

FIGURE 7.112. A spreader is used for lateral gutta percha compression.

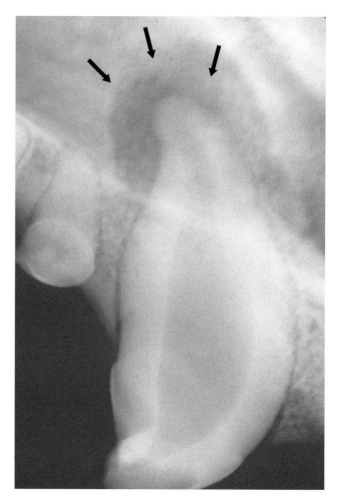

FIGURE 7.113. Periapical lucency secondary to pulpal necrosis.

7. Take a radiograph to confirm a dense apical fill. If absent, spend more time compacting the gutta percha toward the apex. If present, back-fill the coronal portion of the pulp cavity and compact, using cut gutta percha, spreaders, and pluggers (see Figures 7.114–7.117 for examples of conventional endodontic cases).

8. Remove excess gutta percha and root canal cement extending from the access site with
   - An inverted cone or pear-shaped bur on high-speed air-driven handpiece
   - A heated spreader
   - A Touch 'n Heat carrier
   - Iris scissors
   - A spoon excavator to cut the gutta percha and scrape the canal walls clean

Alternative Methods of Obturation

The *McSpadden thermomechanical compaction technique* uses a compactor attached on a slow-speed contra angle. The McSpadden compactor is applied next to the master cone in the root canal to soften and laterally compact gutta percha. Frictional heat forces the gutta percha apically and laterally. Additional points are added until the canal is filled. The main disadvantage of this technique is lack of apical control leading to softened gutta percha extruding beyond the apex. Additionally, heat generated can damage the surrounding soft tissue.

Thermoplastic application of gutta percha for obturation provides a three-dimensional method of filling the canal, often faster and easier than vertical and lateral compaction of conventional gutta percha points.

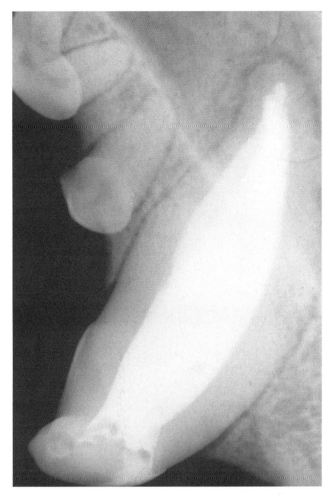

FIGURE 7.114. Periapical lucency resolved 2 months after root canal therapy.

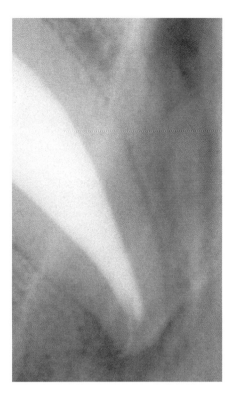

FIGURE 7.115. Properly filled and sealed canine root canal.

Heated gutta percha can be obtained through core carrier or injection techniques.

Core Carrier Techniques

Densfil endodontic titanium and plastic obturators are coated with alpha phase gutta percha for canal insertion. (Caulk/Dentsply: Burns 813-5200, Schein 222-7739) (Figure 7.118).

Densfil uses the following technique:

1. Preheat the DensHeat Oven for 20 minutes (Figure 7.119).
2. Place a working-length Densfil obturator in the heater according to the manufacturer's instructions.
3. Coat the canal with a non-eugenol sealer.

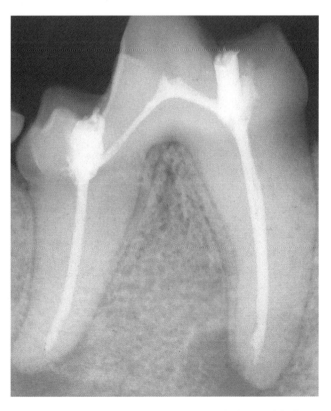

FIGURE 7.116. Properly filled and sealed mandibular first molar.

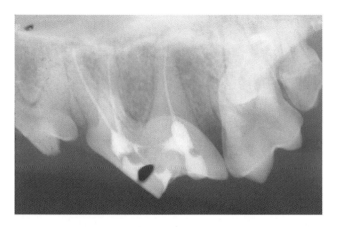

FIGURE 7.117. Properly filled and sealed maxillary fourth premolar.

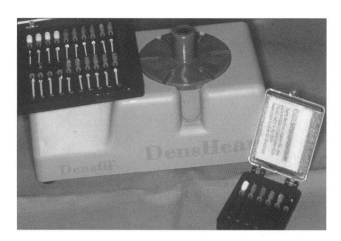

FIGURE 7.119. Densfil system.

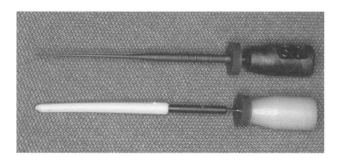

FIGURE 7.118. Densfil plastic obturators.

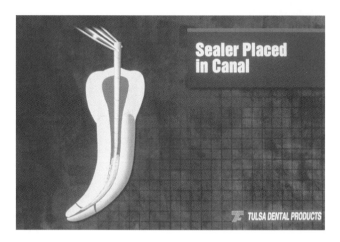

FIGURE 7.120. ThermaFil sealer placed with a paper point.

4. Using firm apical pressure, insert the Densfil obturator to the working length.
5. Sever the shaft with a round, inverted cone or cross-cut fissure bur level with the orifice.

ThermaFil Plus (Dentsply) endodontic obturators are metal or plastic ISO-sized files (carriers) coated with gutta percha. The obturators are available in sizes 20–90, at 25 mm length (Figures 7.121, 7.122).

ThermaFil Plus uses the following technique:

1. Apply zinc oxide eugenol or ThermaSeal Plus sealer to the apex of the prepared canal with paper points (Figure 7.120).
2. Insert a preheated (20 seconds) ThermaFil obturator one size smaller than the master file to the working file depth. Excess gutta percha flows coronally through the groove in the carrier.
3. While stabilizing the carrier with one finger, sever the file handle with a bur at the coronal orifice (Figures 7.123). Compact gutta percha vertically using a plugger. Remove excess gutta percha from the access site and restore the tooth.

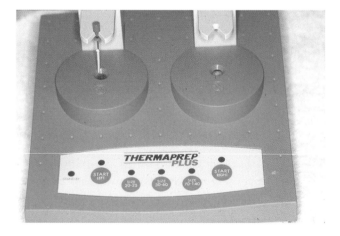

FIGURE 7.121. ThermaFil heater with gutta percha loaded.

SimpliFill (LightSpeed Technology Inc.) uses a 5 mm length of gutta percha placed on the end of a plugger. The plugger, called a *carrier*, allows this 5 mm piece of gutta percha termed the Apical GP Plug to be condensed into the apical portion of the prepared root canal after application of an apical sealer. SimpliFill is used in conjunction with LightSpeed NiTi rotary instruments. The Apical GP Plug diameters correspond with the widths of the LightSpeed instruments. The Apical GP Plug is released from the carrier by turning the handle counterclockwise and removing the carrier from the canal. When the apical portion of the canal is sealed, the remainder of the canal is filled with additional sealer and gutta percha (Figures 7.124–7.126).

SuccessFil titanium cores (Coltene/Whaledent Inc.) are used in combination with SuccessFil gutta percha obturation material. SuccessFil titanium cores are available in sizes 20–80 @ 25 mm length (#20: Burns 844-

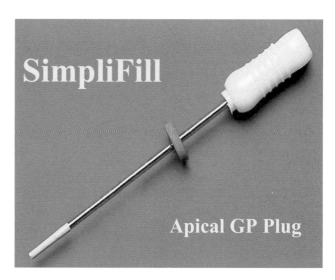

FIGURE 7.124. SimpliFill apical GP Plug (from Lightspeed CD).

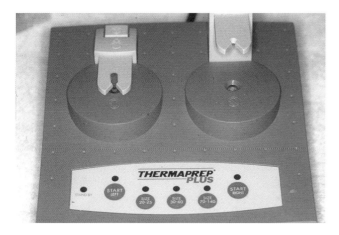

FIGURE 7.122. ThermaFil heater warming gutta percha.

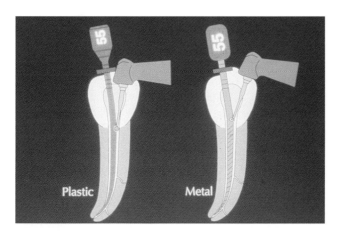

FIGURE 7.123. File handle severed when gutta percha is at apex.

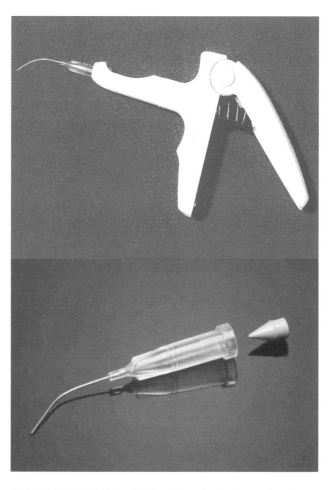

FIGURE 7.125. SimpliFill syringe to load canal sealer.

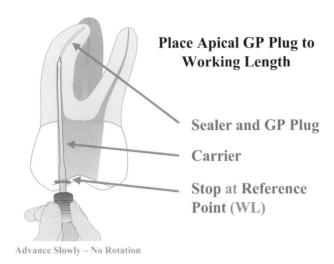

Place Apical GP Plug to Working Length

Sealer and GP Plug

Carrier

Stop at Reference Point (WL)

Advance Slowly – No Rotation

FIGURE 7.126. Placement of Apical GP Plug to working length (human tooth shown).

1878, Schein 547-7689; #25: Burns 844-1880, Schein 547-8273; #30: Burns 844-1882, Schein 547-8355; #35 Burns 844-1884, Schein 547-8566; #40 Burns 844-1886, Schein 547-8642).

The SuccessFil core technique uses these steps:

1. The canals are instrumented in a manner that will result in a flaring preparation from access to apex. After the apical portion of the canal has been enlarged to an adequate size, use additional instrumentation in the coronal portion of the canal to assure the flaring preparation. Final instrumentation should result in a canal in which a file fits snugly in the apical 1–2 mm and loosely in the coronal portion of the canal.
2. Place the SuccessFil syringe into the heater for 15 minutes.
3. Before final placement, insert a preselected (same size as file used for the final apical preparation) sterile titanium core into the canal to the full working length without binding. If binding occurs, select one size smaller.
4. Notch the shaft with a fissure bur at the coronal access length—enough to break at the desired time but still maintain sufficient strength for placement without breaking prematurely (Figure 7.127).
5. Remove the core from the canal and insert into the heated gutta percha syringe. The core is coated with gutta percha from the syringe. After coating, allow the gutta percha to harden (approximately 1 minute).
6. Apply root canal sealer with a paper point to the apex.

7. Immerse the SuccessFil System solid core gutta percha in 5.25% sodium hypochlorite for 1 minute, and then rinse with alcohol and dry with sterile gauze.
8. Warm the precoated core with a flame (Figure 7.128).
9. Insert the core into the canal, twisting the handle counterclockwise until the shaft separates. Discard the shank of the file.
10. Dip a plugger in alcohol and use it to condense the gutta percha into the canal. After all canals are filled, add gutta percha for backfill. Alternatively, a fast set (blue) cannule may be used to fill the canal coronally.

The *Soft-Core System* uses a solid plastic core precoated with gutta percha. The standard length of the obturator is 27 mm from the tip to the handle base. Extra long 18 mm insertion pins are available creating total length of 45 mm. (Soft-Core System, Inc. 888-462-8878).

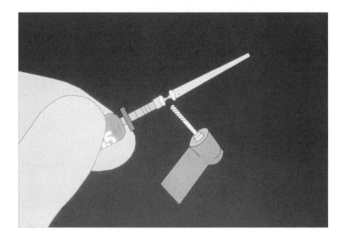

FIGURE 7.127. Notching the shaft before placement.

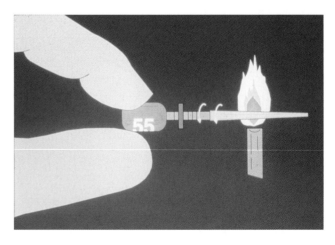

FIGURE 7.128. Gutta percha is softened with flame heat.

The Soft-Core System uses this technique:

1. Following canal preparation, place a size verifier into the canal corresponding to the selected obturator. A slightly loose fit in the apical third is critical to allow clearance for gutta percha back-filling.
2. Insert the selected obturator into a heated oven for 70 seconds attaining 110° C.
3. While the obturator is heating, using the size verifier, carry non-eugenol sealer to the apex.
4. When the oven tone indicates the obturator is ready, remove it and immediately insert it in the canal to the working distance.
5. Allow the gutta percha to cool for 3–4 minutes. A radiograph is taken.
6. Remove the handle and insertion pin by twisting the handle. Use a spreader/plugger to compact the gutta percha. Remove excess plastic core and gutta percha with an inverted cone bur.
7. Restore the tooth.

Injection Techniques

Injection techniques deliver heated, softened, gutta percha into prepared root canals.

Obtura II (Obtura Corporation, SybronEndo) delivers gutta percha heated to 200° C. in an injection pistol. The gutta percha is loaded as preformed bullets placed in the heating chamber of the pistol handpiece. The pistol has a finger control to allow flow of gutta percha through the disposable applicator needles (20 or 23 gauge) into the presealed canal. Unfortunately, the smallest-sized injection needle is 0.6 mm in diameter, necessitating canal preparation to a number 60 file or larger. Plugger compaction follows the gutta percha application. Longer lengths used in veterinary dentistry are available. Obtura II can also be used as a backfill after the apical area has been fitted with a master gutta percha cone (Figure 7.129).

The *ULTRAFIL 3D Injectable Gutta Percha System* consists of a heater, ULTRAFIL syringe, and 22 g disposable cannules of gutta percha. The needle of the cannule is 21 mm long and has a diameter equal to a #70 file. The middle third of the canal must be enlarged to a size #70 file to allow the ULTRAFIL needle to fit in the canal and reach within 6–8 mm of the apex. (Coltene/Whaledent, Inc.: Burns 844-2018, Schein 547-5828) (Figure 7.130).

ULTRAFIL injectable gutta percha cannules are color-coded:

• *Green-Endoset* is used in moderate-to-large canals, those with internal resorption, and retrogrades

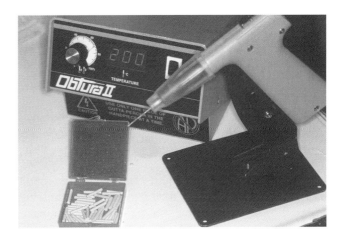

FIGURE 7.129. Obtura II heats gutta percha.

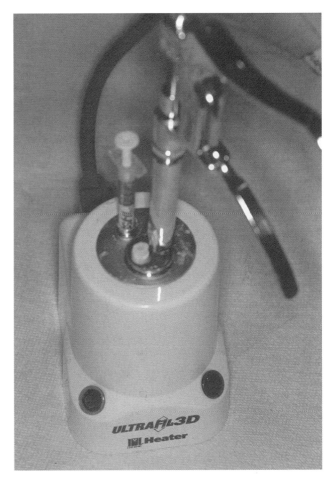

FIGURE 7.130. ULTRAFIL 3D Injectable Gutta Percha System.

where fast compacting is important. Endoset gutta percha has the highest viscosity, is the least flowable, and hardens within two minutes. (Burns 844-2008, Schein 888-6809).

- *Blue-FirmSet* has good flowablility, which makes it suitable for narrow canals and bypassing separated files. FirmSet gutta percha hardens within 4 minutes (Burns 844-2007, Schein 888-8678).
- *White-Regular Set* has excellent flowability but takes 30 minutes to harden (Burns 844-2005) (Figure 7.131).

Regular Set and FirmSet gutta percha have the highest flow properties and are used for injection techniques where the gutta percha will not be manually compacted. Endoset gutta percha is a higher-viscosity gutta percha, with slightly less flow and is positioned for techniques that require condensing using a spreader or plugger.

ULTRAFIL technique:

1. Turn on the heater. The cannules and/or syringes are placed into the heater. The red and green indicator lights illuminate. Within five minutes, the light to the left of the switch will blink intermittently, indicating that the controlled temperature of 90° C. has been reached.
2. Apply an apical sealer (zinc-oxide/eugenol, CRCS) to the apex, using the master file, paper points or a Lentulo spiral filler.
3. Load the preheated cannula and needle into the Ultrafil syringe. To make space for the cannula, pull back the plunger while depressing the plunger release button. A slight amount of gutta percha is extruded to confirm flow. Replace the cannula and syringe in the heater for at least 20 seconds.
4. Place the needle into the prepared root canal (at least to a #70 file size) approximately 8 mm from the apex (Figure 7.132).
5. Compress the trigger three times. Three seconds later, compress it again. With the extrusion of gutta percha, the cannula will appear to be pushed out of the canal. If the operator squeezes the trigger after gutta percha has hardened (cooled down), the cannula will rupture due to tip blockage.
6. Condense the gutta percha with a plugger and spreader to make room for additional injection.
7. Take a radiograph to evaluate the fill and the presence of voids.
8. Replace the carrier and cannula in the heater for 2 minutes and repeat step 5 until the canal is fully obturated. Typically, a 3-year-old medium-sized dog's canine takes 3–5 cannulae to obturate completely.

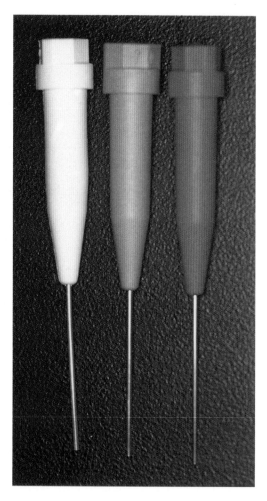

FIGURE 7.131. ULTRAFIL injectable gutta percha cannules.

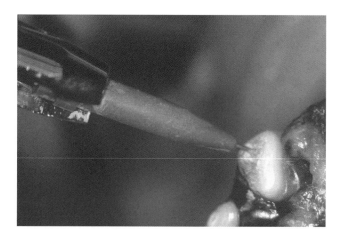

FIGURE 7.132. Injecting ULTRAFIL gutta percha into root canal.

Gutta Percha Carrier Technique

Soft gutta percha syringe techniques have limited use obturating large dog canine teeth because of insufficient length of the applicators. To rectify this shortcoming, #15–25 K files at 45–60 mm lengths can be used as carriers of warm gutta percha into the root canal.

SuccessFil gutta percha is thermaplasticized at 90° C. The SuccessFil syringe contains 0.7 cc of gutta percha. SuccessFil uses this technique after root canal sealer cement has been placed:

1. Place a K file/reamer or H file one size smaller than the last file used to instrument the canal, 2–3 mm inside the heated gutta percha syringe. Without twisting, carry gutta percha from the syringe and insert to the working length of the prepared and sealed root canal. Rotate the file counterclockwise to release gutta percha inside the canal. The number of coatings a syringe provides depends on thickness, shape, and length of gutta percha applied to the carrier (Figures 7.133–7.135).

2. Compact carried gutta percha toward the apex with a plugger. A heated spreader is inserted into the canal to soften and laterally compact the gutta percha before additional compaction. Heat the spreader by external flame or glass bead sterilizer, or use electrically heated spreaders. Between applications, wipe the spreader tip with an alcohol swab. Take a radiograph after the apical third of the canal is filled before continuing.

3. Repeat this procedure until the canal is filled.

Alternatively, fill the remaining portion of the canal with a lower viscosity FirmSet ULTRAFIL gutta percha.

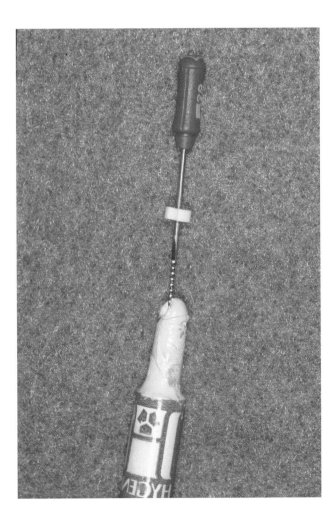

FIGURE 7.133. File used for carrying gutta percha inserted into a heated syringe of SuccesFil.

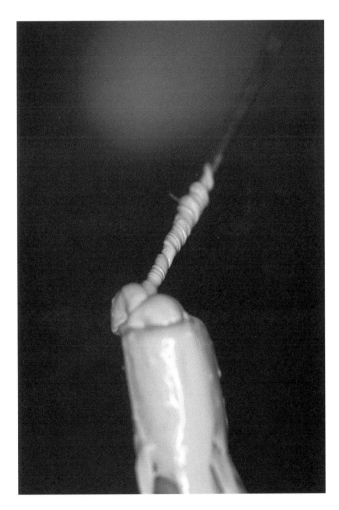

FIGURE 7.134. Rolling the gutta percha around the file.

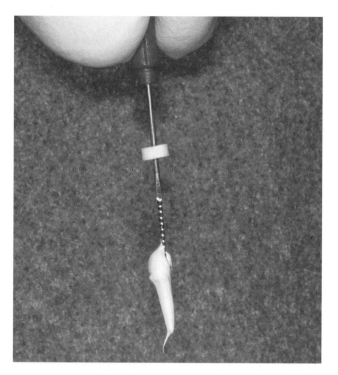

FIGURE 7.135. Coated gutta percha point before insertion into prepared canal.

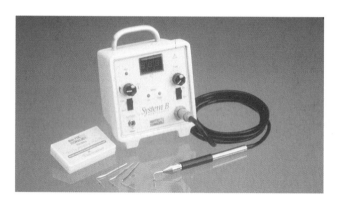

FIGURE 7.136. System B.

SuccessFil technique variations include the following:

- The ULTRAFIL System Master Cone technique uses the standard gutta percha master cone inserted and compacted into the apical third of the root canal, followed by ULTRAFIL gutta percha.
- Insert a gutta percha–coated K file into the canal, followed by severing the file and back-filling with plasticized gutta percha.
- The Trifecta system technique uses a solid core SuccessFil System gutta percha inserted and compacted, followed by injectable ULTRAFIL System gutta percha.

Heated Spreader System

Lateral compaction of warm (heated) gutta percha. A heated plugger pressed apically can be used to warm gutta percha in the canal, creating additional room for more points. When the heat source is a flame, there is uncontrolled heating. Electric heat carriers deliver a precise amount of heat for a specific time. Examples of electronic heat carrier methods are the System B continuous wave technique (Burns 954-3150) (Figure 7.136) and Touch 'n Heat vertical compaction technique (Schein 114-5154) (Figures 7.137, 7.138).

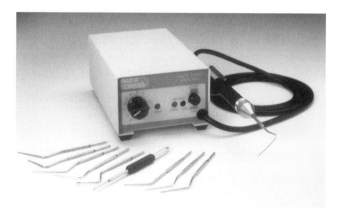

FIGURE 7.137. Touch 'n Heat.

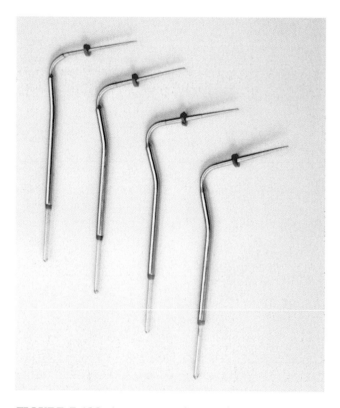

FIGURE 7.138. Assortment of sizes of pluggers for the heated spreader technique.

The heated spreader technique uses these steps:

1. Insert a master gutta percha point into the prepared canal.
2. Evaluate radiographs for proper fit and remove master cone.
3. Apply an apical sealer to the tip of the master gutta percha point.
4. Insert the master gutta percha point and sealer into the prepared canal.
5. Set the Touch 'n Heat to "use" with the intensity at 6. If System B is used, set the power to 10 and the temperature to 200° C.
6. Drive the preheated plugger smoothly through the gutta percha until it stops 5–7 mm short of the working length.
7. Maintain apical pressure as the gutta percha cools during the nonactivation for 10 seconds.
8. Before the spreader removal, apply electrical power. This sets off a surge of heat for 3 seconds, which separates the plugger from the apical mass.

9. Cool the spreader for 1 second before removal.
10. Apply additional gutta percha points until the entire canal is obturated (Figures 7.139–7.145).

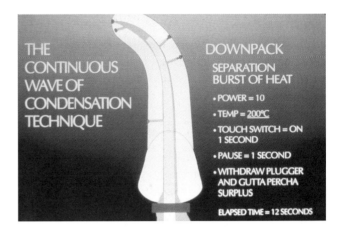

FIGURE 7.141. The continuous wave of condensation technique—Step 2.

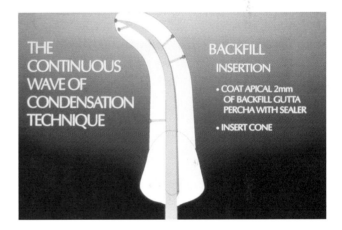

FIGURE 7.142. The continuous wave of condensation technique—Step 3.

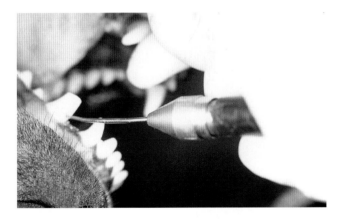

FIGURE 7.139. System B heated plugger in use.

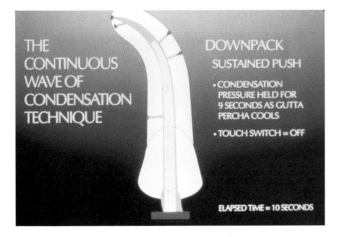

FIGURE 7.140. The continuous wave of condensation technique—Step 1.

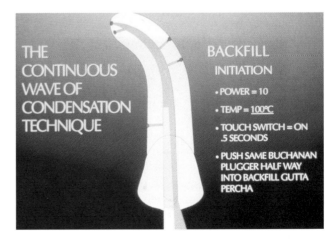

FIGURE 7.143. The continuous wave of condensation technique—Step 4.

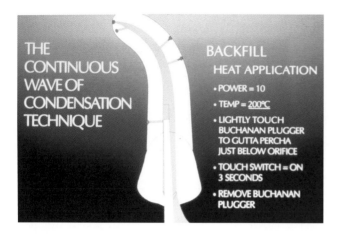

FIGURE 7.144. The continuous wave of condensation technique—Step 5.

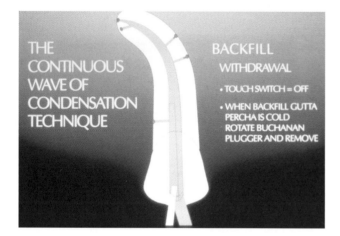

FIGURE 7.145. The continuous wave of condensation technique—Step 6.

ACCESS RESTORATION

Following radiographic confirmation of a complete pulp cavity obturation, the access is restored with glass ionomer cement, light cured composite, or amalgam. If the endodontic sealer contains eugenol (which interferes with polymerization of composite), glass ionomer should be applied between the obturation material and composite:

1. Use a pear-shaped bur to undercut the dentin and remove obturating material from the restoration site (Figure 7.146). With bonded composites, there is little need for an undercut, so the practioner can use a discoid excavator and a long bullet-shaped composite bur to scrape debris off the access site walls.

2. Etch the dentin using polyacrylic acid, rinse, and gently dry.

3. Mix glass ionomer cement according to the manufacturer's directions and apply to the restoration (Figure 7.147).

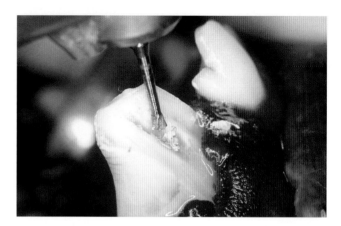

FIGURE 7.146. Inverted cone bur used to prepare crown for restoration.

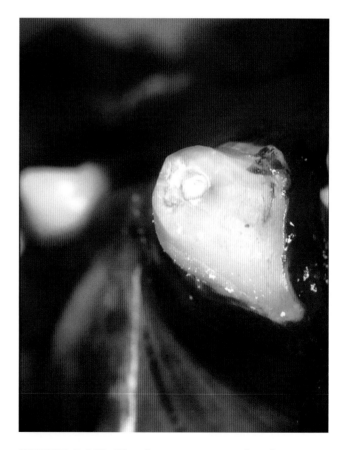

FIGURE 7.147. Glass ionomer cement placed over gutta percha before crown restoration.

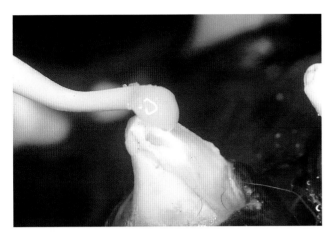

FIGURE 7.148. Composite bonding material placed for crown restoration.

4. After the initial set of 5 minutes, 3 mm of the intermediate restoration is removed, using the pear bur to make room for the composite restoration.
5. Etch the preparation for 20 seconds with 37% phosphoric acid, thoroughly rinse, and dry.
6. Apply bonding agent and composite, or amalgam, according to manufacturer's instructions (Figure 7.148).
7. Finish the restoration with polishing disks.

Cast metal or ceramic crowns may be placed over fractured teeth that have received endodontic therapy to provide additional fracture and wear protection.

Follow-up radiographs are recommended at 4 months and periodically when the animal is placed under anesthesia for other procedures.

SURGICAL ENDODONTICS (APICOECTOMY AND RETROGRADE FILLING)

Apicoectomy is the surgical excision of the apical portion of a tooth root through an opening in the overlying bone and oral mucosal tissues. The goal of the apicoectomy is to perfect a biologic apical seal with a retrograde filling of the apex. Surgical endodontic care is an advanced procedure most commonly performed on the maxillary canine and fourth premolar, and the mandibular canine and first molar.

The following are indications for surgical endodontics:

- Inability to perfect an apical seal with conventional endodontics
- Incomplete apical formation that will not respond to apexification
- Failure of re-treatment or conventional endodontics resulting in periapical inflammation
- Recurrent swelling and/or radiographic evidence of pathology around the root apex
- File separation during the beginning of an endodontic procedure
- Inability to access the apex due to obstruction of the root canal
- Marked apical pathology with root resorption
- Horizontal distal third root fracture with a radiographic periapical lesion

The following materials are used in surgical endodontics:

- High- and low-speed handpieces
- Burs (cross-cut fissure, round, and pear-shaped or inverted cone)
- #2/4 Molt periosteal elevator (Cislak EX-21)
- #85 Lucas bone curette (Burns 843-0559, Schein ST-10 100-3887, Cislak #85)
- Retrograde amalgam carrier (Burns 953-4220, Schein 317-1676) (Figure 7.149)
- Intermediate Restorative Material (IRM) (Burns 813-1530, Schein 222-1135) Super EBA cement (Bosworth: Burns 809-1630, Schein 250-3523), or MTA (mineral trioxide aggregate)
- Suture instruments and absorbable suture material

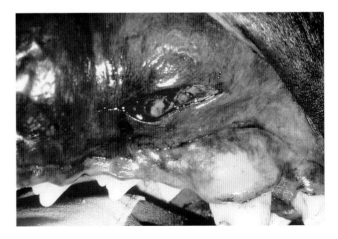

FIGURE 7.149. Semilunar incison made for canine apex exposure.

Procedure

Most root apices can be surgically exposed in the dog. The palatal roots of the maxillary fourth premolar and first molar are not surgically accessible and should be amputated if apicoectomy is performed on these teeth. Conventional endodontic procedures are performed before surgical endodontics:

1. Make a full-thickness semilunar incision over the apex of the tooth. In the dog, the apex of the maxillary canine is typically located dorsal to the mesial root of the second premolar. The apex of the mandibular canine usually lies just lateral and rostral to the caudal border of the mandibular symphysis (access ventral to the mesial root of the second premolar if approached ventrally). Expose the buccal maxillary fourth premolar apices with a wide flap over the apices. Avoid vital soft tissue structures, such as the infraorbital nerves, parotid salivary duct, and blood vessels, while incising the flap for exposure (Figure 7.150).

2. Elevate the periosteum around the apex and retract with a periosteal elevator, exposing cortical bone.

3. Use a sharp curette to probe the density of the cortical plate. If the bone buccal to the periapical lesion is easily perforated, it may be removed with a curette. If the bone is solid, remove approximately a 5 mm circumferential access, using a round bur in a water-cooled handpiece.

4. Amputate 5–8 mm of the apex at a 80–90° angle with a cross-cut fissure bur (apicoectomy), exposing an oval cross section of the root. Gutta percha condensed from conventional endodontics should be observed.

5. Prepare a 3 mm deep retrograde cavity with an inverted cone or pear bur at the root amputation site (Figure 7.151).

6. Use zinc-free amalgam, Super EBA Cement (Bosworth Company), Intermediate Restorative Material (IRM, Densply Caulk), or ProRoot MTA (Densply Tulsa Dental) to fill the cavity preparation using a retrograde amalgam filler or Centrix Syringe (Figures 7.152–7.154).

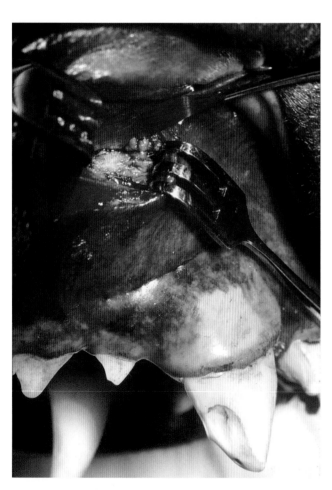

FIGURE 7.150. Flap exposing the periapical lesion.

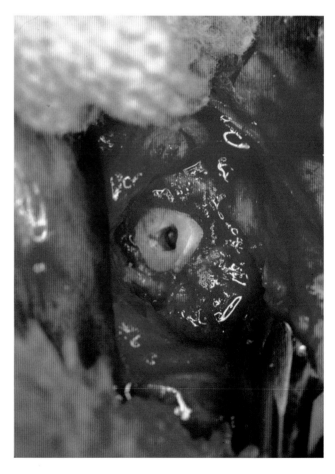

FIGURE 7.151. Amputation and preparation of the apex.

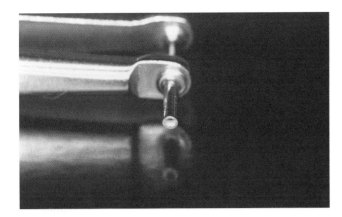

FIGURE 7.152. Retrograde amalgam filler used for applicaton of IRM material.

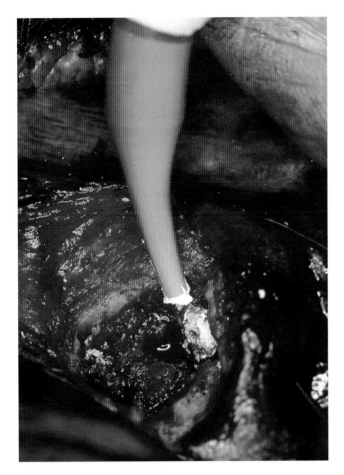

FIGURE 7.153. Centrix syringe tip applying IRM apical cement.

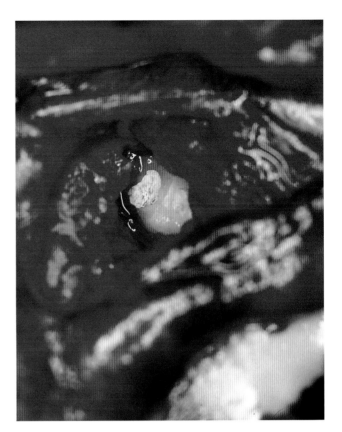

FIGURE 7.154. Sealing cement applied to the apex.

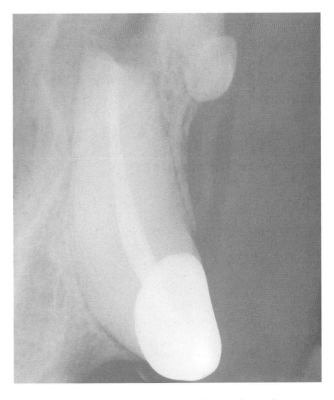

FIGURE 7.155. Post-operative radiograph confirming apical amputation and seal.

7. Take a radiograph to confirm the apical seal (Figure 7.155).
8. Place Consil according to the manufacturer's instructions after the alveolus is cleaned thoroughly.
9. Close and suture the flap.

10. Send the patient home with antibiotics and pain relief medication.

Radiographs are taken at 4 and 12 months postoperatively to monitor healing.

Surgical endodontics of multiple-rooted teeth are treated in a similar fashion. The maxillary palatal root apices of the fouth premolar and molars cannot be surgically exposed and are either hemisected or conventionally instrumented and obturated (Figures 7.156–7.158).

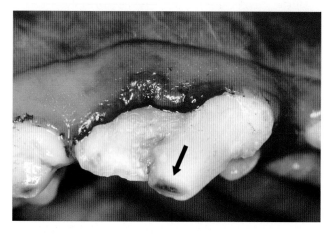

FIGURE 7.156. Fractured maxillary fourth premolar with apparent pulp exposure.

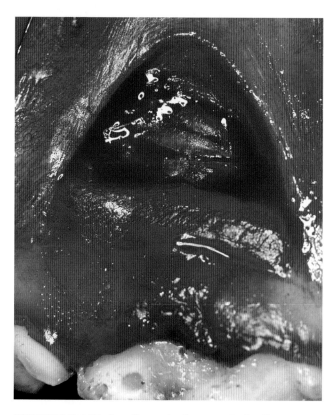

FIGURE 7.157. Semilunar incison made for flap exposure of both buccal maxillary fourth premolar roots.

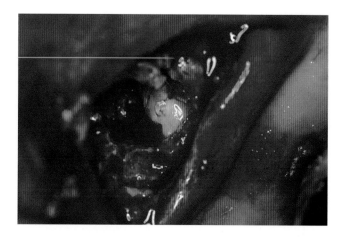

FIGURE 7.158. Apical cement applied to amputated mesiobuccal root.

ENDODONTIC-PERIODONTIC LESIONS

Some animals are affected by both endodontic and periodontal lesions in the same tooth. Communication from the pulp to the periodontal apparatus can originate from the tooth's apex or lateral canal(s). To be classified as an endodontic-periodontic lesion, the tooth must have at least one root with a necrotic pulp and destruction of the periodontal attachment extending from the gingival pocket to the lateral canal or tooth apex. Periodontic-endodontic lesions start as periodontal disease of the tooth, in which bacteria migrates into the endodontic system through lateral canal(s) or through the apical delta.

Endodontic/periodontic pathology classification:

- *Class 0 lesion* is primarily endodontic in origin with minimal or no periodontal involvement (Figure 7.159).
- *Class I endodontic-periodontic (endoperio) lesion* is endodontic in origin and progresses to involve the periodontal tissues. Clinically, there is usually a fractured tooth and a draining canal that exits near the gingival margin. Radiographically, this "J" lesion with the typical periapical radiolucent halo extending a thin radiolucent strip coronally along the root to the gingival margin is pathognomic for endoperio disease (Figures 7.160–7.166).
- *Class II periodontic-endodontic (perioendo) lesion* is periodontal in origin and progresses to invade the pulp. Clinically, a periodontal probe usually extends easily to the apex. Radiographically, there is a marked uniform radiolucent area extending from the gingival margin around the apex of the root.
- *Class III combined endodontic-periodontic lesion* is a combination of independent endodontic and peri-

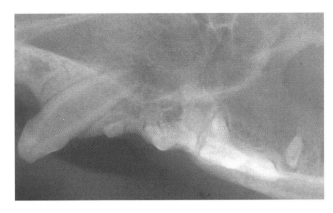

FIGURE 7.159. Class 0 lesion without periodontal involvement.

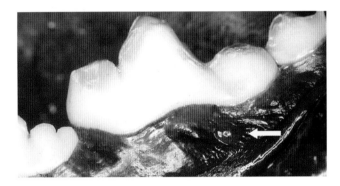

FIGURE 7.160. Mandibular first molar with lesion on the attached gingiva.

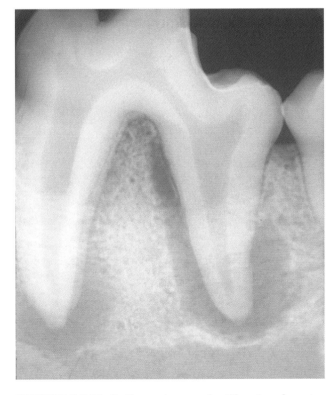

FIGURE 7.161. Radiographs reveal a Class I endoperio "J" lesion.

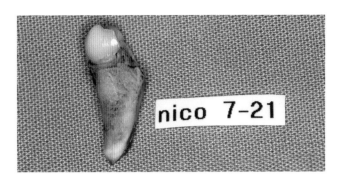

FIGURE 7.162. Hemisected distal root.

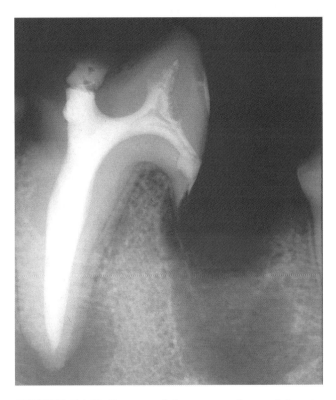

FIGURE 7.163. Root canal therapy on the mesial root of a mandibular first molar in a dog.

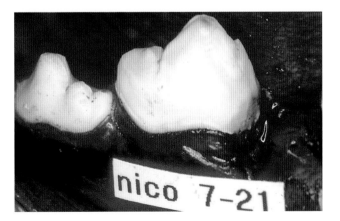

FIGURE 7.164. Post-operative hemisected mandibular first molar.

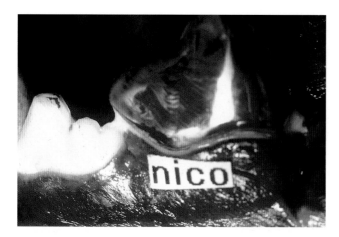

FIGURE 7.165. Crown restoration.

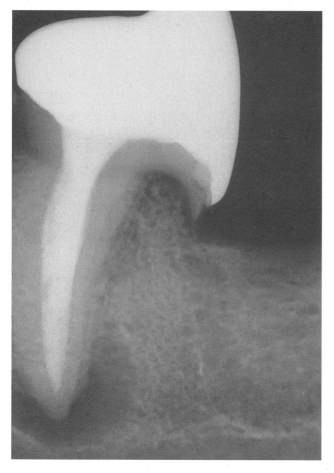

FIGURE 7.166. Three-month post-operative radiograph showing bone fill of distal root defect.

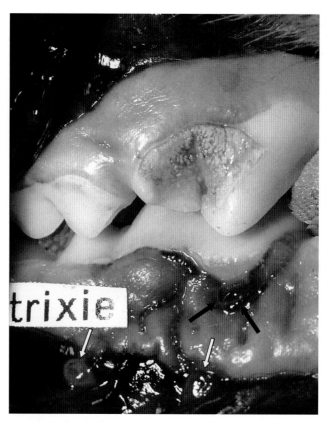

FIGURE 7.167. Clinical appearance of combined endodontic-periodontic lesion (note lesions at the mucogingival line plus gingival recession).

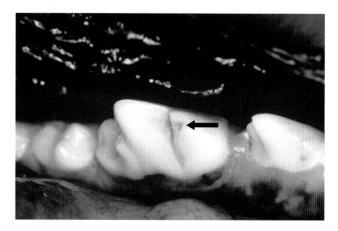

FIGURE 7.168. Fractured mesial cusp of the mandibular first molar in a dog (arrow indicates area of pulpal exposure).

odontic lesions, which are not associated but present on the same tooth. Clinically, there is a fractured tooth, with advanced periodontal disease shown as an easily probed periodontal pocket that extends to the apex (Figures 7.167–7.169).

Therapy for endodontic periodontic lesions depends on the degree of periodontal involvement. In cases of minor involvement (class I), conventional or surgical endodontics is indicated. When attachment loss is marked, extraction of the tooth, or hemisection of the affected half of the tooth plus standard root canal therapy on the remaining root(s) is the treatment of choice.

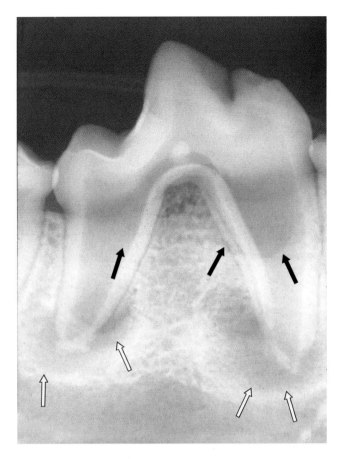

FIGURE 7.169. Radiographic appearance of combined endodontic-periodontic lesion in figure 7.167 (endontic lesions—white arrows; periodontic lesions—black arrows).

ENDODONTIC THERAPY COMPLICATIONS

The best way to avoid endodontic complications and potential failure is to choose cases wisely based on clinical and radiographic findings. Teeth with roots resorbed, vertical root fractures, or those affected with marked support loss are prone to failure even with advanced salvage procedures.

Persistent hemorrhage is usually due to failure to remove all the vital pulpal tissue or perforation of the root. Radiographic examination can confirm perforation if the file is in place.

The following are treatment options in cases where some pulp tissue remains despite best debridement attempts:

- The root canal can be irrigated with lidocaine plus epinephrine 1:100,000, or epinephrine can be introduced into the root with a paper point and allowed to remain 3–5 minutes. Bleeding is re-evaluated with additional paper points.

- Calcium hydroxide powder or paste can be applied to the apex using a paper point.
- A mummifying agent (Formocresol: Burns 951-3876, Schein 102-9994) can be applied to a paper point inserted in the canal (Figure 7.170). The access is then sealed with temporary filler, such as Cavit-G (ESPE America, Inc.) (Burns 878-0360, Schein 378-4404). Two weeks later, the canal is reopened, the paper point(s) removed with a small file and the canal obturated.

Overinstrumentation is the perforation of the apex, root wall, or pulpal floor during debridement. Overinstrumentation occurs from:

- Incorrect bur position when searching for the pulp chamber, which may result in perforating the pulpal floor
- Excessive pressure placed on the endodontic file, especially in a young tooth
- Excessive twisting of the file (usually Hedstrom), acting as a corkscrew perforating the apex
- Perforation can occur with chronic lesions and external resorption of the apical delta.

Clinically, perforation usually results in persistent bleeding. When perforation is suspected, sodium hypochlorite used for irrigation should be discontinued due to the potential soft tissue irritation and severe pain.

Therapy options if perforation occurs include the following:

- A small amount of hard-setting calcium hydroxide cement (Dycal Dentsply International) or MTA can be placed at the apex using the tip of a paper point. After the material sets, obturation using a step-back technique to create a new apical stop for a larger gutta percha point is performed.

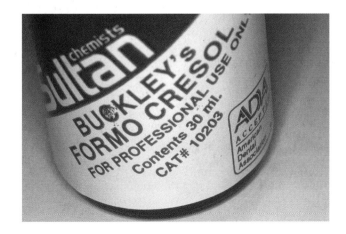

FIGURE 7.170. Mummifying agent.

- Using a calcium hydroxide sealer, the canal is filled with a Lentulo spiral before the master gutta percha point is placed. Some calcium hydroxide will be pushed through the perforation stimulating apical closure.

Incomplete fill is a common endodontic problem, which occurs when the canal is underinstrumented or underobturated. If the pulp cavity is not completely obturated, space or tissue remains, which can lead to further periapical disease from bacterial leakage. When radiographs reveal an incomplete fill, the canal should be reinstrumented to the point of the underfill and refilled (Figure 7.171).

Overfill occurs occasionally, when sealer cement and/or gutta percha extrudes from the apex due to excessive pressure applied in the compaction process, or apical penetration. The extruded sealer is usually resorbed by the periapical tissues (Figure 7.172).

Fractured (separated or disarticulated) files result from:

- Overzealous twisting and/or excessive downward pressure applied on a standard or rotary file.

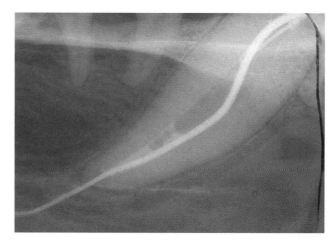

FIGURE 7.172. Gutta percha extending through the apex.

- Excessive use of files leading to weakening and eventual separation.
- Excessive clockwise rotation inside the canal. K files should be rotated only 90° before retrograde pulling; H files should be used in a push-pull stroke without rotation.

If the file fragment is lodged and broken at the beginning of the procedure, it has to be removed to permit complete debriding of the canal. If the file cannot be retrieved, a surgical root canal or extraction is performed. If the file separates after the canal is cleaned past a #30 file, it can be left in the patient and followed clinically and radiographically throughout the patient's life.

Options for broken file removal include the following:

- The separated fragment is hooked with another file or barbed broach and gently pulled backward.
- Cancelliers are stiff, fine, hollow tubes used to gain access to the canal for insertion and retrieval of the separated file (eie Analytic Technology, CK Dental Specialties).
- Mounces are channel-cut ball-ended, stainless steel probes used to retrieve nickel-titanium files (eie Analytic Technology Specialties).
- Fine forceps can be used to remove the fragment (Cislak Peets Forceps #5217).
- Ultrasonic handpiece vibrations, when placed against the fragment, may dislodge the file.
- A paper point can be advanced to engage the file.
- A strong magnet or magnetized file can be used.
- Gravity may make an impact.

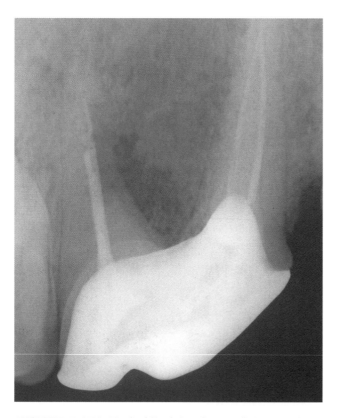

FIGURE 7.171. Underfill of distal root of the maxillary fourth premolar resulted in therapy failure.

FOLLOW-UP CARE

The patient should be reexamined 1 week after endodontic care for evidence of gingival inflammation at the gingival margin or apex. Depending on the case, additional intraoral radiographs are recommended 4, 12, and 24 months post-operatively.

Success is measured by either a decrease in size or resolution of the clinical and radiographic periapical pathology. Failure exists when the observed lesions persist or increase in size.

Causes of failure include:

- Insufficient instrumentation
- Incomplete obturation
- Gross overfill
- Presence of nonobturated additional (lateral) canal(s)
- Fractured root(s)
- Root perforation

Table 7.2 summarizes endodontic care.

Table 7.2. Endodontic care at a glance.

Lesion	Appearance	Diagnosis/Treatment
Enamel fractured	Nick or gouge occurs on the enamel surface.	Radiographs to evaluate the presence of root fractures or periapical pathology. The defect is smoothed with a white stone bur on a high-speed water-cooled delivery system followed by application of a bonding agent.
Enamel and dentin fractured	Yellow dentin is exposed.	If pulp is visualized beneath the dentin, direct/or indirect pulp capping can be performed for pulp protection. If pulp is not observed, depending on the patient's age, crown restoration may protect the pulp if the patient is young (6 years or younger) as long as radiogrphs show the pulp is protected by dentin. Radiograph immediately, and again in 6 and 12 months.
Enamel, dentin, pulp exposure	Pulp shows either as red dot (recent fracture), or as black penetrating hole into pulp chamber (chronic). If pulp is exposed more than 48 hours, it can be considered chronic exposure.	Vital pulpotomy procedure to allow apexogenesis to proceed if the patient is less than 9 months old and the pulp not infected. If infected with an open apex, apexification is the desired outcome, using calcium hydroxide to stimulate hard tissue deposition. Conventional endodontics is performed if the apex is closed and the tooth support adequate. If marked periodontal disease is present, extract. Surgical endodontics if apex is not sealable conventionally.
Endoperio lesions	Inflammatory swelling is noted above and below the mucogingival line, or fractured tooth that is also mobile due to periodontal disease.	If the tooth is salvageable, first care for the endodontic disease and wait for healing; then address periodontal disease if necessary.
Pulpitis	Discolored tooth occurs (off-white, pink, purple, brown, gray).	If less than 9 months and only coronally pink, antibiotics and anti-inflamatories. If the entire tooth is discolored, and apical closure is radiographically not present, fill the tooth with calcium hydroxide mix after removing pulp (apexification). If apex is closed, conventional or surgical endodontics is indicated.
Avulsed tooth	Tooth is completely out of socket due to trauma.	Replace and stabilize tooth in alveolus. Root canal therapy 3–6 weeks after initial treatment. If the owner does not agree to future endodontics, the tooth should not be replaced

8

Restorative Equipment, Materials, and Techniques

Restorative dentistry has the following objectives:

- To return (restore) teeth to optimum form and function.
- To prevent breakdown of the remaining tooth structure.
- To protect pulp tissue from thermal, mechanical, and bacterial insult.
- To create a proper or aesthetic tooth appearance.

Appearance and function conflict often. Restoring a tooth to normal size and color may not make the tooth optimally functional because of its inability to hold up to repeated trauma. In cases of conflict, function should prevail.

Restorative materials include the following:

- Amalgam
- Composite resin
- Glass ionomer
- Metal crown
- Ceramic crown
- Porcelain crown

AMALGAM

Mercury in amalgam is mixed with tin, copper, and zinc to create alloys that form strong surface restoratives (Burns 952-6964, Schein 100-0225) (Figure 8.1). Amalgam has stood the test of time in human dentistry and is still used to restore human occlusal surface carious lesions. Amalgam's use in veterinary dentistry is minimal, because:

- The special handling requirements related to mercury:
  - Amalgam should never be touched with bare hands.
  - Masks must be worn when working with amalgam.
  - The work area must be well ventilated.

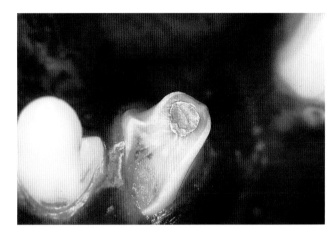

FIGURE 8.1. Amalgam restorative before polishing in a mandibular corner incisor of a dog.

- The need for additional equipment to mix (titrate) encapsulated dental materials (amalgamator: Burns 950-0819, Schein 100-2532)
- Poor cosmetic appearance
- Marginal leakage
- Corrosion
- Amalgam tattooing

COMPOSITE RESINS

Composite resins are tooth-colored plastic–silicon dioxide mixtures used to restore injured teeth.

The following are composite advantages:

- Easy to apply
- Allows conservative cavity preparation, which in some cases leaves the tooth stronger than it would be with amalgam

231

Glossary

Abrasion is the mechanical wearing away of the tooth structure by abnormal stresses.

Adhesive is an intermediate substance that causes two materials to stick together.

Base is a material placed under a dental restoration to insulate the pulp.

Biologic width is the distance physiologically necessary for healthy existence of bone and soft tissue from the most apical extent of a dental restoration.

Bonding is the process of forming an adhesive joint.

Bonding agent is a material used to attach a restorative to the tooth. The bonding agent is applied to the etched enamel or dentin surface, creating a strong micromechanical bond with the tooth surface.

Buccal is the surface of premolar and molar teeth that face toward the cheeks.

Cap (used synonymously with crown) is the restoration of a tooth by the removal of the outer most 1–2 mm coronal surface and replacement with a hard cover.

Cast crown is a metallic restoration that fully or partially covers the visible portion of the tooth.

Chamfer is the tapered finish line or margin placed on the crown preparation frequently used with metal crowns.

Compomer is a combination of glass ionomer with composite resin.

Composite resin is a material used for restorative purposes formed by a reaction of epoxy with an acrylic monomer.

Coupling agent chemically bonds filler to a resin matrix by coating the filler particles with an organosilane compound.

Crown (clinical) is the portion of the tooth covered with enamel inside the oral cavity.

Crown buildup is the process of adding material to cover pins or posts during fractured tooth restoration.

Crown lengthening is a surgical procedure for lengthening the clinical crown to enhance the attachment of a synthetic crown.

Cusp is the tip of the crown.

Dentin is the hard calcified inner layer of tooth structure, immediately covered by enamel and cementum.

Distal is the surface oriented away from the midline of the arch.

Enamel is the hard calcified tissue that covers the anatomic crown of the tooth.

Enamel hypoplasia (hypocalcification) is a developmental lesion, which may affect one or multiple teeth characterized by area(s) of enamel loss. Enamel hypoplasia lesions are caused by an elevated temperature, malnutrition, mechanical trauma, or parasitism resulting in damage to the ameloblasts while the teeth are developing.

Etching is a process used to decalcify the superficial layers of enamel during the restorative process. Etching enlarges the enamel surface for micromechanical anchorage of composite.

Facial is the surface of teeth that face the lips or cheeks.

Gingivoplasty is the surgical contouring of gingival tissues.

Glass ionomer cement is a dental material of low strength and toughness used for small restorations in low stress areas or as an intermediate layer between composite and gutta percha.

Jacket crown is a metal, porcelain, or acrylic resin that covers the clinical crown.

Labial is the surface of an anterior tooth that faces toward the lips.

Lingual is the surface of a mandibular tooth that faces toward the tongue.

Margin is the interface where the restoration meets the natural tooth.

Mesial is the tooth surface closest to the midline of the arch.

Palatal is the surface of a maxillary tooth that faces toward the hard palate.

Polymerization is the process in which resin material is changed from a monomer to polymer state.

Smear layer is a thin coating of organic debris covering the dentin. Removing the smear layer using a dentin conditioner exposes the dentin tubules.

- Can be bonded to dentin and enamel, creating a strong restoration
- Offers pleasing aesthetics
- Offers good wear
- Minimal marginal leakage

Composites commonly contain two components:

- *Organic matrix* (acrylic foundation phase, Type I) is unfilled resin used to coat preparations to prevent microleakage. This resin is not strong enough to be used as a sole dental material. Type I resin bonds to Type II resin.

- *Inorganic fillers* (dispersed phase, Type II) are quartz, glass, and silica particles. The amount of filler and particle size determine strength, wear resistance, hardness, and polish finish of the material:
  - *Macrofilled,* also known as *conventional,* composites contain the largest filler particles, which provide great strength but are dull and rough. Macrofilled composites are used only in posterior restorations, where strength is required to resist fracture. In most cases, hybrids are better choices than macrofilled composites, which do not polish well, are porous, and are plaque-retentive.

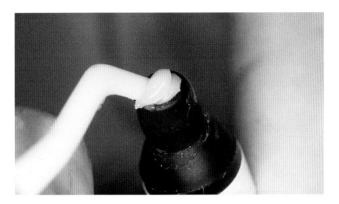

FIGURE 8.2. Hybrid composite material removed with teflon spatula from a restorative compule.

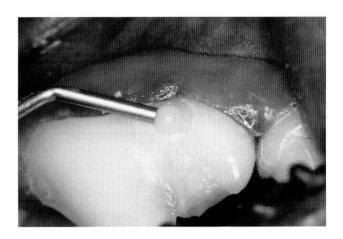

FIGURE 8.4. Flowable composite.

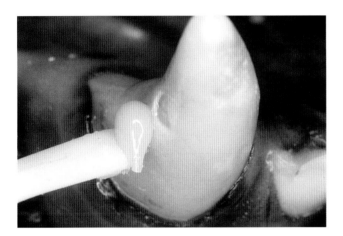

Figure 8.3. Composite material being applied to an enamel defect.

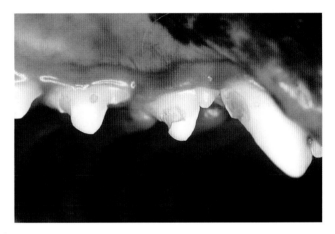

FIGURE 8.5. Maxillary second, third, and fourth premolars affected by enamel hypoplasia.

- *Microfilled* composites use smaller inorganic particles, yielding a highly polishable finished restoration. Microfilled composites are rarely used, because wear and strength are more important than aesthetics in most small animal restorative cases.
- *Hybrid composites* contain both macrofill and microfill particles. The hybrids are more polishable than the macrofilled composites and have greater strength and wear resistance than microfilled. Hybrid composites are most applicable for veterinary dental use (Z-100, Schein 777-2288; Z-250, 3M ESPE) (Figures 8.2, 8.3).
- *Flowable composite resins* are of low viscosity hybrids indicated for areas of low stress, such as non-incisal enamel lesions on anterior teeth typical of enamel hypoplasia lesions (Revolution: Burns 954-1282, Schein 123-2235, Flow-it Jeneric/Pentron) (Figures 8.4, 8.5).

- *Packable, condensable composites* have strength, wear resistance, and are aesthetic. High viscosity of packable composites can result in poor adaptation to cavity walls. Examples include SureFil (Dentsply), Prodigy condensable (Kerr), Alert (Jeneric/Pentron).

Curing

Polymerization (curing) occurs either chemically through mixing or by light activation. Polymerization is an ongoing process that continues even after the material initially hardens.

Self-cured (auto-cured) composites, also called *chemically activated resins,* come as two components (usually two pastes). One paste contains a benzyl peroxide initiator, and the other contains a tertiary amine activator. When the two pastes are spatulated, the amine reacts with benzyl peroxide to form free radicals, which initiate polymerization. The initial curing action proceeds from start to finish within 5 minutes. Self-cured composites should be kept refrigerated; continued exposure to heat can inactivate the catalyst paste.

Light cured resins polymerize when exposed to high intensity (450 nm) blue light generated by a halogen or plasma system. The composite is stored in a lightproof syringe (compule). The paste contains a photoinitiator molecule and an amine activator. Light cured resins do not require mixing. When using light cured composites, the veterinarian has a prolonged amount of working time to shape the restoration before applying the light source (Figure 8.6).

Dual-cured composites polymerize partially as the material is mixed. The final cure occurs when the composite is exposed to the curing light.

The *curing light* consists of a lighted wand, protective shield, handle, and trigger switch. The light is used to activate light cured composites and bonding agents. Most curing lights can penetrate to a depth of 2.0 mm into the composite. The amount of intensity reaching composite is related to the age of the bulb, the condition of the light-guide and wand, distance of the light from the restoration, and time of application (Burns 955-7400, Schein 100-5151) (Figures 8.7–8.9).

Surgery lights should be diverted from the operatory field during light-cured composite placement. Any intense light can initiate the hardening process. Orascoptic (Sybron Dental Specialties) produces a high-intensity light source with a light cure–inhibiting filter.

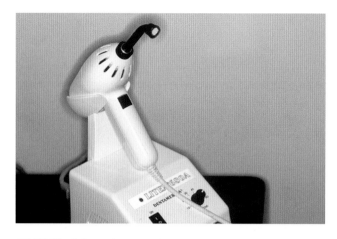

FIGURE 8.7. Light cure "gun."

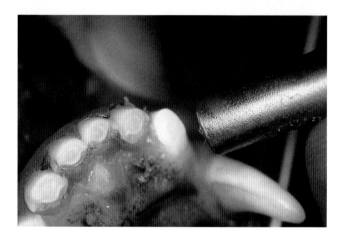

FIGURE 8.8. Curing light wand.

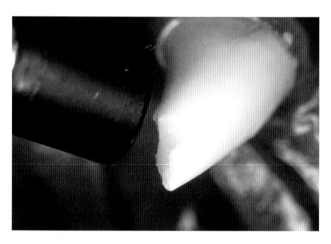

FIGURE 8.6. Light applied to adhesive during the light cure process.

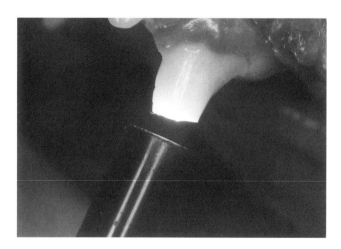

FIGURE 8.9. Correct distance between light wand and restored area.

Curing time depends upon:

- The manufacturer's instructions, most often 20–60 seconds.
- The thickness and size of the restoration. Only that portion of the material exposed to sufficient intensity of light energy will adequately cure. Deep restorations often have to be layered and cured every 1–2 mm.
- The shade of restorative material. Darker shades need longer curing time.

Undercure is a common cause for failure of composite resin restorations. A radiometer should be used when the light is new and monthly to test the light source power, which must be rated at a minimum of 300 milliwatts per meter square (mw/cm^2) to cure properly. If the power rating drops to less than 200 mw/cm^2, curing time should be lengthened, or the bulb replaced. The curing light should be activated for 10 seconds before testing. Test the curing light when it is new (Figure 8.10).

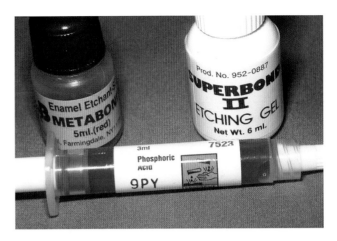

FIGURE 8.11. Etching gel and liquid.

ETCHING

Acid etching is a technique wherein maleic acid or phosphoric acid is placed on the enamel for a short period and then rinsed. Etching is used to increase the enamel bonding surface area and to remove the dentin smear layer. This allows the bonding agent to penetrate into the dentin tubules, creating a micromechanical interlock between the restoration and dentin. Etchants are supplied in either liquid or gel form. Application of the gel allows the etchant to be carefully placed where it is needed (Burns 951-9192, Schein Etch gel 100-4649) (Figure 8.11).

Basic etching procedure includes these steps (follow specific manufacturer's instructions):

1. The surface of the tooth is cleaned and polished with flour of pumice (Figure 8.12).
2. After cleaning, the surface is lightly dried but not desiccated.
3. The prepared tooth is protected with gauze to prevent moisture (saliva) from contaminating the preparation.
4. Etchant is placed and allowed to remain for the time recommended by the manufacturer (30–40 seconds for enamel, 10–15 seconds for dentin) (Figure 8.13).
5. After etching, the surface is thoroughly rinsed for one minute and lightly dried (Figure 8.14).
6. An etched surface appears frosty white. If the surface does not appear chalky, or has been contaminated with moisture, the etching process should be repeated.

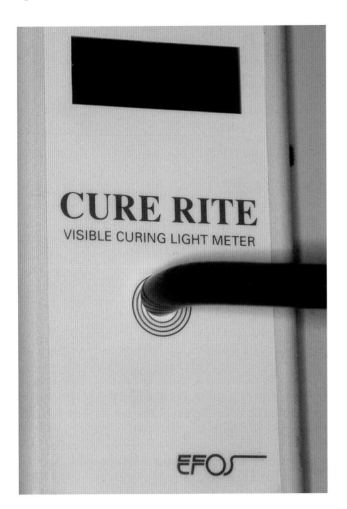

FIGURE 8.10. Curing light meter.

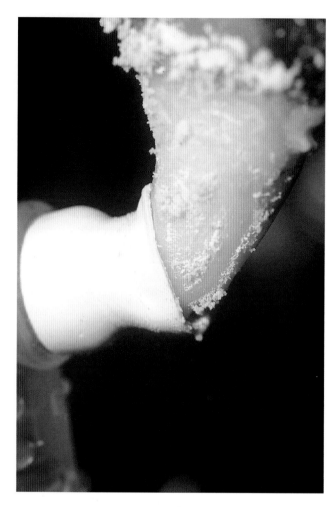

FIGURE 8.12. Application of pumice with a polishing cup on low-speed handpiece.

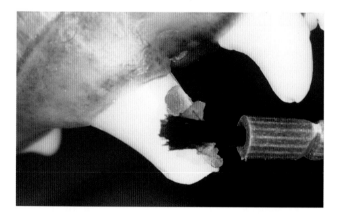

FIGURE 8.13. Application of etchant gel using a brush.

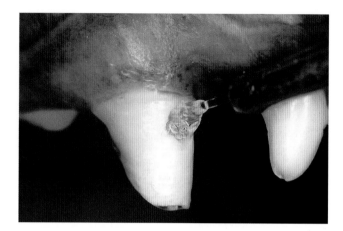

FIGURE 8.14. Rinsing the tooth surface.

BONDING SYSTEMS

Composite resins require bonding agents; glass ionomer cements do not. Bonding improves retention through the creation of a micromechanical attachment between the tooth structure and the restoration.

Bonding systems are available as self-cured, dual-cured, and light cured. Systems use one, two, or three liquids and are either single or multistepped.

During some bonding processes, *etchant* removes the smear layer, *primer* opens the dentin tubules, and *adhesive* flows into the partially opened tubules.

Bonding agents are classified by generations:

- *First generation:* The etchant is applied and washed off to remove the dentin smear layer; primer and adhesive are applied separately.
- *Second generation:* Etchant is applied and washed off to remove the smear layer; primer and adhesive are applied as a single solution.
- *Third generation:* Self-etching primer is applied to dissolve the smear layer and is not washed off. Adhesive is applied separately.
- *Fourth generation:* Self-etching primer and adhesive (total-etch technique) are applied as a single solution, and the surface is left wet to avoid collagen collapse. With fourth-generation bonding systems, the formation of resin tags and adhesive lateral branches completes the bonding mechanism between the adhesive materials and etched dentin.
- *Fifth generation:* There are two different types of fifth generation bonding systems: the one-bottle system, which combines the primer and adhesive into one solution which is applied to etched enamel and dentin; and the self-etching primer bonding system, which reduces the working time, eliminating washing.

- *Sixth generation*: One solution bonds to dentin and enamel. Unfortunately, the first evaluations of this system showed a sufficient bond to conditioned dentin, but the bond with enamel was less effective.

The following are commonly used dentin bonding systems:

- Tenure (Denmat)
- One Step (Bisco)
- All Bond (Bisco)
- Prisma Universal Bond (L.D.Caulk)
- Single Bond (3M ESPE)
- Gluma (Gluma/Miles)
- Clearfil Photo-bond (J. Morita)
- Imperva Bond (Shofu)
- Pertac Universal Bond (Premier)
- Optibond (Kerr)

Materials for light cured composite resin restoration:

- Flour pumice (Burns 907-6002, Schein 100-3821)
- Disposable brushes (Burns 950-3556, Schein 102-9206)
- Phosphoric acid etchant (Burns 951-9192, Schein 100-4649)
- Scotchbond multipurpose dental adhesive 3M ESPE kit (Burns 867-2231, Schein 777-5719)
- Flow-It flowable composite
- Z-100 Restorative syringe refills (Burns 867-7253, Schein 777-4396 A1) (Figure 8.15) (3M Filtek Z250 Universal Restorative as well as other composites can also be used.)
- Plastic, nylon, or aluminum applicators (other metals are contraindicated in composite placement because composite removes metal from the spatula discolor-ing the final restoration) (Burns 953-1733, Schein 100-0049) (Figure 8.16)
- Curing light (Burns 955-7400, Schein 100-5151)
- 12-blade finishing burs 7901 or 7406
- Finishing disc kit (Burns 868-0690, Schein 777-3262), Sof-lex, (3M), Enhance Polishing System (Caulk/Dentsply) (Burns 813-8871)

The following are basic steps in the typical light cure restoration process. Each bonding system is different; manufacturer's directions should be followed:

1. If the restoration area is a cavity or an endodontic access (Figure 8.17), remove 1–2 mm of enamel and dentin using a round or inverted cone bur. A proper preparation leaves no unsupported enamel. Take care to avoid pulp or near-pulp exposure in the vital tooth. Undercutting for composite restorations is controversial, weakens the tooth, and may not be necessary thanks to the advent of newer composite resins (Figure 8.18).

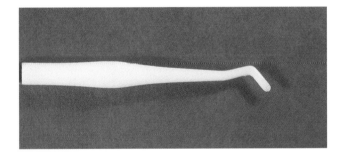

FIGURE 8.16. Plastic spatula to apply composite.

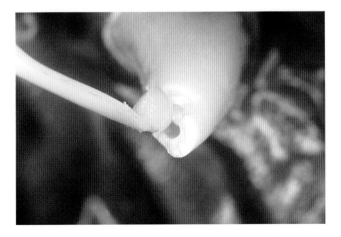

FIGURE 8.15. Composite application.

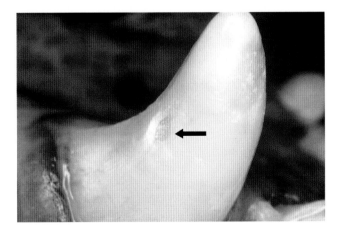

FIGURE 8.17. Enamel defect.

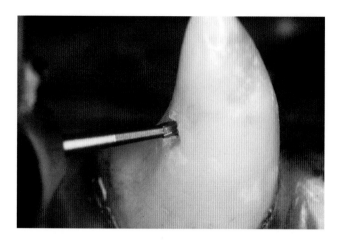

FIGURE 8.18. An inverted cone bur used to undercut the enamel for retention.

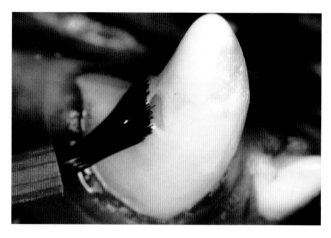

FIGURE 8.19. Primer is applied.

2. Clean the restoration site with fluoride-free pumice. Prepare pumice polish by mixing flour pumice with water. After polishing, rinse and air-dry the residue.
3. Etching procedure:
   a. Place a cotton pellet in a container of 37% phosphoric acid etching solution.
   b. Press the pellet lightly on the enamel margins of the preparation. Take care to avoid swabbing acid on the entire enamel surface.
   c. After approximately 15 seconds (or according to the manufacturer's instructions), rinse the enamel thoroughly and dry it with an oil-free air source. The surface should appear chalky white and left dry but not desiccated. If the tooth becomes overly dry, wet it with a cotton pledget and gently dry.
4. If the tooth is vital, apply a thin layer of *primer* to the exposed dentin. Primer prepares dentin for the adhesive. It is not necessary to apply primer to enamel surfaces. After application, gently air-dry the dentin primer or rinse according to the manufacturer's directions (Figure 8.19).
5. Mix the *bonding agent (dental adhesive)* according to the manufacturer's instructions and place it over the etched enamel. Some bonding agents require light curing immediately after placement (Figure 8.20).
6. Using a plastic or aluminum applicator, or injection device, place 1–2 mm *light cure resin composite* in increments onto the restoration area (Figure 8.21). A clear Mylar strip can be used to compress the composite over the restoration site (Burns 951-6162, Schein 100-8525).
7. Light cure the composite material 20–60 seconds through the Mylar strip according to manufacturer's

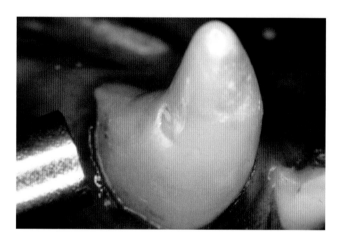

FIGURE 8.20. The adhesive is light cured.

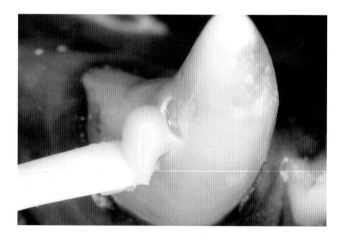

FIGURE 8.21. Composite material is applied on the prepared defect with a plastic spatula.

instructions. Add an additional 1–2 mm of composite and light cure until the defect is slightly overfilled.

When composite is light cured, there is approximately 2% microscopic shrinkage at the curing site. This shrinkage can lead to microfissures and leakage. Slow (pulse-delay) curing results in better marginal adaptation, increasing long-term success. Pulse-delay curing involves using short, low-intensity light exposure at the composite-filled restoration site, finishing the restoration, waiting five minutes, and then curing with full-intensity exposure for the recommended time.

8. Finish the restoration by using 12–30 fluted finishing burs, sanding disks (for flat surfaces), or green stones followed by white stones (Figures 8.22, 8.23). Composite finishing discs attach to a mandrel, which fits into the slow-speed contra-angle or straight handpiece. Disc abrasion ranges from coarse, used to debulk the restoration at the beginning of the finishing process, to extra fine. Examples of composite finishing discs include:

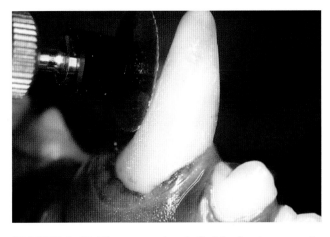

FIGURE 8.22. The restoration is finished using a sanding disc.

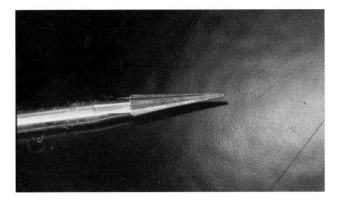

FIGURE 8.23. Finishing bur.

- Sof-lex (3M) (Burns 867-3015, Schein 777-3262)
- Caulk Enhance (Burns 813-8871, Schein 222-5759)
- Moore-Flex (Burns 868-0690, Schein 294-0551)

9. Check the restored tooth for occlusion to make sure there is no interference or abnormal contact.
10. Re-etch and rinse the site, reapply the bonding agent, and light cure over the restoration to give a smooth finish and to seal marginal leaks that developed from polymerization shrinkage.

GLASS IONOMERS

Glass ionomers are hybrids of silicate and polycarboxylate cements. Glass ionomer restoratives bond chemically to enamel, dentin, and metallic materials. This reduces the need for extensive mechanical preparation of the tooth. The bond to enamel is stronger than to dentin. Glass ionomer cements and restoratives generally:

- Release fluoride ions over years. Fluoride has been shown to strengthen enamel, decrease dentinal sensitivity, and provide an antibacterial effect.
- Act as thermal insulators.
- Are relatively non-irritating to the pulp.
- Can be placed in slightly moist environments.
- Can be placed under composite resins to reduce the polymerization shrinkage.
- Gradually harden over years.
- Are technique-sensitive, and if not applied correctly, will fail.
- Have poor compressive strength and do not wear well on occlusal surfaces.

Table 8.1 summarizes the glass ionomer cement classification.

Glass ionomers can also be classified by composition:

- *Glass ionomer cements* consist of an acid-decomposable glass and an acidic polymer that undergo an acid/base reaction when mixed (Figure 8.24). The reaction does not require light to occur. Examples of these products are Ketac-fil (3M ESPE) and Fuji II (GC America).
- *Resin-modified glass ionomers* have a resin added that is activated by light exposure. Examples are Fuji II LC (GC America), and Photac-Fil (3M ESPE).
- *Polyacid-modified composite resin* contains little glass ionomer and requires light to set. Examples are VariGlass VLC (Caulk), Dyract (Caulk) and Geristore (Dent-Mat).

Table 8.1. Glass ionomer cement classification.

Type	Example	Use
Type I	Fuji Cap I (GC America)	Cements for holding crowns, direct-bonded brackets, and orthodontic appliances.
Type II	Fuji Ionomer Type II (GC America) Ketac-Fil (3M ESPE)	Restorative for carious lesions and for restoring areas of erosion near the gingiva. Generally harder and stronger than Type I, Type II is not used for cementation.
Type III	GC Lining Cement (GC America)	Base and liner used under composite restorations.
Type IV	Vitrebond(3M ESPE) XR Ionomer (SDS/Kerr) Zionomer (Den-mat) Fuji Lining LC (GC America), Photac-Bond (3M ESPE)	Visible light-activated liner/base. Hybrid forms resin-modified glass ionomer cement (Fuji II LC Improved (GC America), Vitremer Core Buildup/restorative (3M ESPE), Photac-Fil (3m ESPE) Sets by an acid/base reaction as well as a photo and/or chemical reaction.

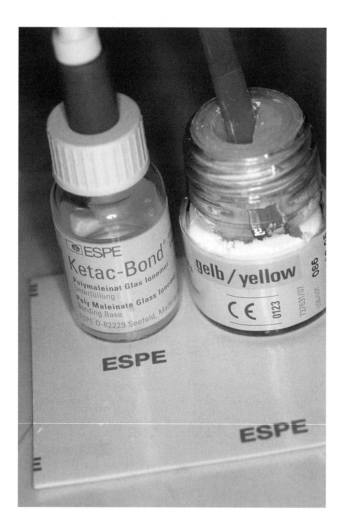

FIGURE 8.24. Type II glass ionomer cement.

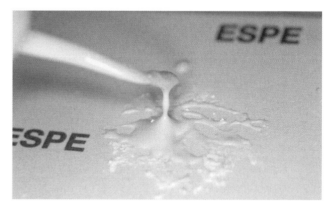

FIGURE 8.25. Mixed Type II non-encapsulated glass ionomer cement.

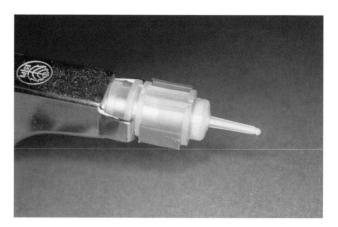

FIGURE 8.26. Encapsulated glass ionomer where the powder and liquid are in one container.

Glass ionomers are available in the following forms:

- *Non-encapsulated,* wherein liquid and powder are mixed with a spatula on a pad to a honey-like consistency before applying (Figure 8.25).
- *Encapsulated,* containing both powder and liquid in one container. The capsules require an amalgamator for mixing and a special applicator to place the mixture on the tooth. (Ketac-Fil and Chelon-Silver, 3M ESPE) (Figure 8.26).

The technique for using glass ionomers in restorations varies by type and manufacturer, when using Ketac-Fil (3M ESPE):

1. Clean the restoration surfaces with flour pumice and water on a polishing cup.
2. Gently dry the surface, but not until desiccated. If the surface is too dry, the bond will be weak. Acid etching is not necessary unless recommended by the manufacturer.
3. If recommended by the manufacturer, a conditioner (polyacrylic acid) is applied, rinsed, and slightly dried to remove the dentin smear layer. By removing the smear layer, the glass ionomer cement bonds to dentin and not to the smear layer.
4. When using the non-encapsulated form, gently shake the jar to fluff the powder before using. Insert the scoop into the jar, overfill with loosely packed powder, and withdraw against the plastic leveler (on the lid) to remove excess powder and obtain a level scoop (Figure 8.27).
5. Dispense the manufacturer's recommended number of drops of liquid onto the mixing pad next to the powder (Figure 8.28).
6. Mix the liquid and powder rapidly with a spatula in a small 1-inch area, which should produce a homogenous glossy liquid in 20 seconds. Place the mixture on the restoration site using a ball applicator, plastic working instrument, or Centrix tube and plug system before it loses its shiny appearance (Figures 8.29–8.33).
7. When the cement is in place, protect it from desiccation and moisture contamination while setting by covering with varnish or unfilled resin. Allow self-cured glass ionomer cement to set and harden for 20 minutes before using finishing burs or sanding disks. Maximum hardness takes place within 24 hours. Light cured glass ionomer cement is exposed to 30 seconds of the light cure unit. Maximum curing depth is 2.0 mm. Thicker applications can be achieved by placing and curing increments separately.

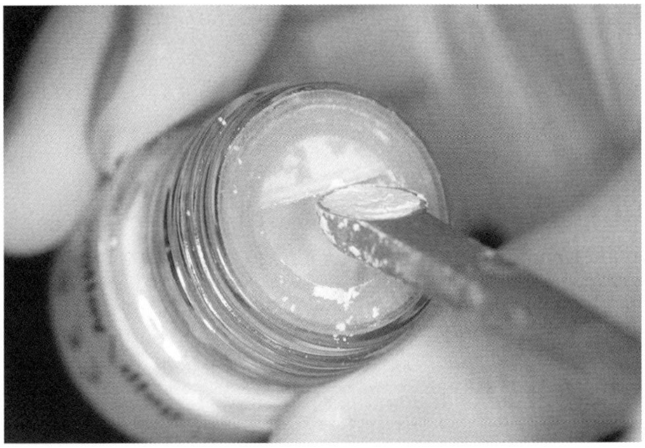

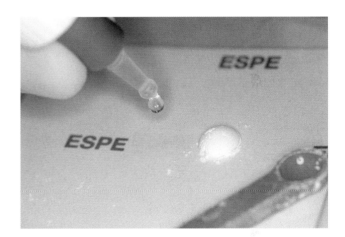

FIGURE 8.28. Liquid placed next to powder before mixing.

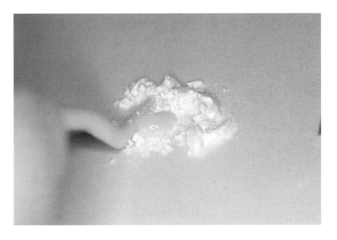

FIGURE 8.29. Using a spatula to mix the liquid and powder.

FIGURE 8.27. Removing a level powder scoop.

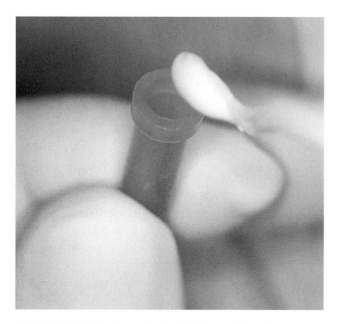

FIGURE 8.30. Mixture is loaded into a Centrix syringe tip.

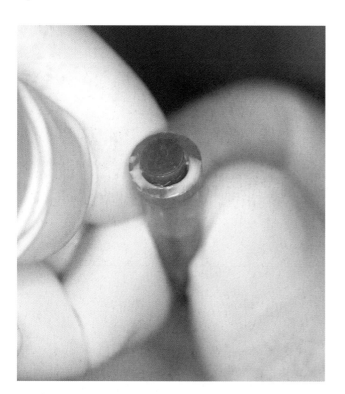

FIGURE 8.31. Cap is placed on top of syringe tip.

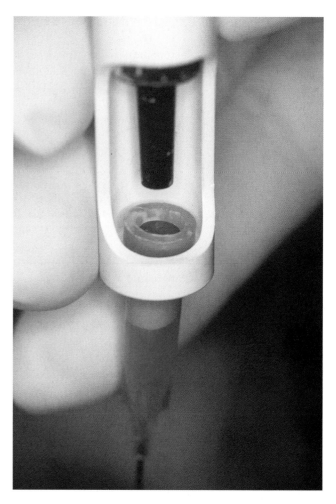

FIGURE 8.32. Filled tip is loaded into Centrix syringe.

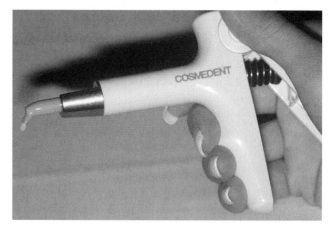

FIGURE 8.33. Loaded syringe before glass ionomer application.

8. Finish the restoration with sanding disks or finishing burs. Use water or cocoa butter as a lubricant when finishing the restoration to prevent overheating. When completed, cover the restoration with a varnish or unfilled light-activated resin to help eliminate water evaporation.

Using Glass Ionomer Restoratives in the Treatment of FORL

Glass ionomer cement may be used to restore some Class 2 *feline odontoclastic resorptive lesions (FORLs)*, which enter the dentin but not into the pulp.

Advantages of using glass ionomer cements for Class 2 restorations include:

- The ability of glass ionomer cement to bond to enamel and dentin
- The advantage of application in a moist environment
- Little to no cavity preparation required
- The release of fluoride slowly over a year, which may decrease plaque and sensitivity

Long-term (2-year) follow-up studies show a low (20%) success rate when glass ionomer cement was used to save teeth affected with feline resorptive lesions. The high failure rate does not lie in the inability of glass ionomer cement to restore the tooth to visible form and function, but the inability to arrest the progression of the resorptive process.

Application of glass ionomer cement in the case of Class 2 FORLs should only be considered after radiographic examination confirms that the resorption has not progressed to Class 3 (endodontic involvement). The practitioner must also consider concurrent periodontal disease, ability to access the lesion, as well as the client's acceptance of 80% failure rate (Figures 8.34, 8.35).

The following steps outline the basic technique for using light cured glass ionomer cement to restore Class 2 FORLs:

1. Scale and polish the affected tooth to remove plaque and calculus.
2. Pack epinephrine-impregnated gingival retraction cord in the sulcus to allow exposure of small marginal lesions. A gingival flap might have to be raised for adequate access to the entire lesion (Figures 8.36, 8.37).
3. Excise hyperplastic gingiva with a scalpel blade, laser, or electrocautery. Perform flap surgery if necessary to allow the free gingiva to lie apical to the restoration.

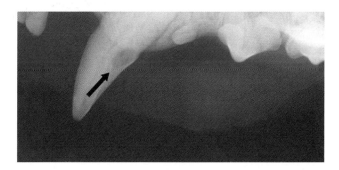

FIGURE 8.35. Radiograph confirming lesion does not radiographically extend into the pulp (Class 3).

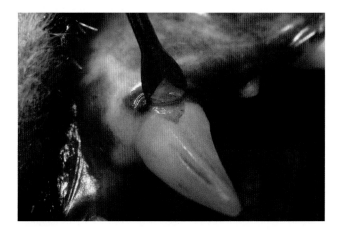

FIGURE 8.36. Molt periosteal elevator used to expose FORL.

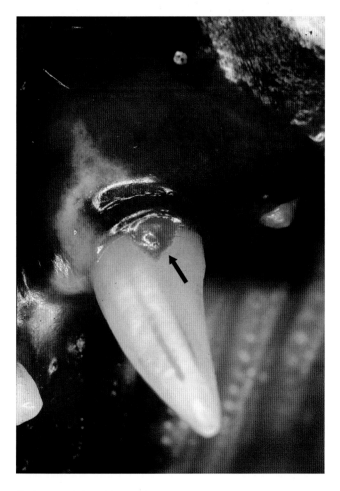

FIGURE 8.34. Class 2 FORL.

4. To remove unsupported enamel, use a No. 1 round bur in a water-cooled high-speed handpiece around the edges of the resorptive lesion.
5. Condition (smear layer removed), rinse, and dry the FORL. Apply Type II glass-ionomer material, following the manufacturer's instructions (Figure 8.38).
6. When the material is hardened, contour the restoration surface with finishing burs.
7. Brush unfilled light cured resin on the restoration and light cure.

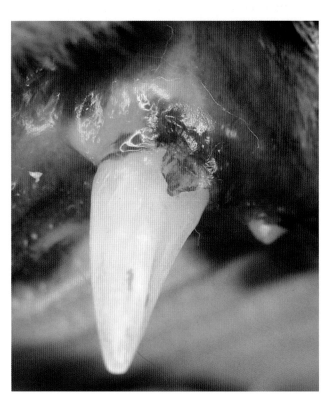

FIGURE 8.37. Prepared FORL for restoration.

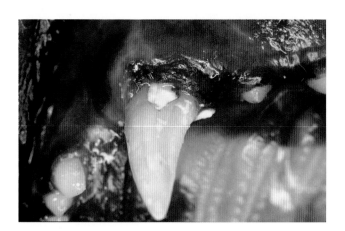

FIGURE 8.38. Glass ionomer restored FORL.

COMPOMERS

Compomers are a combination of composite resin and glass ionomer (as a filler). Compomers are best suited for low stress areas. Compomers are more flexible with less wear resistance than hybrids. Product examples include Dyract AP® (Dentsply), Compoglass F (Ivoclar), and F2000 (3M).

PROSTHETIC CROWN RESTORATION

A prosthetic is used to cover the clinical crown of teeth that have been weakened by decay or damaged by fracture. A restoration helps protect the restored tooth, but does not make it stronger. The purpose of prosthetic crown restoration is to prevent further breakdown of the remaining tooth structure, restore function to the tooth, and—in some instances—create a "normal" aesthetic appearance. In human dentistry, crown restoration is performed after most endodontic procedures, because a significant amount of the crown is removed for access. Human teeth are usually in occlusal contact compared to small animal teeth, which mostly interdigitate. In veterinary dentistry, prosthetic crown restoration is a controversial advanced procedure chosen on a case-by-case basis.

Indications for crown use include the following:

- Restoration of teeth subject to stress following endodontic procedures, especially canines, maxillary fourth premolars, and mandibular first molars
- Crown protection in patients that chew on objects, which continue to injure teeth (abrasion)
- Restoration of teeth affected by enamel hypoplasia
- Protection of the cut surfaces of crown-reduced teeth from fracture or leakage after restoration
- Protection of vital teeth that have enamel and dentin loss with near exposure, potentially decreasing further damage and the necessity for endodontic care

There are several types of crowns:

- *Full cast* or *metal crowns* completely cover the exposed portion of an individual tooth. Metal crowns are manufactured from precious metal (gold), high noble semiprecious metal (gold/alloy mix), or nonprecious (nickel or chromium alloy) materials (Figure 8.39).
- *Porcelain-fused-to-metal (PFM) crowns* are full metal restorations, with the outer surfaces covered with a veneer (thin layer) of a tooth-colored sub-

stance baked onto the metallic framework. The porcelain veneer has the tendency to chip.

- *Porcelain crowns* are constructed from a thin metal shell covered by layers of porcelain built up to resemble the shading and translucence of the natural tooth. Porcelain crowns lack the strength of porcelain-fused-to-metal crowns (Figure 8.40).
- *Sintered ceramic crowns* are porcelain/resin mixtures that are pressed into a corresponding mold and then baked. Sintered ceramics are strong and are manufactured in multiple tooth colors. Examples include In-Ceram Zirconia (Vident) and Procera AllCeram (Figure 8.41).

The following is an overview of crown preparation to installation:

1. Endodontic therapy, if indicated, is performed first, followed by crown preparation, impressions (area-specific and full mouth), and bite registration. Models are made from the impressions.

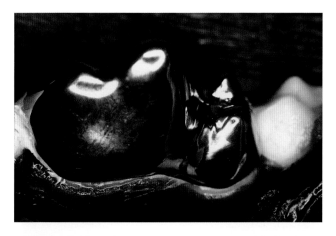

FIGURE 8.39. Full cast crown on the mandibular first molar.

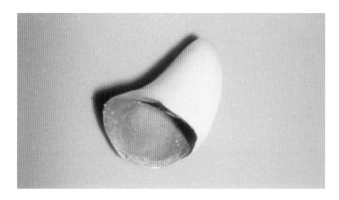

FIGURE 8.40. Porcelain jacket crown.

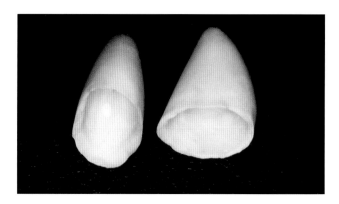

FIGURE 8.41. In-Ceram sintered ceramic crowns.

2. Impressions and models are sent to the dental laboratory to fabricate the crown. The laboratory usually takes between 1 and 2 weeks to deliver the finished crown.
3. The patient is anesthetized for fitting (try-in) and crown cementation. If the crown fits, no adjustments are made and adhesive is applied to the inner crown surface and the tooth for cementation. If the crown does not fit, minor adjustments are made to the crown surface and/or the tooth to improve the mount. If it still does not fit, the tooth is re-prepped, new impressions are taken, and the new models are sent to the lab.

Crown Preparation

Crown preparation provides a smooth, strong junction of the tooth with the cast surface. To accomplish this objective, the height and contour of the tooth are reduced, resulting in a smaller tooth than the original. An impression taken of the prepared tooth provides the laboratory with a negative model for prosthetic crown fabrication.

The preparation setup tray should include the following:

- Gingival retraction cord (Burns 951-4780, Schein 378-0485)
- Retraction cord placer (Burns 950-6563; Cislak CP-G7, CP-113, CP-56; Schein 115-9456)
- Diamond burs (various sizes and shapes)
- Impression tray (various sizes and shapes)
- Bite registration wax (Burns 952-7200, Schein 569-5435)
- Polyvinyl siloxane impression material loaded on two applicator guns—if one runs out of material, the other is ready (Burns 867-1000, Schein 777-8798)

Table 8.2. Width of crown materials.

Materials	Width
Metallic cast crown	0.5 mm
Porcelain fused to metal crown	1.5 mm
Ceramic	1.0 mm

Tooth Reduction

For the crown to fit and properly occlude, the outside dimensions of the tooth are reduced by the width of the crown material (Table 8.2). Reduction should be kept to the enamel (<0.5 mm) if possible, because enamel provides the greatest adhesive bonding surface.

Occlusal Considerations

The *mandibular canines* normally rest between the maxillary canines and corner incisors. The amount of free space remaining between these teeth when the mouth is closed must be accounted for when preparing a tooth for crown restoration. For example, if there were only 1 mm on each side, porcelain fused to metal crown would not fit unless the tooth is reduced 2 mm on all sides (Figure 8.42).

The *palatal surface of the maxillary fourth* premolar occludes closely with the buccal surface of the mandibular first molar. Care must be taken not to overbuild either interface when preparing these teeth. Slab fractures of the maxillary fourth premolar usually result in loss of buccal width, which should not be restored before crown preparation.

Crown Margins

A *margin* is the junction line between the tooth and the restoration. The crown should fit in a flawless fashion over the remaining tooth structure. If the crown is placed over the tooth without margin preparation, excessive plaque would accumulate at the crown/tooth interface predisposing the area to gingivitis and periodontal disease.

Biologic width refers to the combined connective tissue and epithelial attachment from the margin of the alveolar bone to the base of the gingival sulcus. In the normal dog, it is equal to an average of 2 mm. In the cat, the biological width is 0.5–1 mm. Placement of restorative margin 1–2 mm coronal to the epithelial attachment is desirable; therefore, the minimum distance between the alveolar margin and the restorative margin in the dog should be 3–4 mm and in the cat 2–3 mm, allowing 1 mm for the sulcus (Figure 8.43).

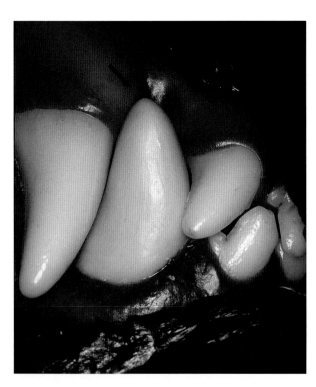

FIGURE 8.42. In-Ceram crown placed on the mandibular canine.

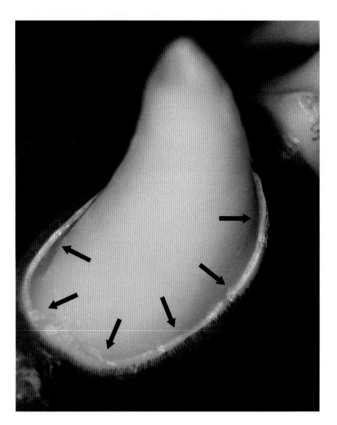

FIGURE 8.43. Buccal view of margin line.

The margin is prepared using a diamond bur powered by a high-speed drill with water irrigation. There are many types of diamond burs available, depending on the veterinarian's choice of marginal finish line. For example, if a chamfer finish line is desired, a chamfer diamond bur is used to prepare the tooth.

Types of marginal finish lines include the following:

- *Feather (knife edge)* margin bevels are angled 70° or greater coronally. The advantage of a feathered margin is ease of preparation and minimal tooth loss. Due to the long slope, the fabricating lab may have difficulty establishing the finish line to determine crown length. In such cases, the veterinarian should indicate where the finish line is on a drawing or instant picture.
- *Chamfer (level)* margin finish is popular for metallic crown restorations. A chamfer finish allows micromovement without damage to the tooth margin. It also permits the lab to make the crown with an ample gingival margin, which is less technically exacting than margins that taper to a fine point (Figure 8.44).
- *Deep chamfer* finishes consist of a 6° taper with a rounded transition area to a 45° margin at the finish line. This prep is used primarily for subgingival finish lines, in cases of subgingival fracture. Exposure is provided by gingivectomy or with an apically repositioned flap (crown lengthening procedure).
- *Shoulder or butt joints* consist of a parallel axial wall (butt) or a 6° taper (tapered shoulder) transitioning to a 90° margin at the finish line. Shoulder margins do not allow micromovement and are recommended when restoring the tooth with porcelain, ceramic, or PFM crowns. A disadvantage of a shoulder margin is the loss of tooth mass to form the joint (Figure 8.45).

Taper

The tooth should be prepared with a taper of 5–6° from the parallel sides. Less taper makes seating and cementing the crown difficult, because air and cement have little room to escape during cementation. Excessive taper reduces surface area available for retention and weakens the crown.

Undercuts

An *undercut* is a defect in the wall of the crown that occurs from the original injury or in the preparation process. Undercuts make it difficult for the lab to remove the wax pattern from the model and for the veterinarian to place the cast metal crown on the tooth.

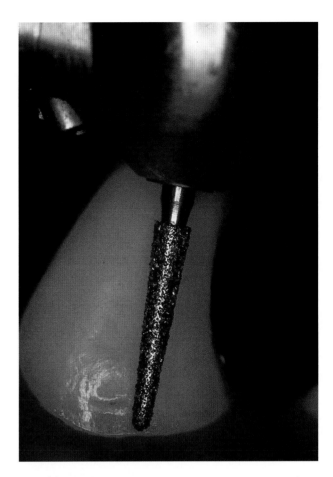

FIGURE 8.44. Rounded taper bur position to produce a chamfer finish line.

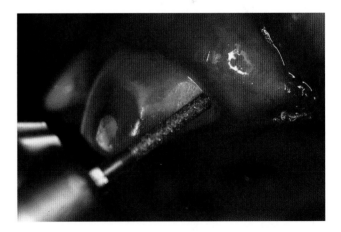

FIGURE 8.45. Diamond bur used to make a butt joint margin line.

When undercuts exist, they should be removed by additional chamfering, or can be filled with composite or glass ionomer before preparation. A completed prepa-

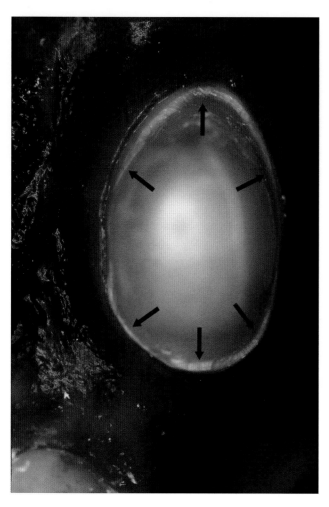

FIGURE 8.46. Birds-eye view of marginal finish surrounding tooth.

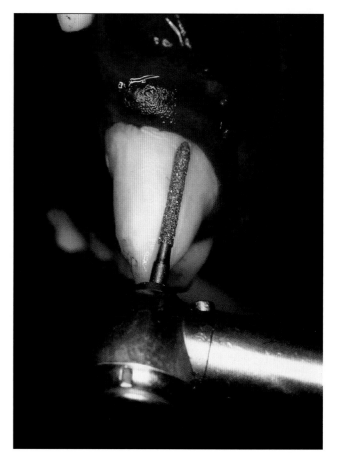

FIGURE 8.47. Diamond bur placement to produce retention groove.

ration without undercuts will enable the veterinarian to view the entire tooth surface and margin while looking straight down the crown with one eye (Figure 8.46).

Rotational Stability

Rotational stability is a concern when there is minimal tooth remaining above the gingiva and the prepared surface approximates a cylindrical cone. To prevent rotation of the crown, retention grooves may be cut in the tooth. These grooves should be parallel to each other and the long axis of the crown. They should be deep enough to offer resistance to rotation while avoiding excessive removal of the natural tooth tissue. Retention grooves weaken the tooth and should be used only when the first attempt at crown restoration has failed because of crown separation (Figures 8.47–8.49).

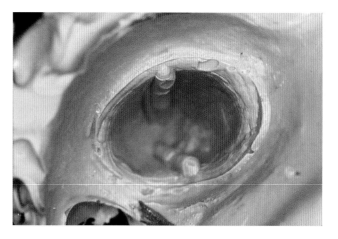

FIGURE 8.48. Impression of retention grooves.

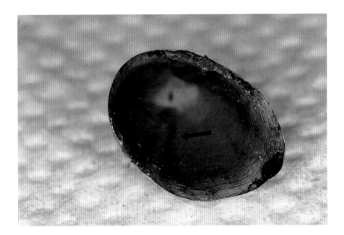

FIGURE 8.49. Cast with retention grooves before cementing.

Crown Color

In veterinary dentistry, most crowns are made from semiprecious metals. If the client requests a tooth-colored restoration, matching the shade of natural teeth can best be accomplished using a shade guide.

The shade guide is held close to the tooth to be restored and moistened to achieve an accurate match. The shade selected is identified by a number and letter, which is noted on the patient's chart and on the laboratory instructions (Figure 8.50).

Crown Lengthening

There should be at least 4–6 mm of sound tooth available supragingivally for crown coverage. Occasionally, fractured teeth have less than 4 mm of crown exposed coronal to the free gingival margin. Additional height of the clinical crown can be achieved by crown lengthening.

Nonsurgical procedures of crown lengthening begin with adding material to the remaining crown, inserting a post and applying core buildup material. A *post* is used as a scaffolding to retain core buildup material. A post is a cylindrical or tapered object that fits into the prepared pulp cavity of a tooth after endodontic care. The ratio of the crown to post depth should be greater than 1:1 (the post depth subgingivally should be greater than the post height supragingivally). In general, the prognosis for crown retention is inversely proportional to the length of post and core buildup.

There are two commonly used posts: *custom*, wherein the post and core buildup (artificial crown mass) are cast together, and *prefabricated*, which can be placed in the canal followed by core buildup.

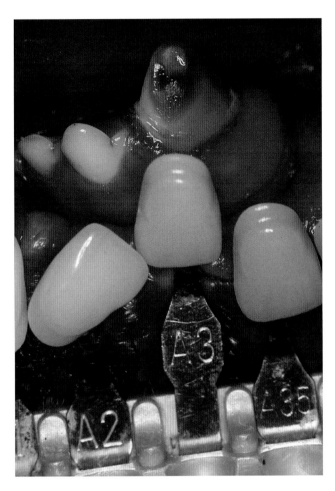

FIGURE 8.50. Shade guide.

Follow these steps for custom post preparation:

1. Treat the patient with conventional endodontics (posts should not be used in surgical endodontic cases).
2. Remove 2/3 of the gutta percha from the pulp chamber with Gates Glidden drills.
3. Select a plastic post (available in various diameters to match the lumen size of the prepared canal and numbered similar to Gates Glidden drills—plastic impression posts, Coltene/Whaledent Intl.). Alternatively, select a universal plastic post, which is placed in heated acrylic before insertion into the canal.
4. After the custom post is formed, leave it projecting from the top of the tooth. Build the core around the post into the desired coronal shape, using two dappen dishes and a brush, with the powder in one container and liquid in another (GC Pattern resin

and Duralay resin, Reliance Manufacturing Inc.). "Build" the core in layers, using "salt and pepper" technique.

5. After it is set, shape the core into the desired tooth shape with a finishing bur.
6. Take an impression of the finished buildup and send it with the post and core to the laboratory, with instructions for the lab to vent the post to allow excess cement to escape.

Prefabricated posts can be placed in the canal, followed by core buildup:

1. Treat the patient with conventional endodontics.
2. Remove 1/2–3/4 of the gutta percha by drilling into the coronal pulp chamber with Gates Glidden drills.
3. Place cement on the apical end of a stainless steel orthopedic nonthreaded pin. Use a hand chuck to place the pin into the pulp chamber and root canal. The post width should be sufficient to fit snugly into the root canal. Avoid excess debridement of the root canal. The inserted post length below the gum line should at least match the clinical crown length or occupy half of the root length, whichever is greater (Figure 8.51).
4. After full insertion, bend the pin to the same angle as the original clinical crown.
5. Cut the post with a pin cutter or diamond bur. The height should be shorter than the same tooth crown on the opposite side of the arch.
6. Apply the core buildup material (composite or core paste) to the exposed post (Figures 8.52, 8.53).

7. When hardened, shape the core material and prepare with margins.
8. Make an impression of the prepared tooth for crown restoration (Figure 8.54).

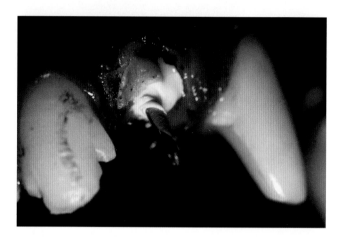

FIGURE 8.52. Pin inserted into fractured tooth pulp chamber after root canal therapy and surgical crown lengthening.

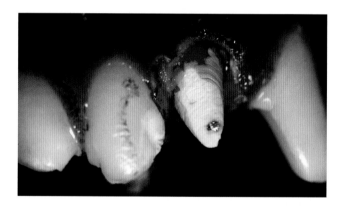

FIGURE 8.53. Core build-up material placed and shaped on pin to form anatomical crown.

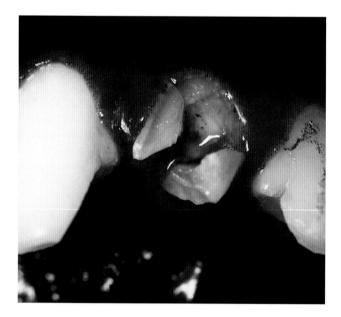

FIGURE 8.51. Subgingival tooth fracture.

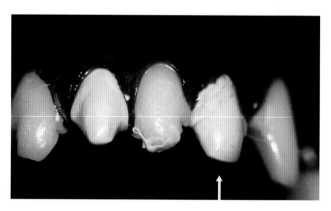

FIGURE 8.54. Cemented crown placed on core build-up, prognosis guarded.

Surgical crown lengthening procedures include the following:

1. Remove a portion of the attached gingiva and alveolar bone, exposing more of the natural tooth structure.
2. Make a gingival incision with a No. 15 blade around the affected tooth, removing 1–4 mm of the attached gingiva exposing the underlying alveolus. At least 2 mm of healthy attached gingiva must remain after gingivoplasty.
3. Remove alveolar bone from the root surfaces using hand chisels (Oschenbein, Wedelstaedt) or a diamond bur on a high-speed drill. The new alveolar crest should be at least 4 mm apical to the new finish line.
4. Alternatively, if insufficient attached gingiva remains, an apical repositioned flap exposing the underlying alveolus and preserving the attached gingival collar can be performed:

    a. Make an intrasulcular incision 360° around the tooth. Vertical releasing incisions are made at the mesial and distal line angles.
    b. Elevate a full thickness mucoperiosteal flap to expose the supporting alveolar bone. A No. 7901 finishing diamond bur on a high-speed handpiece or, preferably, hand chisels are used to remove alveolar bone to the desired height.
    c. Thin out edges of alveolar bone to mimic normal anatomy. Bony ledges are removed with curettes.
    d. Replace the gingiva with gingival margin located 2 mm coronal to the new bone height.
    e. Place sutures to allow gingiva to lie snugly around tooth's circumference.

Often crown lengthening procedures combine gingivectomy, post placement, and core buildup (Figures 8.55–8.58).

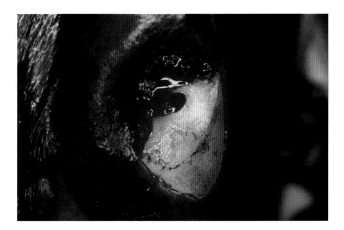

FIGURE 8.55. Class 3b fracture.

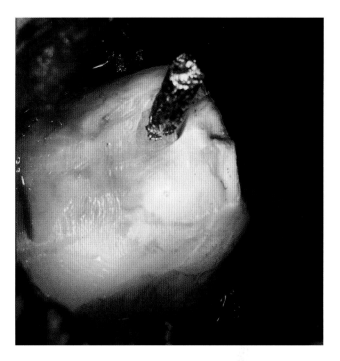

FIGURE 8.56. Post placed in tooth after crown lengthening procedure.

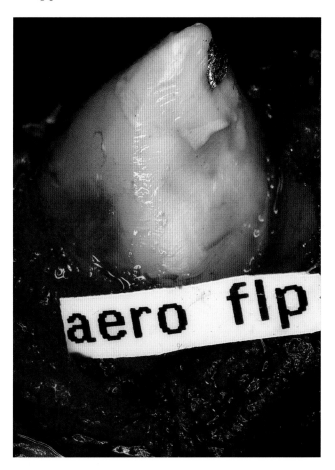

FIGURE 8.57. Crown prepared after core material placed around post.

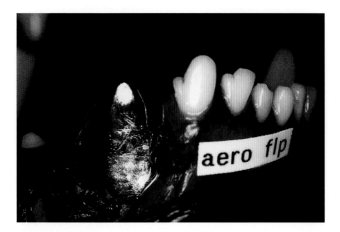

FIGURE 8.58. Cemented metallic crown.

IMPRESSIONS

To fabricate the crown, dental labs request the following:

- Impression of the crown preparation and surrounding soft tissue
- Stone models of the maxillary and mandibular teeth
- Bite registration with bite wax or impression putty to allow articulation of the maxilla and mandibular models

Polyvinyl siloxane—available in heavy, regular, and light-bodied forms—is used in restorative dentistry for area-specific crown impressions. Impression materials are generally supplied in two tubes: base and catalyst. Equal lengths may be dispensed on a paper mixing pad and mixed with a spatula or co-mixed with a special mixing syringe to achieve a homogeneous blend (3M Express, Aquasil, and Reprosil Burns 951-5174, Schein 101-5327)).

Curing is the process of changing the base and catalyst into the final rubber-like material that forms a solid mass in a two-stage process:

- The *initial set* results in a stiffening of the paste without the appearance of elastic properties (Figure 8.59).
- The *final set* begins with the appearance of elasticity and proceeds through a gradual change to a solid rubber mass (Figure 8.60).

The material may be manipulated only during the first stage. Impression material should be in place in the

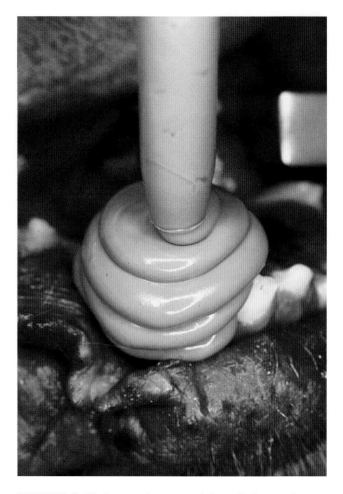

FIGURE 8.59. Impression material applied over the tooth before placing the loaded tray.

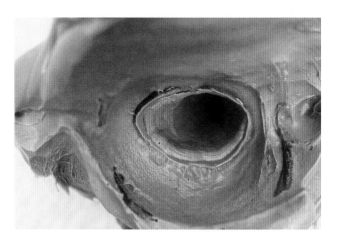

FIGURE 8.60. Elastic final set.

mouth before elastic properties develop. Setting time is affected by temperature and humidity. An increase rise in temperature speeds the set.

Follow these steps for the crown preparation technique and impression process:

1. Obtain alginate impressions and bite registrations of both arches.
2. If a tooth-colored restoration is requested, select the shade, comparing a shade guide to the patient's tooth color.
3. Use a chamfer diamond bur in a water-cooled high-speed handpiece to establish a margin line 1–2 mm coronal to the free gingival margin.
4. A tray is used to hold impression material in the mouth. Trays can be:
   • Commercially purchased pre-formed
   • Fabricated out of impression tray material (3M Express 7312 putty). Mix equal volumes of base and catalyst by hand until a homogenous color is achieved (approximately 30 seconds). The hardening putty is seated on the tooth to be restored and several abutting teeth on either side. The tray material is wiggled around the selected teeth before the putty sets (within 5 minutes) to create an enlarged overimpression. After the putty sets, remove the newly formed tray from the mouth (Figures 8.61–8.67).
   • Made from the bottom of a 6 cc syringe casing
5. Gently place a gingival retraction cord (Burns 951-4780, Schein 115-3925) in the sulcus with the help of a blunt cord-packing instrument (Burns 950-6563, Schein 600-9015). Cut the cord to match the circumferential length of the prepared tooth, loop it around the tooth, and lay it in the sulcus by rocking the instrument backward as it is moved forward to the next loose section of cord (Figures 8.68, 8.69).

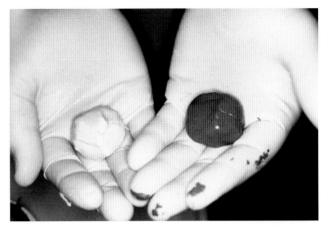

FIGURE 8.62. Equal volumes of base and catalyst obtained for mix (non-latex gloves recommended).

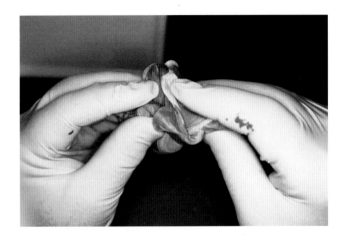

FIGURE 8.63. Mixing base and catalyst.

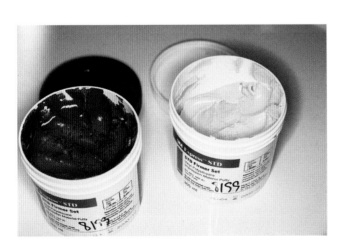

FIGURE 8.61. Base and catalyst containers.

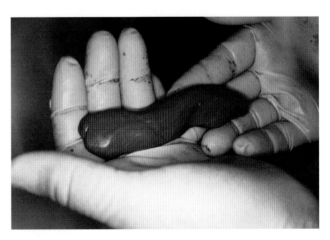

FIGURE 8.64. Homogeneous mixture shaped into an arch while setting.

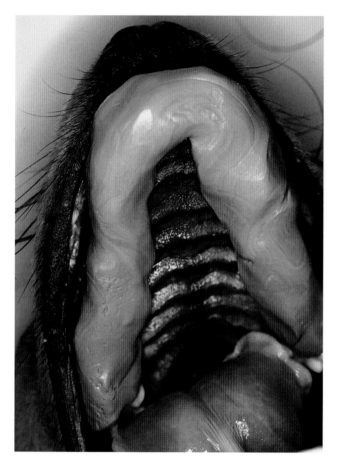

FIGURE 8.65. Hard-bodied material placed over the maxillary crowns.

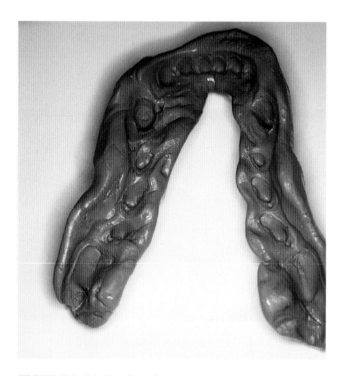

FIGURE 8.66. Hardened negative impression of the maxillary crowns.

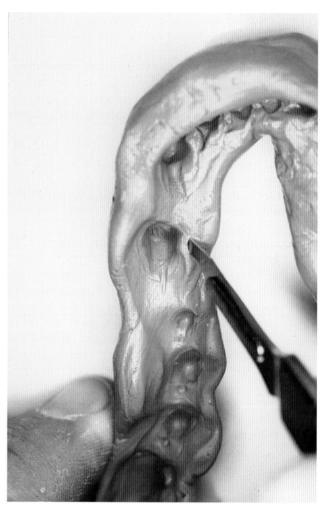

FIGURE 8.67. Space is cut away from the impression to allow room for the light-bodied impression material.

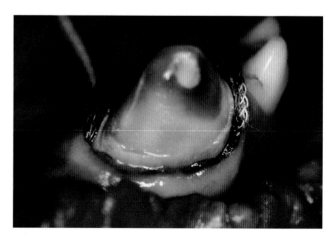

FIGURE 8.68. Gingival retraction cord being applied subgingivally.

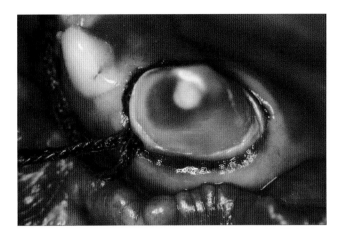

FIGURE 8.69. Gingival retraction cord placement under the canine marginal gingiva.

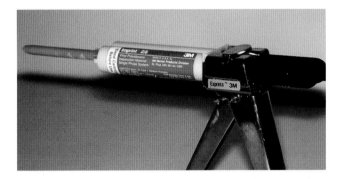

FIGURE 8.70. Express impression material loaded on applicator.

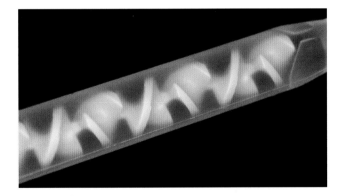

FIGURE 8.71. Close-up of mixing syringe tip.

6. After several minutes, remove the retraction cord, leaving space for the impression material to flow. Thoroughly rinse and dry the crown. All margins should be visible before the impression is seated.
7. Apply polyvinyl siloxine impression material (the light-bodied wash) through an impression syringe. Express a small amount directly into the sulcus, on the crown, and into the tray well (Express System 3M Burns 867-1000, Schein 777-8798) (Figures 8.70–8.76).
8. Use a light stream of air from the air/water syringe to push the impression material into the sulcus.

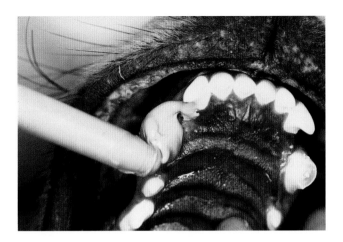

FIGURE 8.72. Impression material placed around the prepared crown.

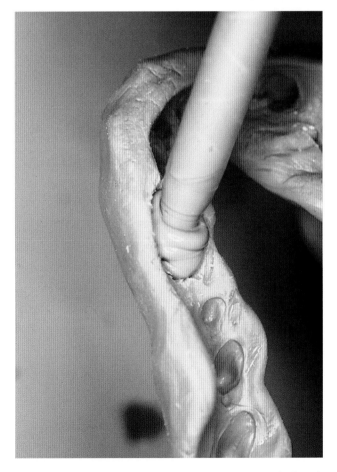

FIGURE 8.73. Light-bodied impression material placed in the hard body over impression.

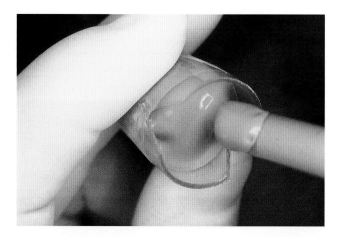

FIGURE 8.74. Light-bodied impression material placed in a syringe holder tip used as a tray.

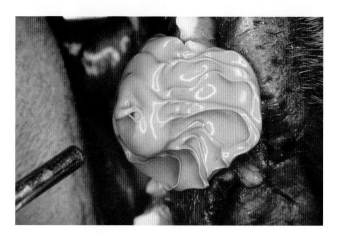

FIGURE 8.75. Light-bodied impression material placed over prepared crown.

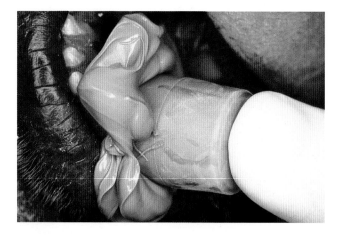

FIGURE 8.76. Pressure placed over syringe tray until impression material hardened.

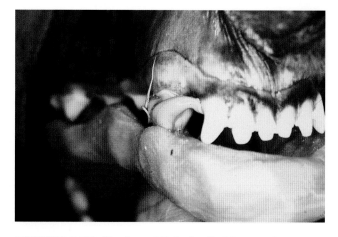

FIGURE 8.77. Hard- and light-bodied impression material compressed on the prepared crown.

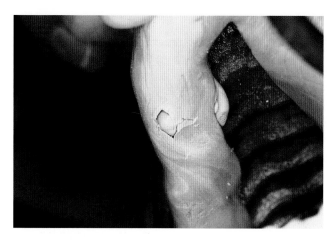

FIGURE 8.78. Excess light-bodied impression material can flow from a release hole.

9. Seat the tray firmly and hold without pressure until the material hardens. After completely set, remove the impression in a rapid downward motion (Figures 8.77–8.79).

10. Inspect the impression for a complete finish line, as well as defects (voids) that may affect the final restoration. If needed, repeat the process (Figures 8.80, 8.81).

11. Take a bite registration and alginate impressions of both arches. The bite registration shows the lab how the maxillary teeth occlude with their mandibular counterparts. This is vital information for the lab to fabricate a crown that will occlude properly. With the help of the dental models, the lab can determine whether the tooth to be crowned has been reduced adequately to allow for sufficient clearance.

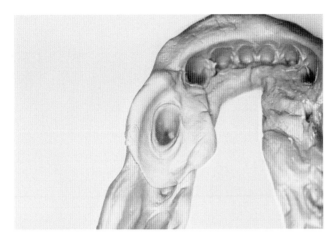

FIGURE 8.79. Completed light- and hard-bodied impression.

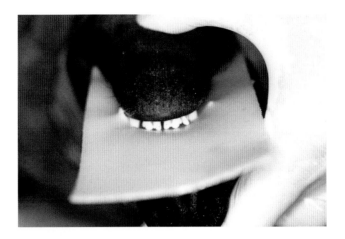

FIGURE 8.82. Bite registration.

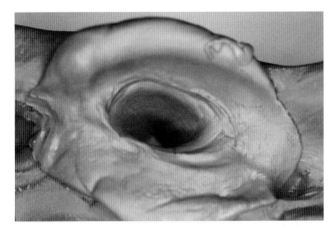

FIGURE 8.80. Impression inspected for voids in crown and margin line before sending the impression to the laboratory.

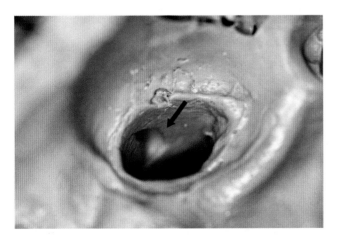

FIGURE 8.81. Appearance of impression void necessitating repeat impression.

12. Send the impression, the stone model, and the bite registration to the laboratory with instructions (prescription). The laboratory chosen to fabricate the crown should have experience working with small animal cases.

Bite Registration

Materials for bite registration include the following:

- Warm water
- Bite wax (Kerr Set Up Wax)

Follow these steps to make a bite registration:

1. Soften bite wax in warm water for a minute.
2. After induction before intubation, place the tongue in the caudal part of the mouth.
3. Place the softened wax sheet over the mandibular anterior dentition, and close the mouth to capture incisors and canine teeth (Figure 8.82).
4. Open the mouth to remove bite wax.
5. Allow cool water to flow over the wax, which will rapidly regain its original rigidity.
6. Mark the maxillary side of the wax with an arrow pointing rostrally; mark also right and left sides.

Crown Cementation

Many materials are available to permanently attach a crown to the tooth. The author prefers C & B Metabond adhesive cement (Burns 875-0390, Schein 186-5548) and Panavia 21 (Burns 955-6409, Schein 721-2341).

After the animal is anesthetized, place the crown on the tooth. If it does not fit, identify areas that can be altered on the crown or tooth to improve the fit. If

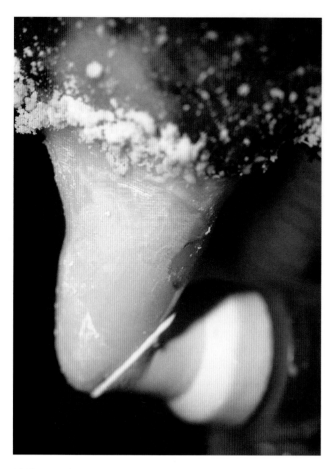

FIGURE 8.83. Tooth cleaned with pumice.

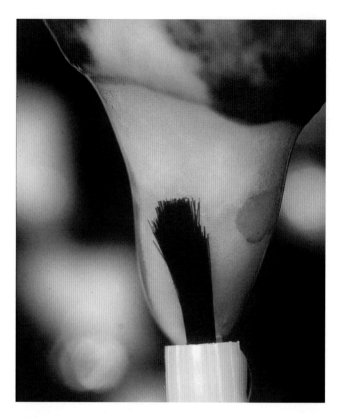

FIGURE 8.84. Etchant applied.

changes cannot be made, pour another impression for the lab to remake the crown.

Follow these steps to prepare the tooth surface for crown cementation using C & B Metabond:

1. Clean the tooth surface with fluoride-free pumice; rinse and dry the surface (Figure 8.83).
2. Etch the enamel surface for 30 seconds with an etchant-saturated foam pledget (Figure 8.84).
3. Rinse the etchant and dry the tooth (Figure 8.85).
4. If the tooth is vital and dentin exposed, apply a dentin primer for 10 seconds (Figure 8.86).
5. Rinse and dry the tooth.

When cementing the crown, using C & B Metabond, the internal surface of the metallic crown should be pre-etched or sandblasted to enhance retention. To cement the crown on the prepared tooth:

1. Remove the ceramic mixing dish from the storage box or freezer. Dispense four drops of C & B

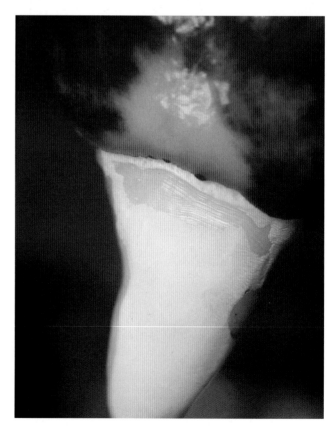

FIGURE 8.85. Etchant rinsed and tooth dried.

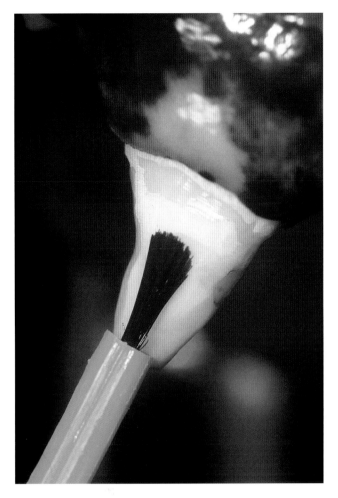

FIGURE 8.86. Primer applied to the tooth.

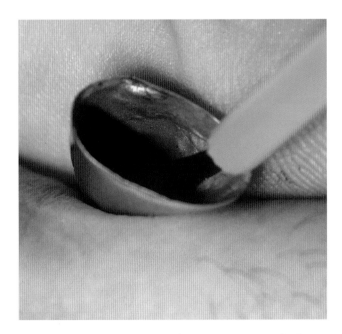

FIGURE 8.87. Base and catalyst mixture is applied to the inside of the crown.

Metabond base (brown bottle) into one well of the mixing dish.

2. Add one drop of catalyst to the base liquid and stir the mixture.
3. Paint the internal surface of the crown with the mixture (Figure 8.87).
4. Prepare an identical mixture of base and catalyst in the second well. Add two scoops of powder.
5. Stir the second well's contents to a creamy consistency. Apply the mixture with a brush to the inside of the crown and to the outside tooth surface (Figures 8.88, 8.89).

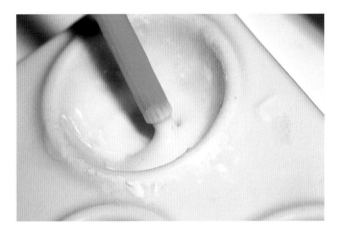

FIGURE 8.88. Cement mixture in dappen dish.

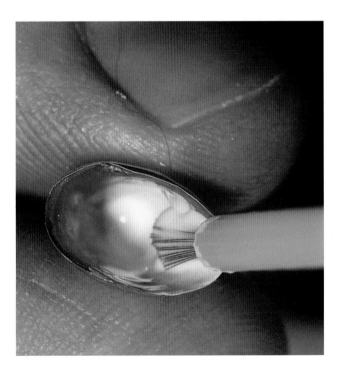

FIGURE 8.89. Cement applied on the inside surface of the crown.

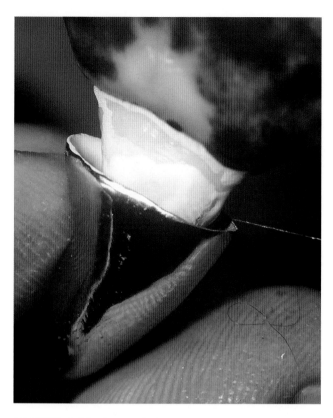

FIGURE 8.90. Crown delivery.

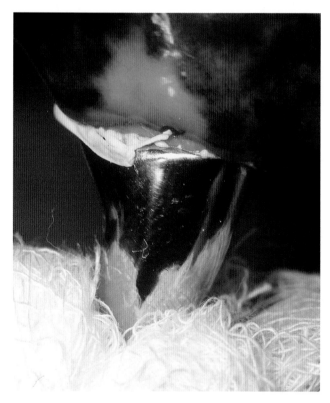

FIGURE 8.91. Pressure applied with gauze sponge, excessive cement is removed before it hardens.

6. Seat the restoration on the tooth and use pressure to hold it in place until the cement dries (5 minutes) (Figure 8.90).
7. Remove excess cement with a gauze sponge before it hardens (Figure 8.91).

Crown Failure

Occasionally, crown restorations fail to remain on the tooth (crown separation). Restoration failure can be due to one or more of the following:

- Crown problems caused by flawed impressions or laboratory errors
- Mistakes in the cementation process or cement material failure
- A restoration area insufficient for long-term retention
- Patient chewing on hard object(s), which dislodges the crown

Occasionally, the tooth refractures with the crown attached to the coronal segment (Figure 8.92).

RESTORING TEETH AFFECTED BY DENTAL CARIES

Caries, or cavities, in humans are infections of the dental hard tissues caused primarily by *Streptococcus mutans*, *Steptococcus sanguis*, and lactobacilli, which demineralize enamel, promoting enzymatic digestion of dentin. The pulp can become inflamed in the process

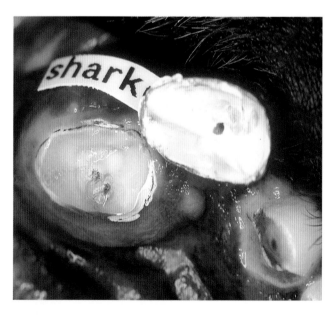

FIGURE 8.92. Restoration fracture.

from substances that diffuse through the dentinal tubules.

In dogs and cats, carious lesions are not common, because of the shape of teeth and higher oral pH, which suppresses the growth of cariogenic flora. When present, caries occurs predominately in larger-breed dogs, in the pit and fissures of the maxillary first molar. Smooth surface, dentin, and root caries occurs, but less frequently. Clinically, the advanced carious lesion is softer than healthy dentin, allowing a dental explorer to stick on compression. Healthy underlying dentin offers greater resistance. Occasionally, the carious lesion extends into the pulp, leading to pulpal necrosis and periapical pathology (Figure 8.93).

The following are therapy options to treat dental caries:

- *Indirect pulp capping* is indicated in cases where radiographs reveal normal endodontic and periapical anatomy. Use the following steps to perform indirect pulp capping:

1. Remove the carious lesion initially with a round bur on a high-speed water-cooled handpiece. Presence of healthy dentin can be felt as increased resistance. A sharp spoon excavator can also be used to remove remaining soft dentin.
2. Irrigate and dry the cavity floor, and line it with a fast-setting calcium hydroxide base. Use of calcium hydroxide is controversial because it may weaken the restoration and be of no particular benefit.
3. Overlay the calcium hydroxide with an intermediate restorative material: 1–2 mm of zinc oxide eugenol paste or a Type II glass ionomer cement. Place a restoration, using composite or amalgam (Figure 8.94). A full metal crown restoration is recommended in affected teeth that occlude.
- *Conventional* or *surgical* endodontics followed by crown restoration should be performed when pulpal exposure has occurred, if the tooth is not affected by end-stage periodontal disease (Figures 8.95, 9.96).
- *Extraction*

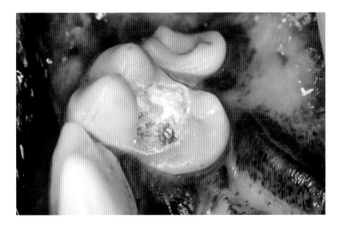

FIGURE 8.93. Carious lesion affecting the maxillary first molar without pulpal exposure.

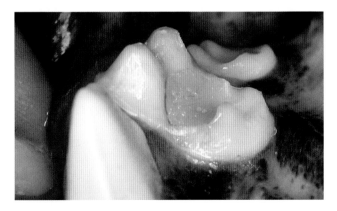

FIGURE 8.94. Composite resin applied before curing and polishing.

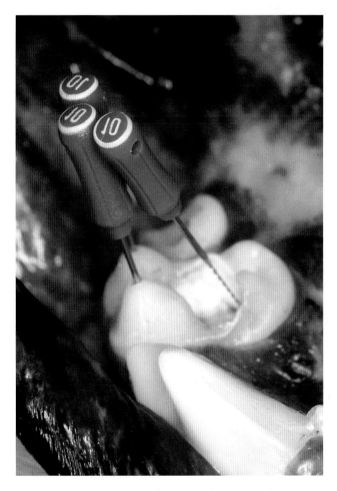

FIGURE 8.95. Root canal therapy for carious lesion that extended to the pulp.

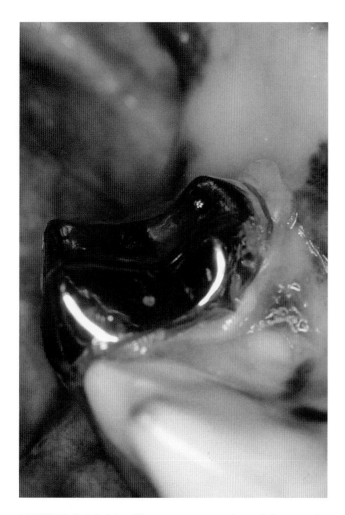

FIGURE 8.96. Metallic crown restoration of the maxillary first molar in a dog.

9
Orthodontic Equipment, Materials, and Techniques

Orthodontics is the branch of dentistry that deals with the development and correction of tooth malpositions and malocclusion. In mesocephalic (medium-sized muzzle) and dolichocephalic (long, narrow muzzle) breeds, the dentition is normally arranged to create a self-cleaning mechanism, which pushes food away from the teeth and gingiva. If the teeth are not aligned properly, food may be retained. Abnormally positioned teeth may impinge on oral structures, causing the patient pain, discomfort, and trauma, while predisposing them to periodontal disease.

Teeth that are crowded, rotated, or positioned at abnormal angles can result in:

- Early onset and increased severity of gingivitis and periodontal disease.
- Damage to the soft tissues due to penetration of the gingiva (*example:* lingually displaced mandibular canines might perforate the hard palate).
- Excessive wear when abnormally aligned teeth grind against each other (attrition). Continued attrition will lead to dentin and possible pulp exposure.

OCCLUSION

Many factors are evaluated when determining normal occlusion in the long- and medium-muzzled dog and cat breeds:

- The mandibular teeth should occlude lingual to the maxillary teeth (Figure 9.1). The mandibular incisor cusps should rest on the cingulum on the palatal side of the maxillary incisors.
- The mandibular canine crowns should lie equally between the maxillary third incisors and the maxillary canines (Figure 9.2).
- The mandibular premolar crown tips should point to the interproximal spaces between the crowns of the maxillary premolars. Each mandibular premolar

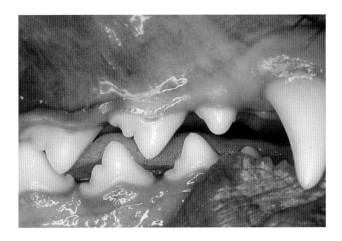

FIGURE 9.1. Normally, the mandibular premolars lie lingual to their maxillary counterparts.

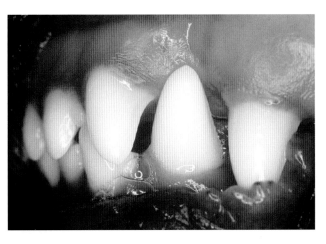

FIGURE 9.2. The mandibular canine lies equidistant between the maxillary canine and lateral incisor.

should be positioned rostral to the corresponding maxillary premolar.

263

Glossary

Alginate is an irreversible hydrocolloid material used to make dental impressions for orthodontic models.

Anterior cross bite is a condition where one or more of the anterior mandibular incisors are positioned rostral to their maxillary counterparts.

Articulator is a mechanical device to join models of the maxilla and mandible to mimic patient occlusion.

Attrition is the wearing of the crown due to mastication or chewing.

Base narrow canines are lingually displaced mandibular canines.

Bite registration provides a record of jaw relations when aligning models.

Brachygnathia (retrognathism) is a short mandible relative to he maxilla.

Distocclusion (Class II malocclusion) occurs where the mandible is relatively shorter than the maxilla.

Edgewise bracket system is a method of moving teeth using bonded brackets with a rectangular slot for placement of a round or rectangular arch memory wire.

Extrusion is the movement of the tooth farther out of the alveolus, typically in the same direction as normal eruption.

Inclined bite plane is an orthodontic appliance designed to make contact with the cusps or incisal edges of the teeth of the opposing occlusion to encourage tooth movement directed by the incline.

Interceptive orthodontics is early intervention to control orthodontic problems that might worsen if left untreated. Interceptive orthodontics involves extraction or recontouring of the primary or secondary teeth that interfere with normal jaw growth or alignment of the permanent dentition.

Intrusion is the movement of the tooth farther into the alveolus.

Lance canines (canine mesioversion) occur when the maxillary canine teeth are directed mesially, decreasing the interpoximal space between the maxillary canine tooth and maxillary third incisor.

Level bite exists when the incisor teeth meet edge to edge, or the premolars occlude cusp to cusp.

Malocclusion is a deviation from the normal relationship of the maxillary and mandibular teeth.

Mesiocclusion (Class III malocclusion) occurs when the mandible is relatively longer than the maxilla.

Occlusion is the contact between the maxillary and mandibular teeth in a functional relationship.

Oligodontia is a condition in which some teeth are missing.

Open bite occurs when part or all of the teeth are prevented from closing to normal occlusal contact.

Overbite (vertical overlap) is an excessive vertical overlap of the rostral maxillary teeth. With an overbite, the caudal teeth will be in normal occlusion.

Overjet (overjut, overshot, or horizontal overlap) is the horizontal projection of the maxillary teeth beyond mandibular teeth measured parallel to the occlusal plane.

Polyodontia occurs when an animal has extra (supernumerary) teeth.

Posterior cross bite exists when one or more posterior mandibular teeth bucally occlude with its maxillary counterpart.

Prognathism (underbite) is a long mandible, usually resulting in a horizontal overlap of the mandibular rostral teeth in relation to their maxillary counterparts.

Retrusion occurs when the teeth and/or jaws are located caudal to their normal position.

Scissors bite is the normal relationship where the maxillary incisors overlap the mandibular incisors. In a scissors bite, the incisal edges of the mandibular incisors rest on the cingulum of the maxillary incisors.

Stone models (casts) are a positive likeness of a part or parts of the oral cavity reproduced in a durable hard material.

Underbite generally refers to a Class III malocclusion.

Undershot occurs when the mandible protrudes relative to the maxilla.

Wry bite (mesiodistocclusion) is a condition where one or more of the jaw quadrants are out of proportion to the other three, causing a facial deviation from the midline.

- In the dog, the maxillary fourth premolar cusps should lay buccal to the mandibular first molars and occlude with the mesio-buccal surfaces of the mandibular first molars. (Figure 9.3).
- The space between the maxillary and mandibular cusps should have level horizontal alignment.
- The distal occlusal surfaces of the distal mandibular first molars should occlude with the occlusal surfaces of the maxillary first molars.

- The angle of the temporomandibular joint, the coronoid process, and the body of the mandible should form a right angle.

In brachycephalic dogs and cats that have short and wide muzzles, a reverse scissors bite or underbite is considered normal. The mandibular incisors are positioned rostral to the maxillary incisors. The mandibular canines and premolars are shifted forward.

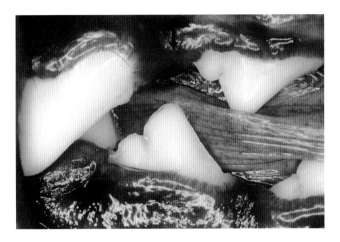

FIGURE 9.3. The mandibular fourth premolar cusp points to a space between the maxillary third and fourth premolars.

Occasionally this "normal" occlusion results in abnormal tooth-to-tooth or tooth–to–soft tissue contact.

The mandible is smaller than the maxilla at birth. Mandibular growth occurs in a downward and forward direction at a faster rate than maxillary growth.

ANGLE CLASSIFICATION

The Angle classification system based on tooth relationships used in human dentistry has been adapted to categorize veterinary dental occlusion and malocclusion. In the Angle classification, the following divisions are listed:

- Class 0 refers to normal occlusion.
- Class I neutrocclusion occurs when both jaws occlude properly, but individual teeth are misaligned. Examples of Class I malocclusions include cross bite (anterior or posterior), lingually displaced (base narrows) canines, mesoversion of the maxillary canines, rotated incisors, and crowded incisors.
- Class II distocclusion exists when there is either a short mandible or an elongated maxilla and/or a wry bite.
- Class III mesiocclusion occurs when there is either a long mandible or short maxilla and/or a wry bite.
- Class IV mesiodistocclusion is a special classification of wry bite where one jaw is in Class II and the other in Class III.

MALOCCLUSION

Abnormal tooth alignment occurs from jaw length discrepancy (skeletal malocclusion), tooth malposition (dental malocclusion), or a combination of both.

Skeletal malocclusions exist when one jaw is longer, shorter, or angled abnormally. Examples of skeletal malocclusions:

- An *overbite (distocclusion, Angle Class II malocclusion, overshot, parrot mouth, shark bite, overjet, mandibular retrognathism, maxillary prognathism)* occurs when the maxillary premolars are displaced rostral to their normal location in relation to the mandibular premolars. In the pure sense, an overbite is a vertical malocclusion, and an overjet occurs when there is an excessive horizontal protrusion of the maxillary incisors. An overbite malocclusion is never considered normal in any breed and is a genetic fault. Most commonly affected breeds are those with the elongated muzzles (collies, Shetland sheepdogs, dachshunds, rottweilers, and Russian wolfhounds) (Figure 9.4).
- An *underbite (mesiocclusion, Angle Class III malocclusion, undershot, under jet, monkey mouth, mandibular prognathism, maxillary brachygnathism)* occurs when the mandibular teeth protrude in front of the maxillary teeth. It is abnormal for an underbite to occur in a medium- or long-muzzled dog. Some short-muzzled breeds normally have an underbite (classified as Angle Class 0 [Normal] Type 3). Excess "freeway space" may be observed due to mandibular bowing (Figures 9.5–9.9).

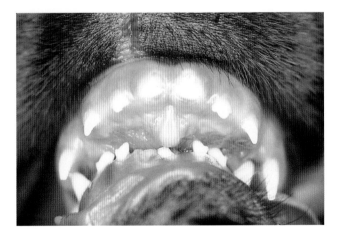

FIGURE 9.4. Mandibular brachygnathism in a puppy.

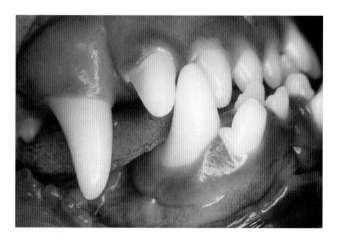

FIGURE 9.5. Mandibular prognathism (canine) Class III malocclusion.

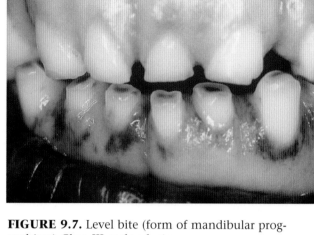

FIGURE 9.7. Level bite (form of mandibular prognathism) Class III malocclusion.

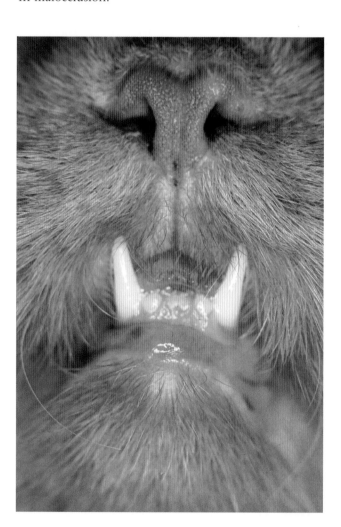

FIGURE 9.6. Mandibular prognathism (feline) Class III malocclusion.

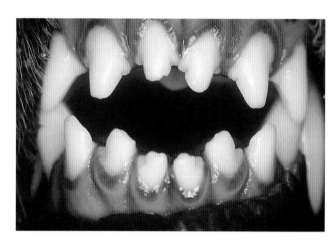

FIGURE 9.8. Open bite.

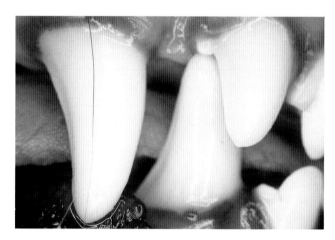

FIGURE 9.9. Mandibular canine interferring with arch closure.

- *Angle Class IV (wry bite)* exists when one side of the skull develops at a different rate than the adjacent side, creating a triangular defect. Clinically there will be an abnormal matchup between the maxillary and mandibular midlines Figures 9.10, 9.11). Note that a Class IV malocclusion is a special classification of wry bite (one jaw is in mesioclusion and the other is in distoclusion). A "simple" unilateral wry bite refers to a Class II or III malocclusion.

Dental malocclusions (Class I or neutrocclusions) occur when there are normal maxillary and mandibular jaw lengths, but one or more teeth are out of alignment or rotated. Some examples of dental malocclusions are:

- *Anterior cross bite,* where one or more of the anterior mandibular incisor teeth lies in front of its maxillary counterpart (Figure 9.12).
- *Posterior cross bite,* where one or more of the posterior mandibular premolars lies bucally to its maxillary counterpart. Posterior cross bite is a rare inherited condition presenting most commonly in long-muzzled dog breeds (collies, greyhounds). Treatment entails extraction or crown amputation and vital pulpotomy of the affected teeth if they are causing trauma, pain, or periodontal disease (Figure 9.13).
- *Incisor crowding* (Figure 9.14).
- *Lingually displaced (base narrows) canines* (Figure 9.15).
- *Mesioverted (lance) canines* (Figure 9.16).

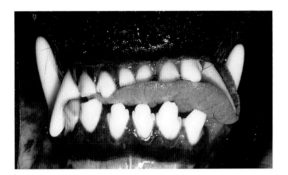

FIGURE 9.10. Simple wry bite Class III malocclusion (canine).

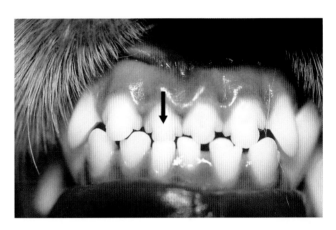

FIGURE 9.12. Anterior cross bite.

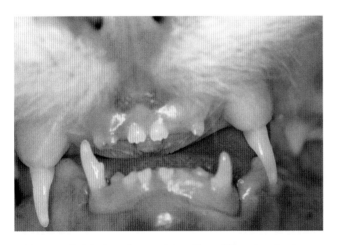

FIGURE 9.11. Simple wry bite Class III malocclusion (feline).

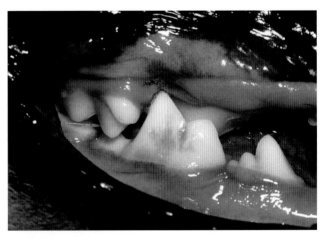

FIGURE 9.13. Posterior cross bite.

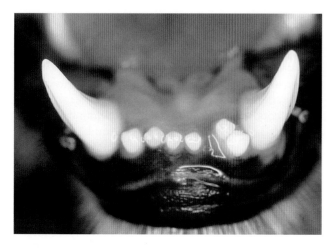

FIGURE 9.14. Incisor crowding (linguoversion of the left mandibular intermediate incisor).

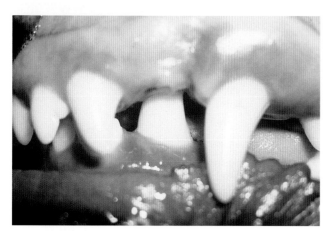

FIGURE 9.15. Lingually displaced (base narrow) mandibular canine causing palatal trauma.

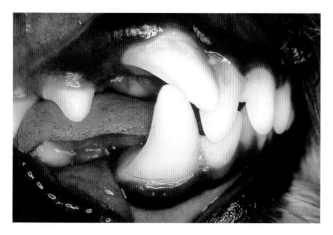

FIGURE 9.16. Mesioverted maxillary (lance) canine.

Etiology of Malocclusion

Occlusion is controlled by:

- Genetics
- Nutrition
- Trauma
- Environment
- Mechanical forces generated by an interlock of the maxillary and mandibular teeth

To appreciate the etiology of malocclusion, an understanding of the growth patterns of the maxilla and mandible is essential. The maxilla and mandible are divided into quadrants. The quadrants grow independently and in spurts. If the animal has an infection, trauma, or poor nutrition during one of the spurts, that part of the jaw might not grow normally, producing a developmental malocclusion.

To determine whether the likelihood of a malocclusion is genetic in origin, interdigitation of premolars can be studied. In the normal medium- and long-muzzled dog or cat, the premolars meet in a "pinking shears" fashion, where the tips of the mandibular premolars point to the interproximal spaces between their maxillary counterparts. (Example: the medium- to long-muzzled dog, the tips of the mandibular third premolars are positioned equally between the crowns of the maxillary third and fourth premolars.) If the cusp tip of one premolar points to the tip of another, or if there is an increased space between the cusps of the maxilla and mandible, the malocclusion probably is due to genetic influence. Skeletal malocclusions are generally considered genetic or traumatic in origin, and dental malocclusions are either genetic or developmental (Figure 9.17).

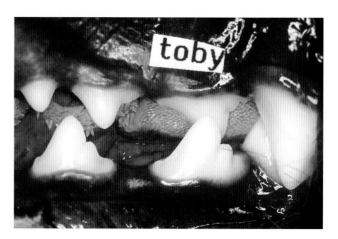

FIGURE 9.17. Malpositioned premolars (posterior cross bite) indicating skeletal malocclusion with genetic implications.

Ethics of Performing Veterinary Orthodontics

The shape and size of the skull and the number and position of teeth are genetically controlled. Occasionally, owners of show dogs seek orthodontic care to correct abnormal tooth placement. The American Kennel Club does not allow a dog that has had orthodontic care to compete in the show ring.

Animals that have pain or periodontal disease secondary to orthodontic abnormalities deserve care to alleviate lesions and make the mouth comfortable. Often extraction or crown height reduction is chosen over tooth movement based on the degree of difficulty and time needed for proper tooth movement. Clients that agree to orthodontic care must understand that there is potential injury to the teeth and gingiva, the process may take months, and that the outcome is often a functional bite rather than a perfect bite. Orthodontic treatment release forms are essential.

TOOTH MOVEMENT PRINCIPLES

Teeth are anchored to the alveolar bone by the periodontal ligament fibers. Orthodontic tooth movement properly occurs as the result of light, persistent pressure resulting in bone remodeling. Orthodontic tooth movement involves at least three variables:

- Magnitude of force
- Direction of force
- Duration of force

There are SIX basic tooth movements in orthodontics:

- *Tipping* involves single force applied to the crown, which causes the tooth to pivot around its center of resistance. The crown moves in one direction and the apex in the opposite direction. It is the most common movement in veterinary orthodontics.
- *Bodily movement (translation)* occurs when the crown and apex move in the same direction.
- *Rotation (torsion)* moves the tooth in one direction around its long axis.
- *Extrusion* moves the tooth out of the alveolus.
- *Intrusion* moves the tooth into the alveolus.
- *Radicular (root)* movement is tipping from the opposite end of the tooth (i.e., the root moves the greatest distance in relationship to the crown).

Extrusion is the easiest to accomplish, followed by tipping. Intrusion is the most difficult.

Force must be applied at least 6 hours each day for proper orthodontic tooth movement. Orthodontic appliances result in different types of forces:

- *Intermittent force* can be applied with rest periods characterized by an abrupt decline of force to zero every time the load is released. An inclined plane would be an example of an intermittent force appliance.
- *Continuous force* produces effective tooth movement when light forces are used. Orthodontic buttons and elastics applied to an anchor and target tooth would be an example of continuous force orthodontic movement.

Pressure of the tooth against bone, caused by orthodontic devices designed to push or pull teeth, causes blood vessel compression on the pressure side. This compression leads to cell death within hours. Through biological feedback, the body increases osteoclastic activity on the side of increased pressure and increases osteoblastic activity on the side of decreased pressure (tension side). The result is a shift in the position of the alveolar socket in the direction of applied force. With sustained light force, movement usually begins in 2 weeks.

Excessive force might cause interference with the periodontal ligament and alveolar bone blood supply, which can lead to pulpal and bone necrosies. Damage to the periodontal structures may produce tooth mobility, external root resorption, ankylosis, and possible exfoliation.

INSTRUMENTATION FOR BEGINNING ORTHODONTIC CARE

A *rubber mixing bowl* is a green soft-sided rubber basin used to mix impression or stone material before placement on impression trays (Burns 951-3151, Schein 547-4106) (Figure 9.18).

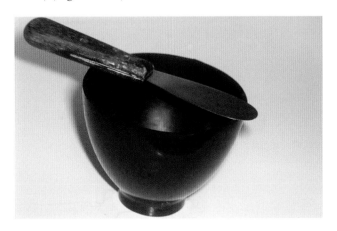

FIGURE 9.18. Rubber mixing bowl with beavertail spatula.

A *buffalo spatula* is a large mixing instrument made of nylon, metal, or plastic used to combine alginate and water (Burns 810-1230, Schein 100-3035).

A *dental vibrator* is used to remove air bubbles from the mixture of water with plaster or die stone. The vibrator helps move bubbles to the surface during the initial mixing and immediately after the stone is poured into the impressions (Burns 810-1568, Schein 365-3554) (Figure 9.19).

Etching solution, adhesive, and *brush* for orthodontic button placement may be purchased as a kit (Consise Orthodontic, ESPE 3M) (Figure 9.20).

Metal/resin buttons are bonded onto the teeth (Ormesh curved lingual pad with button, Ormco Corp.; Burns 070-5233, Schein 106-7408) (Figures 9.21, 9.22).

The *elastic Masel chain* is used as a source of force (Burns 005-1050, Schein 106-0335, O.S.E. 0188-180) (Figure 9.23).

Bracket placement tweezers are long-tipped reverse action instruments with fine serrated beaks used to carry and place brackets (buttons) to be bonded on teeth (Burns 091-4300, Schein 106-6184).

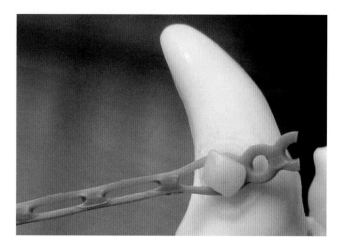

FIGURE 9.21. Light-cured resin button (Ortho Arch).

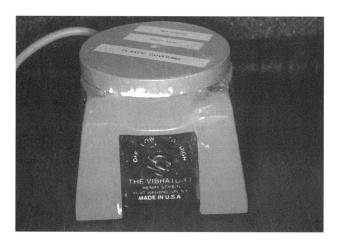

FIGURE 9.19. Vibrator to mix dental stone.

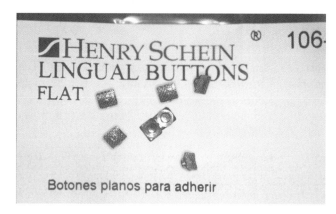

FIGURE 9.22. Curved rectangular base orthodontic buttons.

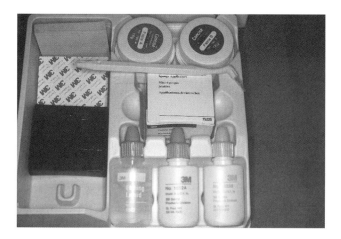

FIGURE 9.20. Concise orthodontic cement kit.

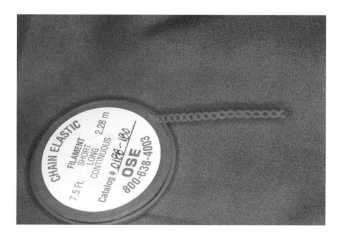

FIGURE 9.23. Masel chain.

ORTHODONTIC MATERIALS

Alginate is an irreversible hydrocolloid material used to make dental impressions for orthodontic study models. A paste-like mixture of water and powder is prepared in a rubber mixing bowl according to the manufacturer's instructions. The mixture is poured onto a tray placed in the mouth and compressed around the teeth for molding. In minutes, the alginate solidifies and the tray is removed from the mouth. Dental plaster or stone is then poured into the impression, creating a permanent model.

Alginate can be purchased as Type I (*fast set*) that gels within 1 or 2 minutes after mixing with water, or Type II (*normal set*) that takes 2–4 minutes to gel. The temperature of the water and environment affect the setting time. Heat speeds up the rate; cold slows it down. There is no difference in the completed impression between the two setting types of alginates.

It is imperative to accurately measure the alginate powder:water ratio. To help ensure accuracy, the manufacturer supplies a plastic scoop for dispensing bulk powder and a plastic cylinder for measuring water. The typical ratio is one scoop of powder to one measure of water.

The setup for obtaining an alginate impression requires the following:

- Alginate (regular set, Burns 950-0460, Schein 100-5292; fast set: Burns, 950-0465, Schein 100-5455) (Figure 9.24)
- Powder measure
- Water measure
- Medium-sized rubber mixing bowl (Burns 951-3151, Schein 547-4106)
- Beavertail-shaped wide-blade spatula (flexible: Burns 810-1230, Schein 365-7743; rigid: Burns 810-1225, Schein 365-0211) (refer to Figure 9.18)
- Impression tray (Shipp Laboratories) (Figures 9.25, 9.26)

The procedure for preparing an alginate impression begins with anesthetizing and intubating the animal, and cleaning the teeth. An impression tray is used to hold the alginate material. The tray is a rigid or semi-rigid device that is either prepurchased and reusable or custom-fabricated to specifically match the dog or cat's mouth.

Follow these steps:

1. Before loading the tray with alginate, test it for fit in the patient's mouth. A proper tray fit should:

- Cover all the teeth of interest and extend past their gingival margins. Occlusal surfaces and incisal edges of teeth should not contact the impression tray.
- Be sufficiently rigid to hold and support the material during tray placement and removal.
- Maintain an even distribution of 3–4 mm of the impression material between the tray and teeth.

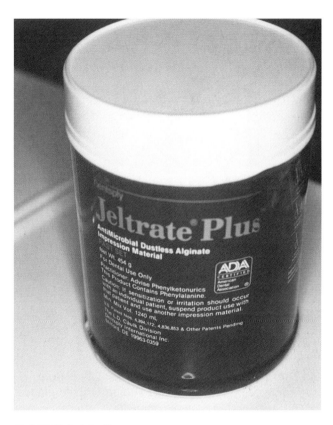

FIGURE 9.24. Alginate.

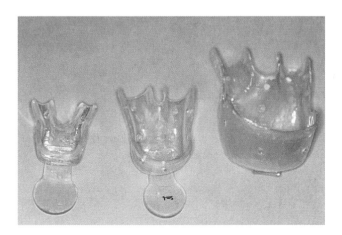

FIGURE 9.25. Commercial impression trays.

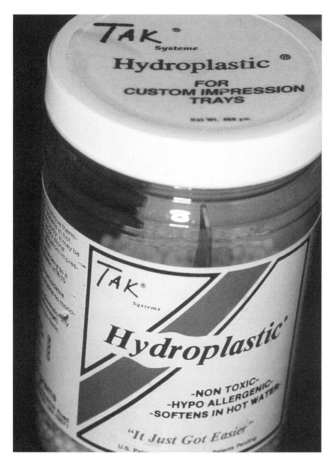

FIGURE 9.26. Custom tray material.

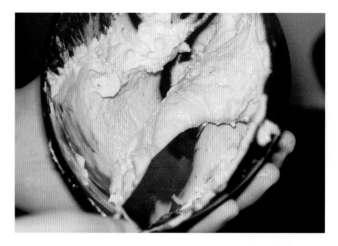

FIGURE 9.27. Alginate and water combined in mixing bowl.

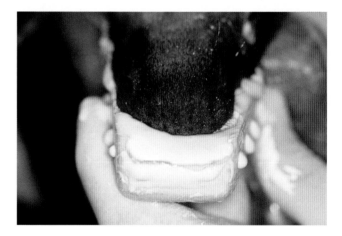

FIGURE 9.28. Alginate mixture loaded on to tray.

2. Fluff the alginate by gently rolling and inverting the storage container. Alginate should not be inhaled. As with other dental procedures, the operator should wear a surgical mask. After fluffing, slowly remove the storage container lid. Use the scoop provided to pour a predetermined amount (based on the size of the impression tray) of alginate into the flexible mixing bowl. An appropriate amount of water recommended by the manufacturer is combined in a green mixing bowl.

3. With a broad flexible spatula, mix the powder and water to a homogeneous consistency and load it on the impression tray. Level the surface of the tray (Figures 9.27, 9.28).

4. Place the loaded tray into the animal's mouth and seat distally first, then rostrally. The lips are retracted to avoid inclusion in the impression. The tray is held steady in the mouth until the alginate hardens (2–4 minutes depending on the type of alginate, the water, and environmental temperature) (Figures 9.29, 9.30).

5. Gently remove the tray by pulling away from the teeth. Examine the impression for significant voids or air bubble defects. If the impression is defective, repeat steps 3–5 (Figure 9.31).

6. Prepare two impressions of the maxilla and mandible. Dental laboratories prefer two master stone models of the arches; the primary is used for fabrication, and the backup model is used for fitting and adjusting. Backup models are also used by the laboratory when the case arrives damaged from shipping, or when the master model is found to have undesirable artifacts that would compromise the quality of the fabricated appliance.

7. Take a wax bite registration immediately after removing the endotracheal tube (see the section "Impressions," in Chapter 8, "Restorative Equipment, Materials, and Techniques").

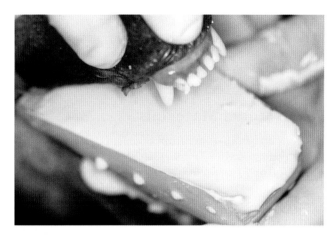

FIGURE 9.29. Tray placed inside of mouth, distal teeth first.

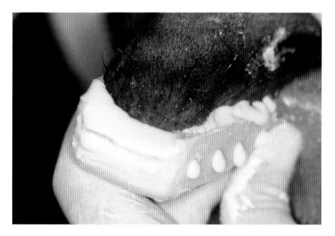

FIGURE 9.30. Mandible pressed into setting alginate.

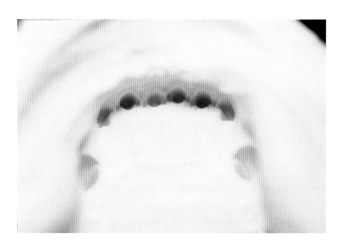

FIGURE 9.31. Negative alginate impression.

8. To avoid distortion of the alginate impression, pour the plaster or stone material immediately. If there is more than a 20-minute wait, wrap the impressions in damp paper towels and place in a covered container or plastic bag for storage up to 12 hours before pouring.

STONE MODELS

Dental models serve to permanently record occlusion. Dental models also help for:

- Preparation of a treatment plan
- Consultation with a colleague
- Fabricating orthodontic devices in the laboratory
- Comparison at follow-up examinations

The quality of the final orthodontic appliance can be no better than the quality of the stone models (Figure 9.32). Any geometric defect in the impression will be translated to the stone model and ultimately onto the appliance, which might not fit the patient. The stone model may be poured by staff in the veterinary office or by the laboratory if the alginate impression can be delivered within hours after fabrication.

Use the following setup for pouring stone models:

- Alginate impressions
- Model plaster or dental stone (Burns 985-1690, Schein 569-3164) (Figure 9.33)
- Water at room temperature
- Water measure
- Flexible bowl (Burns 951-3151, Schein 547-4106)
- Blunt-ended spatula (Schein 365-3203)

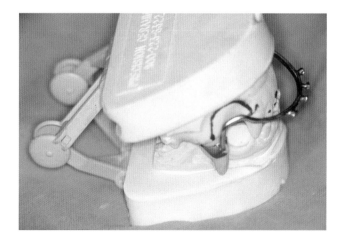

FIGURE 9.32. Stone model returned from laboratory with mounted orthodontic appliance.

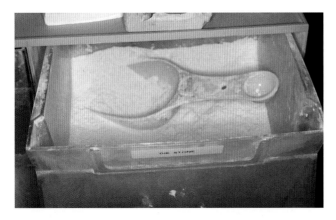

FIGURE 9.33. Dental stone with scoop.

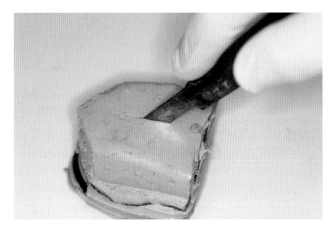

FIGURE 9.34. Laboratory knife incising alginate over the poured model.

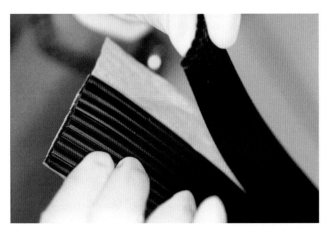

FIGURE 9.35. Utility wax round strips.

- Dental vibrator (Burns 952-2140, Schein 365-3554)
- Laboratory knife (Burns 951-5120, Schein 600-9130) (Figure 9.34)
- Boxing wax supplied in strips measuring 1–1½ inches wide, 12–18 inches long, and 1/8-inch thick, soft and

pliable at room temperature, may be further softened by passing through an open flame (Burns 854-0750, Schein 922-8232) (utility wax round strips may also be used for this purpose) (Figure 9.35)
- Brass pins (Pindex-Coltete Whaledent)

Stone Model Materials

Gypsum is the dihydrate form of calcium sulfate. When the gypsum powder is mixed with water, it hardens. Three forms of gypsum are used in pouring up stone models (Note: Type I impression plaster is too soft and Type V high-strength high-expansion dental stone is too hard to use in the veterinary setting):

- *Type II model plaster*, also called laboratory plaster of Paris, is used for pouring the primary impression, making study models, and repairing models. Type II plaster is weaker (low compressive and tensile strength) compared to dental stone because of the increased amount of space left by the evaporating water.
- *Type III dental stone* crystals are denser than those of model plaster. Dental stone does not require as much water to mix as the Type II plaster. The resulting product is harder, stronger, and more expensive than model plaster (Burns 985-1690, Schein 569-3164).
- *Type IV high-strength dental stone* requires less water than the other forms of gypsum, resulting in a stronger model (Tru-Stone: Miles, Inc., Schein 569-0883).

Water/Powder Ratio

The lower the water:powder ratio (more powder and less water), the greater the setting strength and hardness of the product. The optimal water:powder ratios for different types of dental stone and plaster differ markedly. If less than the minimum amount of water is used making the mix, a dry, crumbly, useless mixture results. When the mix is too thin, more powder should be added. If mix is too thick, more water is added. Common water:powder ratios for gypsum products include the following:

- Type I: 40–75 ml of water to 100 g of powder
- Type II: 45–50 ml of water to 100 g of powder
- Type III: 28-30 ml of water to 100 g of powder
- Type IV: 22–24 ml of water to 100 g of powder
- Type V: 18-22 ml of water to 100 g of powder

There are two commonly used techiques to pour stone models: Single pour and double pour. Follow these steps to mix and pour stone:

1. Premeasure 100 g of plaster and 50 ml water, or 100 g of dental stone and 25 ml water.

2. Place water in a green mixing bowl and hold the bowl in the palm of one hand. With the spatula in the other hand, slowly stir in one direction to avoid spilling powder. Mix the powder and water for approximately 20 seconds.

3. Place a cover over the platform of the vibrator to protect the rubber surface. When the mix is homogenous, place the bowl on the vibrator platform with the speed turned to low or medium.

4. Slightly press and rotate the flexible bowl on the vibrator to permit bubbles to rise to the surface. The total time for mixing and vibration of the model plaster should not exceed 2 minutes.

The following steps outline the double-pour method:

1. Place the alginate impression on the vibrator platform, angled forward. Set the vibrator at low to medium speed.

2. Place the mix near the vibrator. Dip a spatula into the bowl to pick up small increments of the mix.

3. Place a small mass of mix in the molar area of the alginate impression. Material poured into the impression on the vibrator will flow into tooth indentations slowly, forcing the mass forward.

4. Place additional small increments of the mix in the same area to provide gravitational flow. Because of the possibility of creating trapped air bubbles, do not place large amounts of the mixture on top of the flowing mass.

5. Rotate the tray slowly from side to side, providing continuous flow of the mix throughout.

6. After filling the indentations within the impression, place larger increments of the mix until the entire impression is filled.

7. Turn off the vibrator.

8. To prevent breakage of the large canine teeth, small brass pins (Pindex) can be inserted in the canine spaces before the model solidifies.

9. Repeat the process with the opposing arch and let dry.

Preparing a Base for Each Cast

Before sending the cast to the laboratory, a base is prepared. Commercial rubber molds are available for making bases, providing symmetry to the cast and reducing the need for trimming. Alternatively, a base may be made using boxing wax as a frame for additional plaster pour. There are multiple methods to construct the base:

With the insertion method:

1. The poured impression is allowed to set 5–10 minutes.

2. Additional plaster is mixed, adding 10% more powder than water to achieve a slightly thicker mixture. The combination is placed on a glass slab in a mound approximately the size of the impression and one inch thick.

3. The maxillary or mandibular cast is inverted onto the base of the new mix.

4. A spatula is used to drag the plaster base mix up onto margins of the initial pour.

With the box and pour method:

1. Alginate impressions are trimmed with the laboratory knife to remove alginate overlying the tray.

2. Boxing wax is attached and pressed in place around the impression, providing a "box" to contain the mix of plaster or stone. Boxing limits the flow of plaster or stone and makes a neat base for the cast (Figure 9.36).

3. Plaster/stone is poured as indicated in the previous procedure. The mix is added to the rim of the box to complete the pouring process (Figure 9.37).

In two hours, the model is ready for alginate removal. To separate the cast from the alginate impression:

1. If boxing wax is used, cut and gently pull the model away from the cast (Figure 9.38).

2. Use a laboratory knife to cut away the alginate in small pieces from the stone. Alginate should not be removed in a side-to-side fashion. That motion might fracture teeth on the cast (Figures 9.39, 9.40).

3. If a crown does fracture, replace and cement it with instant glue.

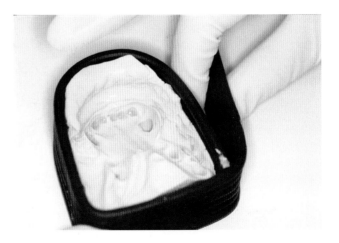

FIGURE 9.36. Boxing wax applied around prepared alginate impression.

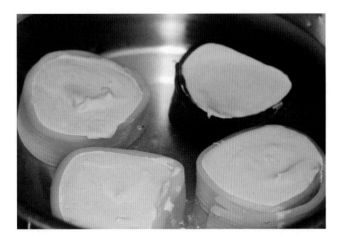

FIGURE 9.37. Dental stone poured on boxed impressions.

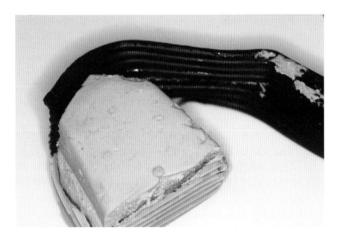

FIGURE 9.38. Removal of boxing wax.

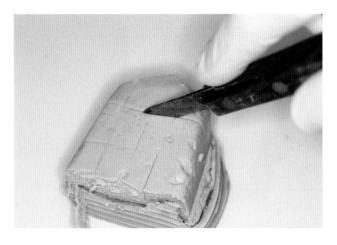

FIGURE 9.39. Laboratory knife used to incise alginate on stone model.

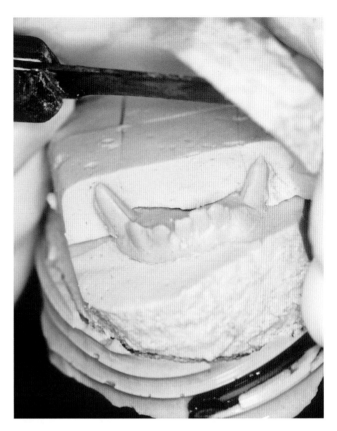

FIGURE 9.40. Removal of a section of alginate exposing stone model.

Trimming the Cast for Case Presentation

Casts should be trimmed geometrically to present an aesthetic appearance. The finished cast consists of two sections: the *anatomic portion*, representing the teeth and gingival attachment, and the *art portion*, which is the base or pedestal. When the bite impression is matched, both arches can be articulated and placed on the model trimmer at the same time to remove excessive plaster or stone (Figure 9.41). Articulation can be done in the office or by the dental laboratory.

Occlusion Alignment Marking

It is important to provide marked alignment points on the bite registration for the laboratory:

- At the midline
- At the left side (Figure 9.42)
- At the right side

Figure 9.43 is an example of an orthodontic prescription form.

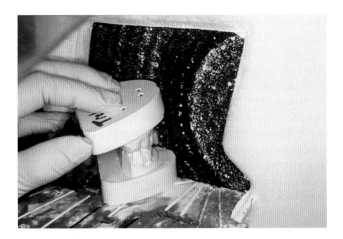

FIGURE 9.41. Model trimmer.

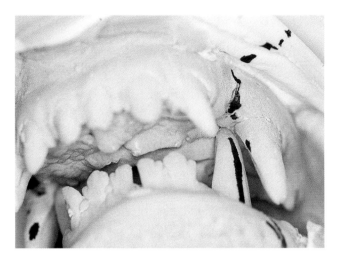

FIGURE 9.42. Model marked where the mandibular canine occludes with the maxilla.

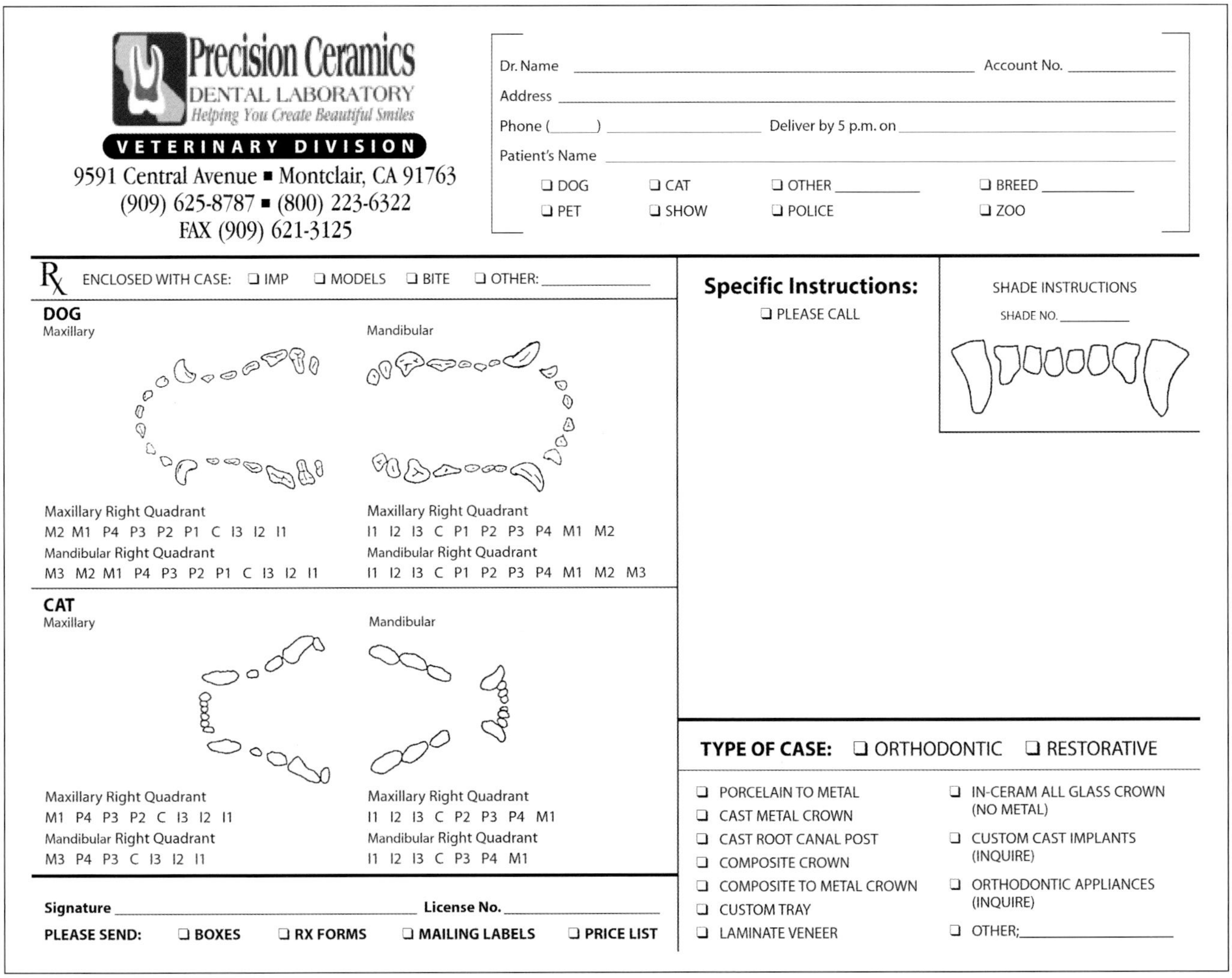

Precision Ceramics
DENTAL LABORATORY
Helping You Create Beautiful Smiles
VETERINARY DIVISION
9591 Central Avenue ■ Montclair, CA 91763
(909) 625-8787 ■ (800) 223-6322
FAX (909) 621-3125

Dr. Name _____ Account No. _____
Address _____
Phone (_____) _____ Deliver by 5 p.m. on _____
Patient's Name _____
❏ DOG   ❏ CAT   ❏ OTHER _____   ❏ BREED _____
❏ PET   ❏ SHOW   ❏ POLICE   ❏ ZOO

℞ ENCLOSED WITH CASE: ❏ IMP ❏ MODELS ❏ BITE ❏ OTHER: _____

DOG
Maxillary   Mandibular

Maxillary Right Quadrant
M2 M1 P4 P3 P2 P1 C I3 I2 I1
Mandibular Right Quadrant
M3 M2 M1 P4 P3 P2 P1 C I3 I2 I1

Maxillary Right Quadrant
I1 I2 I3 C P1 P2 P3 P4 M1 M2
Mandibular Right Quadrant
I1 I2 I3 C P1 P2 P3 P4 M1 M2 M3

CAT
Maxillary   Mandibular

Maxillary Right Quadrant
M1 P4 P3 P2 C I3 I2 I1
Mandibular Right Quadrant
M3 P4 P3 C I3 I2 I1

Maxillary Right Quadrant
I1 I2 I3 C P2 P3 P4 M1
Mandibular Right Quadrant
I1 I2 I3 C P3 P4 M1

Signature _____ **License No.** _____
PLEASE SEND: ❏ BOXES ❏ RX FORMS ❏ MAILING LABELS ❏ PRICE LIST

Specific Instructions:
❏ PLEASE CALL

SHADE INSTRUCTIONS
SHADE NO. _____

TYPE OF CASE: ❏ ORTHODONTIC ❏ RESTORATIVE

❏ PORCELAIN TO METAL
❏ CAST METAL CROWN
❏ CAST ROOT CANAL POST
❏ COMPOSITE CROWN
❏ COMPOSITE TO METAL CROWN
❏ CUSTOM TRAY
❏ LAMINATE VENEER

❏ IN-CERAM ALL GLASS CROWN (NO METAL)
❏ CUSTOM CAST IMPLANTS (INQUIRE)
❏ ORTHODONTIC APPLIANCES (INQUIRE)
❏ OTHER;_____

FIGURE 9.43. Orthodontic prescription form.

Shipping

Models must be protected from breakage during shipping. Wrapping the separate arches in bubble wrap and placing them in Styrofoam popcorn is generally sufficient.

When the appliance returns from the laboratory, it should be placed on the model to make sure the laboratory filled the prescription properly. The animal is then anesthetized, the appliance fitted, and the endotracheal tube removed to check occlusion. If it fits, the patient is re-intubated and the appliance cemented in place. If the appliance does not fit well, adjustments are made to make it functional, if possible, or it is sent back to the laboratory to be refabricated.

ORTHODONTIC CONDITIONS AND PROCEDURES

Case selection is critical in choosing patients to perform orthodontic care, especially if the case involves tooth movement. The client must be willing to return for rechecks and provide home care for prolonged periods of 6 months or longer.

Persistent Primary (Deciduous) Teeth

Normally, the primary tooth roots are resorbed as the secondary teeth erupt. The mechanism that causes resorption of the primary roots is not fully understood; neither is the mechanism that leads to failure of the roots to resorb. When resorption fails, the secondary teeth occupy the same alveolus as the primary teeth. Double sets of teeth may overcrowd the dental arch,

moving the secondary teeth to abnormal locations and causing malocclusion (Figure 9.44). Double sets of roots may also prevent the normal development of the alveolus and periodontal support around the permanent tooth, resulting in early tooth loss.

A persistent primary tooth should be extracted as soon as the secondary permanent tooth starts to erupt in the same socket. If extraction is performed early, the abnormally positioned permanent tooth usually moves to its normal location.

When a wait-and-see approach is taken to see whether the persistent primary tooth is exfoliated on its own accord, the secondary tooth often becomes permanently malpositioned, requiring orthodontic movement, crown reduction, or extraction.

Extra Teeth

Extra (supernumerary) teeth, depending on the size of the teeth and the arch, may cause periodontal disease from crowding and displacement of normal teeth. Supernumerary teeth should be extracted if crowding or gingival impingement exists. Supernumerary teeth are considered genetic faults (Figure 9.45).

Missing Teeth

Missing teeth (hypodontia) usually occurs in the premolar area, but any tooth in the mouth may be absent. The clinically absent tooth may be present below the gingival margin. Dental radiographs are indicated to determine whether the tooth is not present, nonerupted, or the crown missing with a fractured or resorbing root positioned subgingivally. True missing teeth are considered genetic faults.

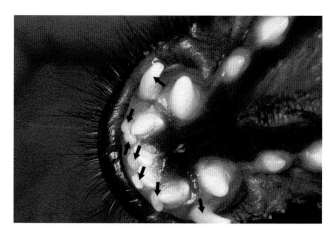

FIGURE 9.44. Multiple persistent primary mandibular canine and incisor teeth.

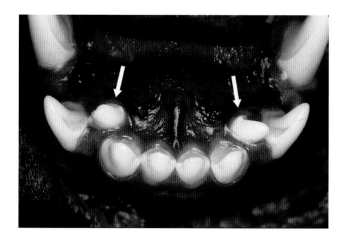

FIGURE 9.45. Supernumerary secondary maxillary incisors.

Maxilla Penetration by the Primary Mandibular Canines

Generally, any time there is a significant lesion caused by the primary dentition, the teeth causing the lesion should be extracted. When the maxilla is penetrated by the mandibular primary (deciduous) canines, the offending mandibular teeth should be extracted. Progress re-exams are necessary to make sure that the secondary canines do not follow the same path, necessitating additional attention (Figure 9.46).

Some breeders "trim" the primary canine tooth crowns in hopes they will shed early, preventing orthodontic problems. *"Trimming" is NOT a recommended procedure because it results in pulp exposure, pain for the animal, and the subsequent infection can affect the developing permanent tooth bud.*

Interceptive Orthodontics

Most dogs and cats are born overshot. This occlusion allows the neonatal animal to nurse effectively. As the animal grows, the mandible normally goes through a growth spurt. Occasionally the primary teeth erupt during the accelerated growth, resulting in the mandibular canines erupting distal and lingual to their normal positions, causing an interlock with the maxillary canines.

A dental interlock might prevent normal rostral growth of the maxilla or mandible. Even genetically normal dogs can occasionally develop malocclusion because of this interlock. Extraction of the affected primary mandibular canines and incisors before the dog or cat becomes 3 months old removes the interlock, allowing the jaws to continue to grow independently to their genetic potential.

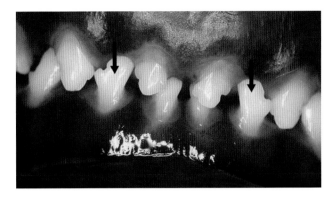

FIGURE 9.47. Intermediate primary incisors in an anterior cross bite occlusion.

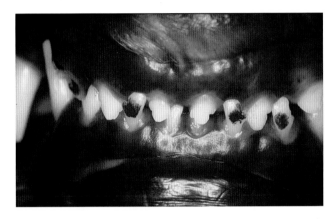

FIGURE 9.48. Mandibular teeth marked for extraction for interceptive orthodontics.

This procedure, called *interceptive orthodontics*, allows correction of a small percentage of the interlocked malocclusions by the time the secondary teeth erupt. Extraction does not stimulate jaw growth; it removes the mechanical barrier to genetic control of the growth process (Figures 9.47, 9.48).

Using Orthodontic Appliances for Tooth Movement

The following are steps of orthodontic therapy using appliances:

1. Diagnosis and discussion of client expectations, commitment, and genetic issues, if relevant
2. Alginate impression of the maxilla and mandible under general anesthesia (animal awoken from anesthesia after the impression is made)
3. Stone models poured in the veterinary office or dental laboratory
4. Laboratory appliance fabrication
5. Fit the appliance to the model.

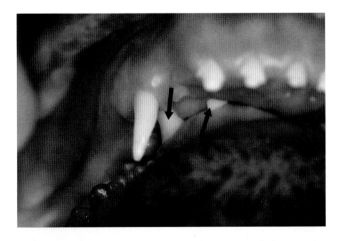

FIGURE 9.46. Primary mandibular canine (left arrow) and corner incisior penetrating maxilla (right arrow).

6. Fit the appliance to the patient under general anesthesia.
7. Cement the appliance into the patient's mouth
8. Activation of the appliance
9. Re-examination and adjustment visits, based on the type of orthodontic appliance, until the desired result has been achieved
10. Retention
11. Removal of the appliance under anesthesia, and teeth cleaning
12. Follow-up consultation

Underbite/Overbite

Therapy decisions to treat skeletal malocclusions are based on the ultimate goal to decrease or eliminate dental trauma, allowing the patient to have a functional and pain-free occlusion. Treatment options include crown reduction and restoration, movement of teeth with elastics attached to orthodontics buttons and/or appliances, or extraction are common options (Figures 9.49–9.61).

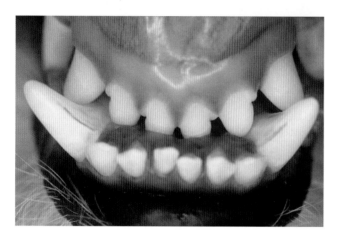

FIGURE 9.49. Maxillary incisors penetrating mandibular gingiva due to prognathism.

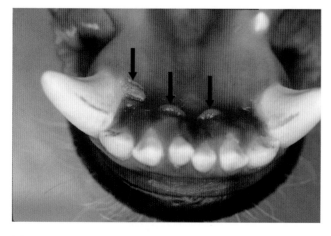

FIGURE 9.50. Mandibular ulceration caused by maxillary incisor impingment in the dog pictured in fig. 9.49.

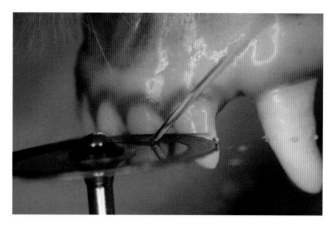

FIGURE 9.51. Maxillary incisor crown reduction using a diamond disk.

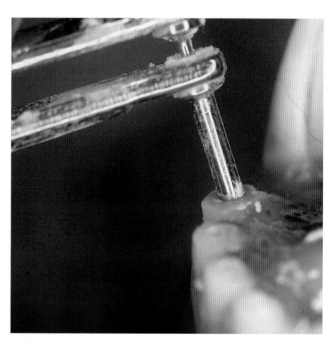

FIGURE 9.52. Calcium hydroxide applied on top of vital pulp tissue.

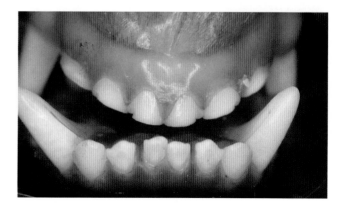

FIGURE 9.53. Crown reduced and restored incisors alleviating mandibular penetration.

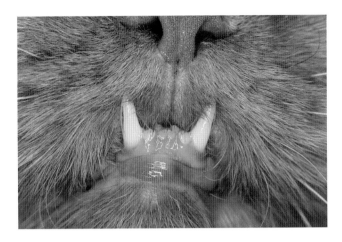

FIGURE 9.54. Mandibular canines protruding due to marked prognathism (Class III malocclusion) in a cat.

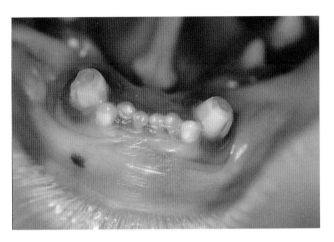

FIGURE 9.57. Composite restoration of crowns after direct pulp capping of the reduced canines.

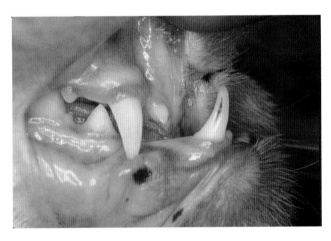

FIGURE 9.55. Lateral view of prognathic malocclusion.

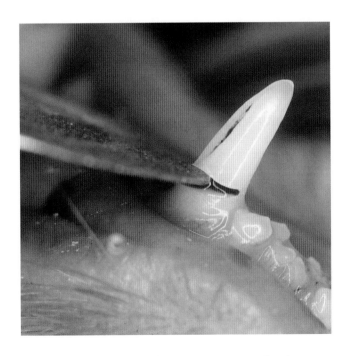

FIGURE 9.56. Mandibular canine crown reduction.

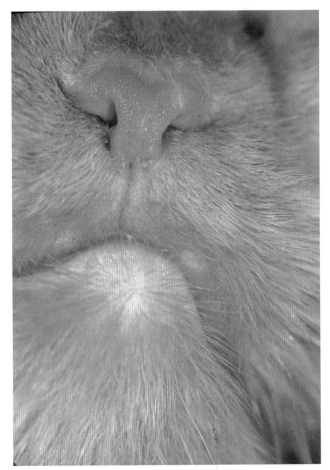

FIGURE 9.58. Lips close normally after crown reduction, vital pulpotomy, and direct pulp capping.

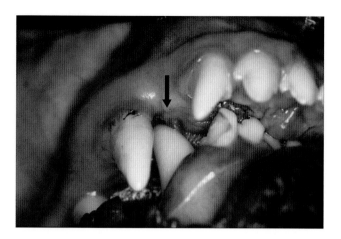

FIGURE 9.59. Mandibular canine penetration of the maxilla from brachygnathism (Class II malocclusion).

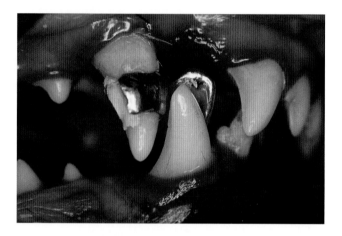

FIGURE 9.60. Mann inclined plane used to move the mandibular canine rostral and labial (in the above patient).

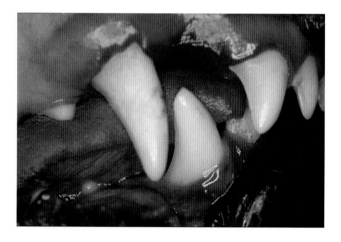

FIGURE 9.61. Mandibular canine moved to a functional occlusion.

Level Bite

When the maxillary and mandibular incisor, canine, or premolar teeth meet each other edge to edge, the occlusion is termed *even* or *level* (Fig 9.62). Level bite is considered normal in some breeds, although it is an expression of mandibular prognathism. A level bite produces increased contact between the maxillary and mandibular incisors, which will lead to attrition and may lead to uneven wear, traumatic pulpitis, trauma to the periodontal ligament, pulpal exposure, and early tooth loss. Orthodontic correction can be accomplished using an arch bar, attached to the maxillary canines extending rostral to the incisors, and orthodontic buttons cemented to the palatal surface of the incisors. Elastics are attached to the buttons and the arch bar to pull the maxillary incisors forward.

Anterior crossbite occurs when one or more mandibular incisors are positioned rostral to the maxillary incisors (Figs. 9.63, 9.64). This condition can be caused by persistent maxillary primary incisor teeth, trauma in the neonate or juvenile causing displacement of the permanent tooth bud, skeletal malocclusion

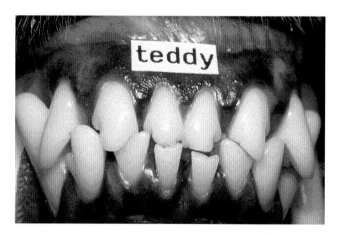

FIGURE 9.62. Level bite.

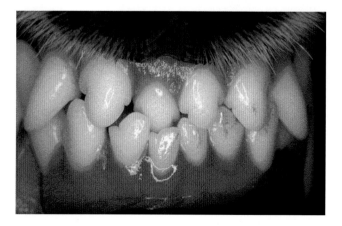

FIGURE 9.63. Anterior crossbite.

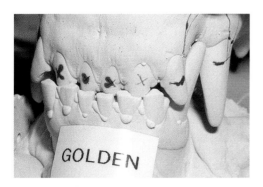

FIGURE 9.64. Stone model of Golden retriever with corner incisors in scissors and the remaining incisors in an anterior cross bite.

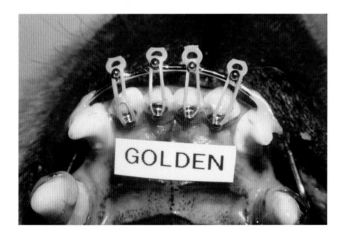

FIGURE 9.65. Maxillary arch bar affixed to canines and corner incisors with buttons and elastics attached to the central and intermediate incisors.

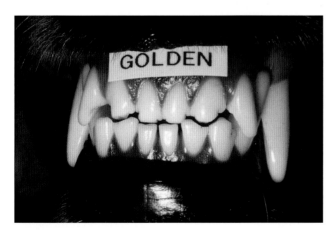

FIGURE 9.66. Improved occlusion after orthodontic movement.

(Angle Class III malocclusion), overzealous tug-of–war games, or impacted roots.

Options to correct rostral crossbite include the following:

- Labial movement of the affected maxillary teeth through placement of a maxillary arch wire cemented to the maxillary canines. Buttons bonded on the palatal surface of the affected incisors are attached by elastics to the arch wire leading to rostral tooth movement (Figs 9.65, 9.66).
- Movement of the mandibular incisors lingually with elastics attached to an arch bar cemented to mandibular canines.
- Maxillary arch wire with finger springs to push the abnormally placed teeth forward (Figure 9.67).
- Maxillary acrylic appliance with expansion screw device (Figure 9.68).
- Surgical repositioning of the affected teeth to a functional state.

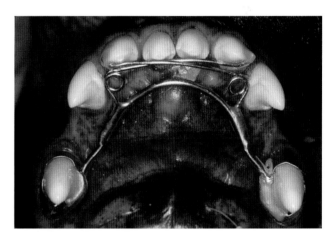

FIGURE 9.67. Maxillary arch wire with finger springs.

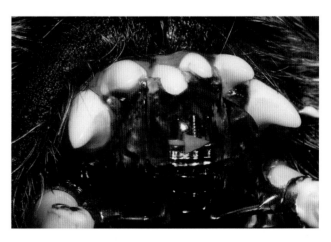

FIGURE 9.68. Maxillary acrylic screw appliance.

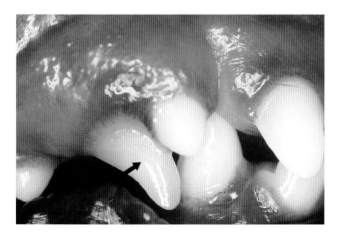

FIGURE 9.69. Dental linguoversion of the mandibular canine caused by persistent primary teeth.

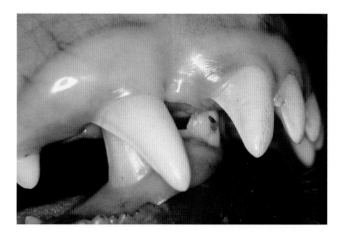

FIGURE 9.70. Linguoverted mandibular canine secondary to skeletal malocclusion.

Base Narrow Canines

Base narrow (lingually displaced, lingual inclined, lingual tipped, linguoverted) canines occur when the mandibular canine teeth impinge on the maxilla. Base narrow canines can result from:

- *Dental linguoversion*, which occurs when the mandibular canine(s) appears upright and impinges on gingiva between the maxillary third incisor and the canine, or contacts the palate. In cases of dental linguoversion, the rest of the occlusion is normal, including the incisor relationship, premolar alignment, and molar occlusion. The most common etiology for linguoverted mandibular canines is persistent primary mandibular canine teeth (Figures 9.69, 9.70).
- *Skeletal linguoversion* can occur when the mandible is underdeveloped (mandibular brachygnathia or micrognathia). In these cases, the mandible is too narrow, and/or short, resulting in the mandibular canines traumatizing palatal tissues (Figure 9.71).

Base narrow canine teeth can be classified is as follows:

- *Class I*: The mandibular canine tip is directed *toward* a line connecting distal face of maxillary canine and corner incisor.
- *Class II*: The mandibular canine tip is directed *palatal* to a line connecting the distal face of maxillary canine and corner incisor.
- *Class III*: The mandibular canine tip lies palatal to maxillary canine.
- *Class IV*: The mandibular canine tip impinges the palate distal to the maxillary canine.

Lingually displaced canines may be treated by:

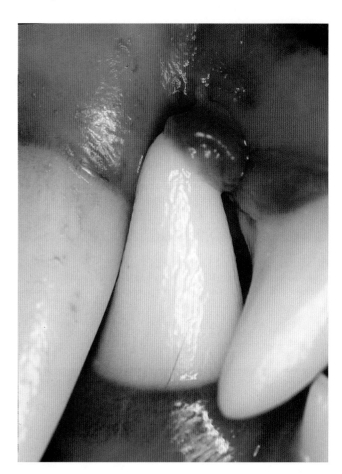

FIGURE 9.71. Lingually displaced mandibular canine impinging on the maxillary gingiva.

- *Extracting* the persistent primary mandibular canines in cases of dental linguoversion, allowing the secondary canines the oppprtunity to erupt laterally (interceptive orthodontics).

- *Gingivoplasty (surgical incline plane),* where a wedge of gingival tissue is excised between the permanent maxillary canine and corner incisor in minor cases. The gingivoplasty may allow movement of the mandibular canines into normal position while they are erupting (patient is 5–8 months old), and contacting the auto incline plane (Figures 9.72–9.73).
- *Mandibular canine crown reduction, vital pulpotomy, direct pulp capping, and restoration,* where the affected tooth is reduced in height, removing palatal contact. After crown reduction, a partial coronal pulpectomy with direct pulp capping is performed and the tooth restored (Figures 9.74–9.77). The main advantages of crown reduction are decreased therapy time, less aftercare, and lower expense compared to tooth movement procedures. The treatment is completed within one or two visits (if the tooth is restored with a laboratory-prepared crown, the patient needs to be anesthetized twice). Yearly fol-

low-up radiographs are recommended to check for endodontics disease Disadvantages of crown reduction and restoration lie in exposure of the pulp, possible future restoration leakage, and failure to maintain a vital tooth.
- *Extracting the maxillary canine(s)* in cases where the mandibular canines are directed palatally to the

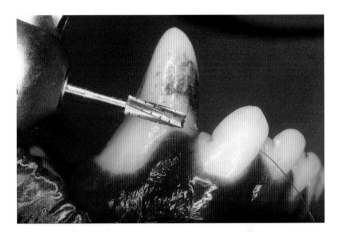

FIGURE 9.74. Cross-cut fissure bur used for crown reduction.

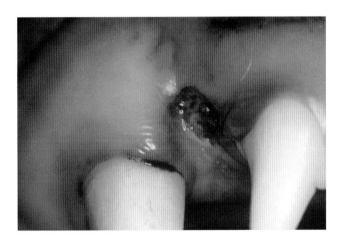

FIGURE 9.72. Laser gingivoplasty.

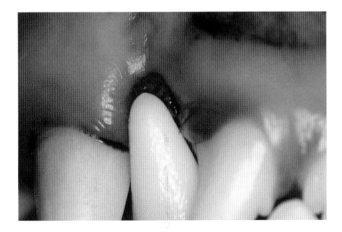

FIGURE 9.73. Correction of gingival penetration due to lingually displaced canine.

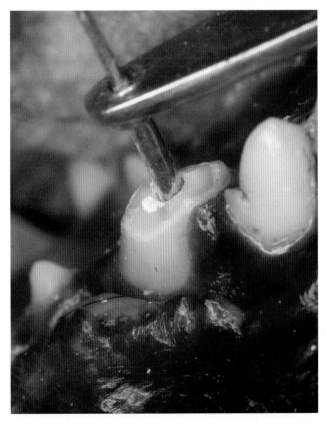

FIGURE 9.75. Calcium hydroxide applied on vital pulp.

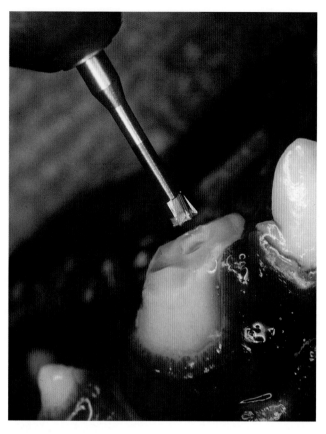

FIGURE 9.76. Inverted cone bur used to prepare access for composite restoration.

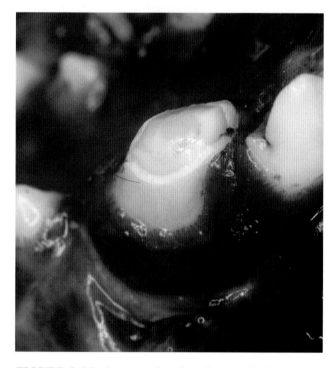

FIGURE 9.77. Crown reduced and restored alleviating palatal trauma.

maxillary canines. Mandibular canines are more "important" than the maxillary canines for oral function. When the maxillary canines are removed, the mandibular canines usually fit functionally into the void that is left. After the procedure, the dog will still have use of the maxillary incisors, which occlude with the mandibular canines to pick up objects.

- Cementing an acrylic, composite, or cast metal telescoping *inclined bite plane* on the maxillary canines to move the mandibular canine teeth labially or facially. Orthodontic movement to treat lingually displaced canines should start between 9 and 12 months old, before the roots are fully developed. Over time (weeks) gradual lateral pressure usually moves the canine(s) to functional positions. An *acrylic or composite inclined plane* is useful for minor movements. The acrylic plane is either fabricated on a stone model and installed during a secondary anesthetic event, or fabricated directly on the patient's maxilla (preferred). (When using Jet acrylic, an exothermic reaction takes place that may injure the gingiva; Protemp Garant does not produce an exothermic reaction.) Non-telescopic acrylic bite planes restrict maxillary growth because of their rigid nature. Food debris also lodges under the bite plane, causing localized gingivitis. Careful toothbrushing, twice-daily home care, and application of 0.12% chlorhexidine flushes are recommended (Figure 9.78, 9.79).

The following are materials used to fabricate an acrylic or composite appliance (Figure 9.80):

- Jet acrylic orthodontic powder and liquid (Burns 859-1001, Schein 125-1546) or ProTemp Garant (Burns 878-0534)
- Rope wax (Burns 952-2420, Schein 547-0200)

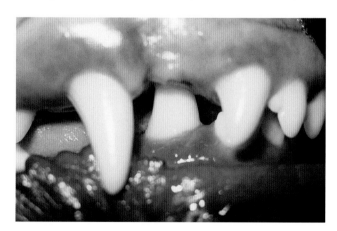

FIGURE 9.78. Lingually displaced right mandibular canine penetrating the maxillary gingiva.

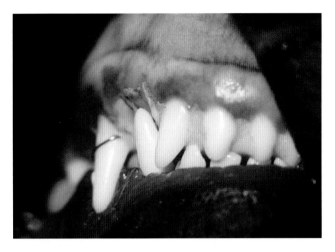

FIGURE 9.79. Orthodontic correction, afrer three weeks of treatment, using an acrylic inclined plane.

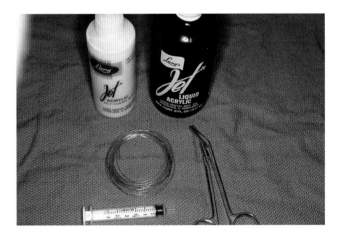

FIGURE 9.80. Materials needed to fabricate an acrylic inclined plane.

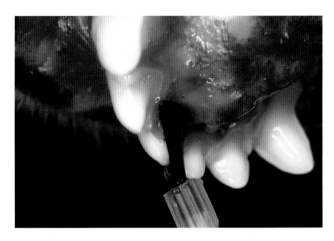

FIGURE 9.81. Liquid etchant applied to incisial palatal surfaces.

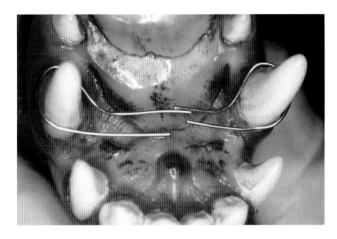

FIGURE 9.82. Orthodontic wire placed before acrylic placement.

- 21 gauge orthodontic wire
- Orthodontic cement

To directly fabricate an acrylic inclined bite plane appliance on the maxilla, first anesthetize, place the animal in dorsal recumbency, and intubate. Pack the pharynx with gauze. (*Note:* if using Jet acrylic, the exothermic reaction generated may injure gingival tissues.) Then use the following steps:

1. Clean, polish (using fluoride-free polish), acid-etch (according to the manufacturer's directions), rinse, and air-dry the palatal surfaces of the incisors, canines, and first premolars (Figure 9.81).
2. Brush a layer of unfilled composite resin bonding agent on the etched enamel and light cure.
3. Place rope wax around the periphery of the appliance area at the gingival level to serve as a dam to contain the material (rope wax not pictured in example figures)
4. Cut and bend orthodontic wire. Loop it around the maxillary canines and place it against the palatal surface of the maxilla (Figure 9.82).
5. Sprinkle a light coating of the powder polymer on the rostral maxilla (Figure 9.83).
6. Add drops of the liquid portion to the powder until a gel consistency is formed (Figure 9.84).
7. Place more powder, followed by more liquid ("salt and pepper"), until a 2–4 mm thickness is achieved.
8. Before the acrylic hardens, extubate the animal and occlude its jaws to create indentations in the acrylic; these serve as starting points for the incline plane. Form the inclined plane by rolling a rounded instrument (Steinman pin, pen tip) from the impingement point to the space between the canine and corner incisor. Fabricate the incline deeper laterally (Figure 9.85). Fine adjustments of angulation

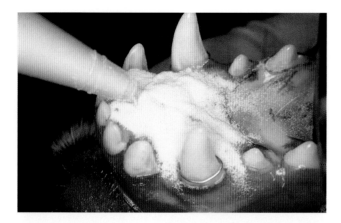

FIGURE 9.83. Powder polymer applied.

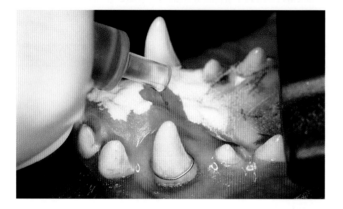

FIGURE 9.84. Liquid applied to initiate acrylic hardening.

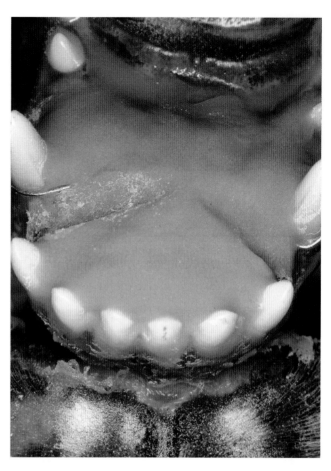

FIGURE 9.86. Hardened acrylic inclined plane.

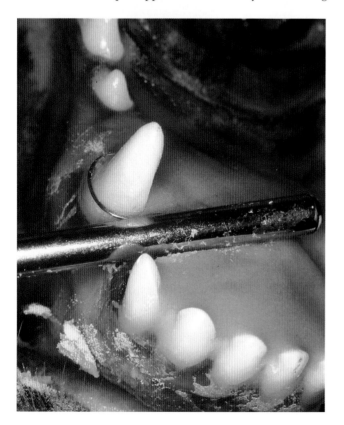

FIGURE 9.85. Steinman pin used to make incline.

and direction can be achieved with a white stone bur attached to a low-speed handpiece after the acrylic hardens or finishing bur on a high-speed handpiece (Figure 9.86).

9. Cement the retention wires placed around canines with glass ionomer, C&B Metabond, Panavia, or Concise orthodontic cement. *Note:* The acrylic incline dose not allow for maxillary growth and should only be used for a period of one or two weeks in a growing patient.

The *Mann inclined plane* has a telescoping connecting bar between the sides of the appliance. As the skull grows in width, the appliance expands. Even if only one mandibular canine is lingually displaced, both mandibular canines should be included—one incline plane to move the displaced canine and the other to prevent shifting of the mandible (Figures 9.87–9.91). To fabricate a Mann inclined plane, the laboratory needs orthodontic casts and bite registrations of the maxillary and mandibular incisors and canines.

Composite restorative bite planes can be fabricated between the maxillary canines and corner incisors (Figures 9.92, 9.93).

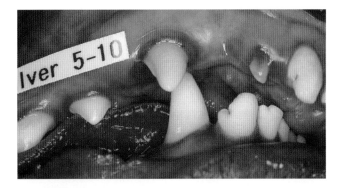

FIGURE 9.87. Mandibular canine impinging on palate in a brachygnathic weimeraner.

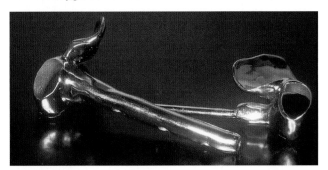

FIGURE 9.88. Cast metal inclined plane with telescoping bar.

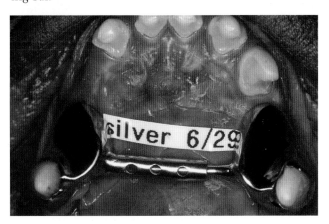

FIGURE 9.89. Telescoping inclined plane cemented to the maxillary canines after extraction of the maxillary corner incisor.

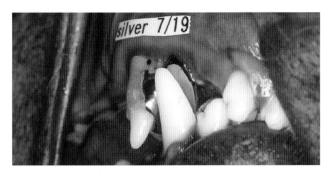

FIGURE 9.90. Lingually displaced canines after 3 weeks of orthodontic correction.

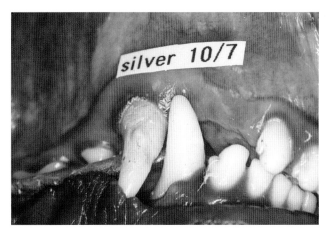

FIGURE 9.91. Right mandibular canine moved labially by inclined plane (maxillary canine moved distally).

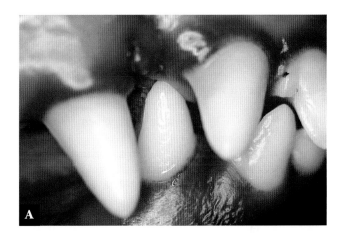

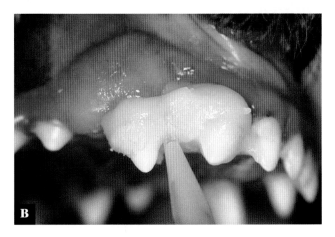

FIGURE 9.92. (A) Lingually displaced mandibular canine; (B) composite applied to fabricate an inclined plane between the maxillary canine and corner incisor.

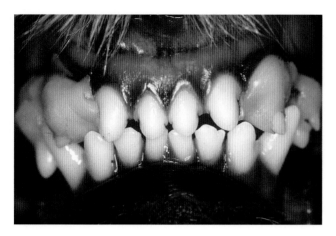

FIGURE 9.93. Mandibular canines (of the patient in figure 9.92) moved labially after three weeks of orthodontic care.

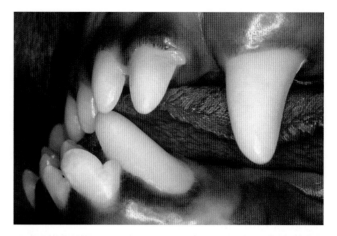

FIGURE 9.94. Rostroverted mandibular canine.

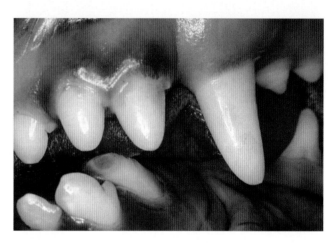

FIGURE 9.95. Crown reduction, vital pulpotomy, direct pulp capping, and restoration of a mandibular canine alleviating interference.

Attention must be given to prevent accumulation of debris between the orthodontic appliance and the gingiva. The client is instructed to daily apply a 0.12% chlorhexidine solution and gently brush the pet's teeth. When the teeth have reached their designated position, which takes from weeks to months, the animal is anesthetized, the appliance is removed by gentle rocking or use of a high-speed dental drill, the cement removed, and the teeth polished.

An *activated "W" wire* or Unitek expansion screw device cemented on the mandibular canines can push the mandibular canines laterally. The screw device should be activated every 4–6 days, slowly moving the mandibular canines laterally.

Rotated Teeth

Rotated teeth occur most often in short-muzzled (brachycephalic) dogs. Selective breeding creates an undersized mouth that cannot accommodate 42 teeth in normal alignment. The maxillary third premolar is most commonly affected. In the case of multiple-rooted teeth, the rotated tooth root closest to the palate is prone to support loss. Daily toothbrushing may help save a rotated tooth. Often the tooth will be extracted due to periodontal disease.

Rostral Displacement

Rostral displacement (mesioversion, lance, spear teeth) of the maxillary or mandibular canine teeth may be caused by persistent permanent tooth buds, genetic influence (especially Shetland sheepdogs and Persian cats), or skeletal abnormalities (Figures 9.94).

Treatment for rostral canine displacement includes the following:

- *Crown reduction, vital pulp therapy, and restoration* (Figure 9.95).
- *Orthodontic movement with elastics.* The best time for this treatment is between 9 and 18 months. Tooth movement to a functional position takes 2–6 months.
- *Custom-made brackets and elastics* from impressions of the target and anchor teeth can be fabricated by a dental lab (Figure 9.96).

TOOTH MOVEMENT WITH ORTHODONTIC BUTTONS AND ELASTICS

Tooth movement with elastics and buttons involves anchor and target teeth. Anchor teeth with greater surface area are chosen to provide higher resistance to the

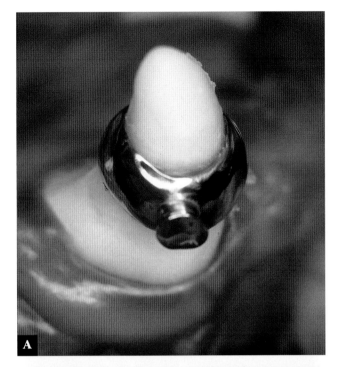

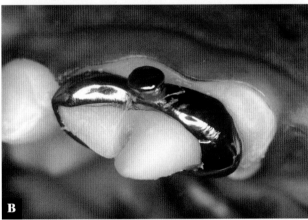

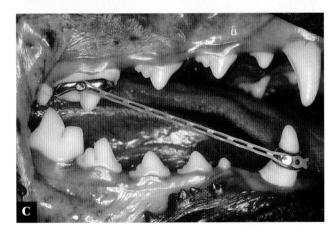

FIGURE 9.96. Custom brackets (A) and (B), and elastic chain (C) move the mandibular canine distally. (Ideally more than one anchor tooth is used.)

move compared to the *target tooth*. Ideally, the anchor tooth remains stable, allowing the target tooth to move. Healthy anchor teeth and periodontal support is critical for successful target tooth movement. Commonly, the maxillary fourth premolars and first molars are used together as anchors to move rostrally deviated canines distally.

Direct Bonding of Orthodontic Buttons

Orthodontic brackets or buttons are cemented on teeth to provide attachment for elastics, wires, or springs. Elastic chains are used as a source of force for many appliances.

Use the following setup for bracket application and elastic placement:

- Right-angled handpiece (Burns 951-4635, Schein 100-8643)
- Rubber polishing cup (Burns 951-8500, Schein 100-5078)
- Fine pumice (Burns 990-2705, Schein 312-2547)
- Cotton pliers (Burns 951-8225, Schein 100-3313)
- Etching solution, adhesive, and brush (may be purchased as a kit from Consise Orthodontic)
- Metal brackets, Ormesh curved lingual pad with button (Ormco Corp.) (Burns 070-5233, Schein 106-7408)
- Elastic Masel chain, flattened elastic with an arrangement of holes to allow attachment to buttons or brackets (Burns 005-1050, Schein 106-0335, O.S.E. 0188-180)
- Bracket placement tweezers (Burns 091-4300, Schein 106-6184)

Affixing the Orthodontic Buttons

Follow these steps to prepare the tooth:

1. Polish the tooth surfaces free of plaque and debris using a rubber cup on a prophy angle and slurry of pumice/water. Fluoride paste should not be used, because the fluoride might prevent the etching process of the enamel.
2. Thoroughly rinse the teeth for at least 30 seconds.
3. Dry the teeth to be bracketed with oil-free compressed air.
4. Apply etching solution or gel according to the manufacturer's instructions on the enamel surface where the bracket is to be affixed. After etching, rinse and air-dry the tooth surface (Figure 9.97).
5. After etching, the tooth surface should appear dull and chalky. If not, repeat the etching process.

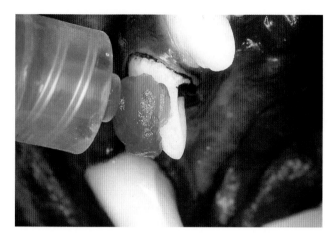

FIGURE 9.97. Etchant applied to enamel surface.

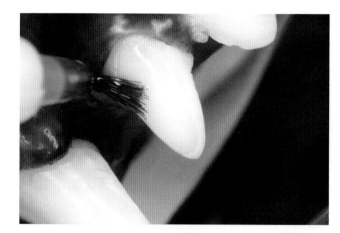

FIGURE 9.98. Sealant and accelerator brushed on etched enamel.

To affix buttons or brackets using Concise Orthodontic (3M):

1. Place a drop of sealant, the accelerator, and equal portions of adhesive material and hardener in separate locations on a paper pad.
2. With a small absorbent square cotton pellet attached to cotton pliers, or a brush, mix the sealant and accelerator; paint the mixture on the etched surfaces of one or more teeth (Figure 9.98). Choose the location for button placement to provide a straight line between the anchor and target tooth.
3. Mix the adhesive and hardener with a plastic instrument or spatula.
4. Select metal orthodontic brackets with bracket forceps or college tipped pliers.
5. Apply the adhesive/hardener mixture to the base of the bracket (Figure 9.99).
6. Position the bracket on the tooth and press into the adhesive. Remove excess bonding material with a hand scaler (Figure 9.100).

Elastics may be placed on the buttons approximately 10 minutes after cementation (Figure 9.101). Some cases may need the addition of composite on the molars to open the bite (bite block) sufficiently for mandibular and maxillary canines to pass without occlusal interference. The use of posterior bite blocks in young animals may cause intrusion of the treated teeth. To place elastics, apply light force to the elastic power chain. If the bracket does not come off the tooth, pull the chain to test the bond. If the bracket is dislodged, it can be reap-

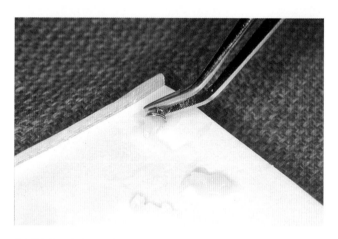

FIGURE 9.99. Adhesive mixed and applied on the bracket base.

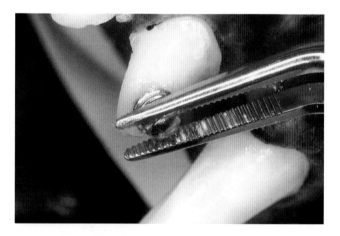

FIGURE 9.100. Bracket placement.

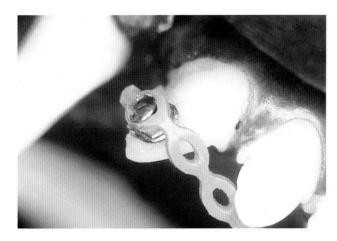

FIGURE 9.101. Masel chain applied to cemented bracket.

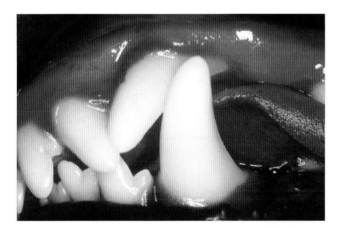

FIGURE 9.102. Rostrally deviated maxillary canine.

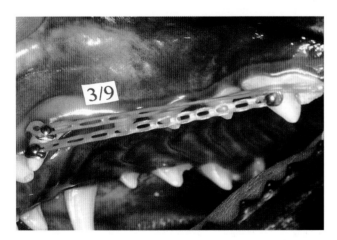

FIGURE 9.103. Orthodontic buttons and elastics affixed to the maxillary canine (target tooth) and maxillary fourth premolar and first molar (anchor teeth).

plied using the adhesive/hardener mixture.

Check the patient weekly to monitor progress and replace elastics. Tooth movement is not expected in the first 2 weeks, because it takes that long to recruit osteoclasts and osteoblasts. Movement in the first 2 weeks would be secondary to bone necrosis, not remodeling, indicating excessive force and potential failure. The goal is slow movement over 2–4 months. At the recheck appointment, anchor tooth movement should also be checked and if present, elastics removed or additional anchor teeth added (Figures 9.102–9.111).

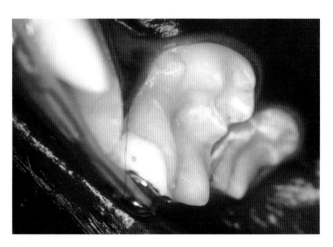

FIGURE 9.104. Maxillary fourth premolar before bite block fabrication.

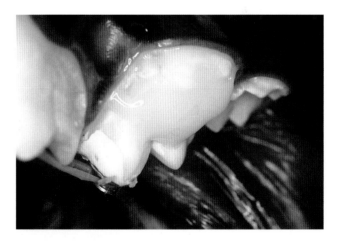

FIGURE 9.105. Acrylic resin bonded to the maxillary first molar occlusal surface to provide a bite block to open the mouth for the maxillary canine to pass the mandibular canine.

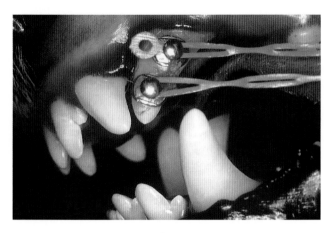

FIGURE 9.106. Resulting open bite after bite block placement.

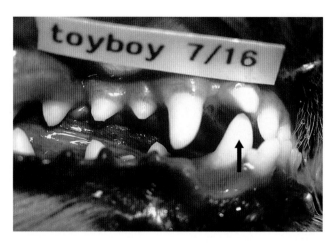

FIGURE 9.109. Mandibular canine interfering with the maxillary corner incisor in a brachygnathic Maltese.

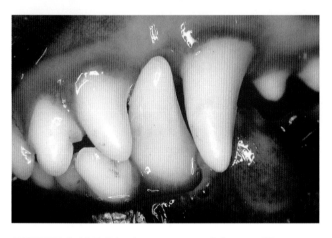

FIGURE 9.107. Distal movement of the maxillary canine achieved in 3 months.

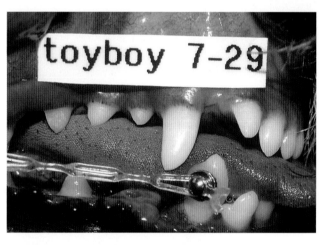

FIGURE 9.110. Orthodontic buttons and elastics 13 days after application.

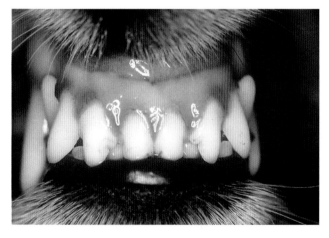

FIGURE 9.108. Mandibular canine moved to functional occlusion without further orthodontic intervention.

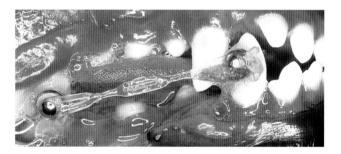

FIGURE 9.111. Functional occlusion achieved 21 days after after buttons and elastics were applied and continuous active force orthodontics was begun.

Extraction of the Malpositioned or Impinged-upon Tooth

In some malocclusions, extraction of the offending or impinged-upon tooth is performed to allow a functional pain-free bite. The advantages of extraction compared to orthodontic movement include less total treatment time, less expense, and less anesthetic procedures to accomplish therapy. The disadvantage of extraction is loss of a permanent tooth (Figures 9.112, 9.113).

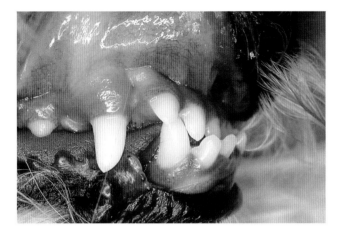

FIGURE 9.112. Mandibular canine interferring with the maxillary corner incisor.

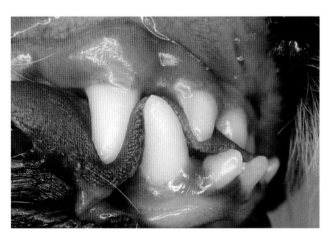

FIGURE 9.113. Maxillary corner incisor extracted alleviating the interference.

EDGEWISE BRACKET SYSTEM

Arch wire shaped as a horseshoe can be applied to edgewise brackets to move teeth. The wire has memory providing sufficient force to move teeth gradually to the normal arch form. Round wires (in cross section) are used initially to correct crowded and crooked teeth. Square wire can be used during the final stages of treatment to position the crown and root in the correct alignment. Edgewise bracket system therapy is considered an advanced dental procedure (Burns 981-1042, Schein 106-0439) (Figure 9.114).

Table 9.1 summarizes orthododontic care.

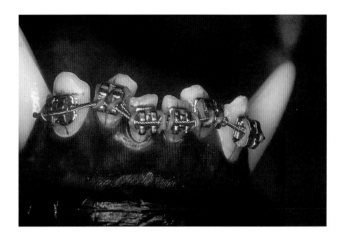

FIGURE 9.114. Edgewise bracket system.

Table 9.1. Orthodontic care at a glance.

Diagnosis	Clinical Significance	Treatment
Persistent primary teeth	Two teeth in the same alveolus at the same time result in abnormal secondary tooth position.	Extraction of the persistent primary tooth
Dental interlock	The mandibular canines or incisors impede the forward growth of the maxilla.	Extraction of the teeth interfering with the maxillary forward growth (usually the impinging teeth of the shorter jaw)
Class II occlusion	Mandibular canines may traumatize the hard palate.	Crown reduction and vital pulp therapy of the mandibular canines, orthodontic movement of the affected teeth into a functional occlusion, or extraction
Class III malocclusion	Maxillary incisors or canines may contact the mandibular gingiva lingually.	Crown reduction if mandibular penetrations are ulcerated
Anterior cross bite	One or more mandibular incisors located rostral to the maxillary incisors may cause increased trauma to misaligned teeth.	Orthodontic correction with arch wire and elastics or extraction of the malpositioned teeth
Base narrow mandibular canines	Mandibular canines impinge on the hard palate.	Mandibular crown reduction with vital pulp therapy and restoration, inclined plane (metal or acrylic) attached to maxillary canines to push the mandibular canines into functional occlusion, or extraction
Rotated third premolars	Periodontal disease affecting the palatal side of rotated tooth or crowding.	Extraction if pathology noted or prophylactically to prevent bone loss with periodontal disease
Rostral displacement of maxillary or mandibular canines	Canines positioned rostrally may interfere with other teeth.	Crown reduction with vital pulp therapy and restoration, orthodontic movement using buttons and elastics, or extraction
Supernumerary teeth	Extra secondary teeth may result in crowding, which predisposes these teeth to periodontal disease.	Extraction of the extra tooth if crowding occurs

10
Oral Surgical Equipment, Materials, and Techniques

EXTRACTIONS

Dental extractions are the most commonly performed surgical procedures in general practice. The objectives of extractions are to:

- Remove the tooth and its root(s) with minimal trauma to the alveolar bone and surrounding soft tissues.
- Eliminate periodontal and periapical lesions.
- Prepare the alveolus for proper healing.

Indications for extractions include the following:

- Persistent primary (deciduous) teeth interfering with the normal eruption of permanent teeth. When persistent primary canines are not extracted, the maxillary secondary canine teeth may be diverted mesially, or the mandibular canines diverted lingually (Figures 10.1, 10.2). When the persistent primary teeth are extracted early, the secondary teeth usually return to their normal location.
- Abnormal location of primary or secondary teeth, causing trauma to opposing teeth or oral soft tissues (Figure 10.3).
- Dental overcrowding predisposing to periodontal disease(Figure 10.4).
- Retained or fractured root fragments (traumatic or pathological) (Figure 10.5).
- Impacted and unerupted teeth. When left untreated, a dentigerous cyst might form affecting adjacent structures (Figures 10.6–10.9).
- Periodontal disease where >50% of the tooth support is lost and/or the owner does not consent to procedures to try to save the tooth.

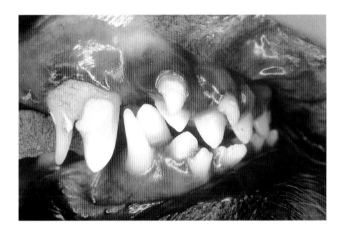

FIGURE 10.1. Persistent primary maxillary and mandibular canine and incisor teeth.

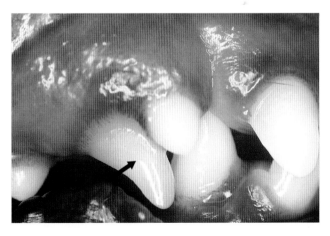

FIGURE 10.2. Persistent maxillary primary canine tooth displacing the secondary canine.

Glossary

Alveoloplasty (Alveoplasty) is the surgical shaping and smoothing of the tooth socket margins after extraction.

Ankylosis is the fusion of the cementum or dentin and alveolar bone.

Avulsion is the separation of a tooth from its alveolus.

Caries is a demineralization and loss of tooth substance, common in humans and rare in dogs and cats. Caries begin on the external tooth surface by demineralization of enamel or exposed cementum.

Dentigerous cyst is an epithelial-lined sac, which forms around the crown of an unerupted tooth.

Dilaceration refers to a sharp bend, curve, or angulation in the root or crown of a tooth from developmental causes.

Elevator is a dental hand instrument used to elevate teeth and/or section roots to remove them from the alveoli.

Embedded tooth is covered with bone.

Epulis is the clinically descriptive term denoting any growth on the gingival margin.

Faucitis is the often-used incorrect term to denote caudal stomatitis lateral to the palatoglossal folds.

FORL(s) is an abbreviation for *feline odontoclastic resorptive lesion(s)*.

Frenectomy is the surgical detachment of a frenulum.

Frenulum is a fold of mucous membrane attaching the cheeks and lips to the maxillary and mandibular arches and limiting the movement of an organ (tongue).

Hemisection is the surgical separation of a multirooted tooth through the furcation.

Impacted tooth is a tooth that is not completely erupted and is fully or partially covered by bone or soft tissue.

Implantation is the return of an avulsed tooth into its alveolus.

Interdental refers to the space between adjacent teeth.

Interproximal surface refers to the surface of a tooth that is nearest to the adjacent tooth in the same arch.

Juga is the prominence in the bone overlying a root.

Luxation is the partial or complete displacement of a tooth into the alveolar socket (intrusive luxation), out of the alveolar socket (extrusive luxation), or laterally (lateral luxation).

Luxator is a dental hand instrument with a wide, sharp, delicate blade used to sever the periodontal ligament when extracting a tooth.

Non-odontogenic tumors arise from structures of the oral cavity excluding the dental tissues.

Odontogenic tumors arise from cellular components of the developing tooth structure classified as epithelial, mesenchymal, or mixed.

Operculectomy is the removal of dense fibrous tissue covering an impacted immature tooth to allow further eruption.

Pericoronitis is an inflammation of the gingival during eruption or tissue flaps over a partially erupted tooth.

Primary teeth are the first set of teeth. Primary teeth are also referred as *deciduous teeth* or *baby teeth*.

Subluxation is an incomplete dislocation of a joint, loosening the tooth without displacement.

Supernumerary refers to any extra tooth in addition to the normal secondary dentition.

Surgical extraction is a removal of a tooth or teeth requiring flap exposure.

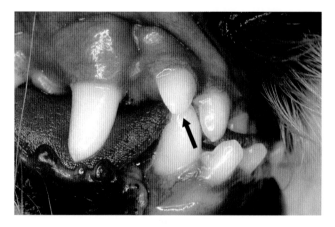

FIGURE 10.3. Mandibular canine interfering with the maxillary corner incisor. Extracting the incisor alleviates the interference.

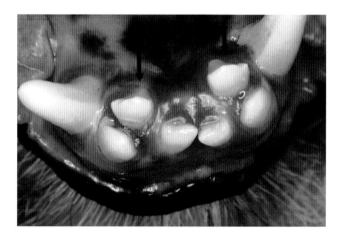

FIGURE 10.4. Malpositioned (linguoversion) second (intermediate) mandibular incisors.

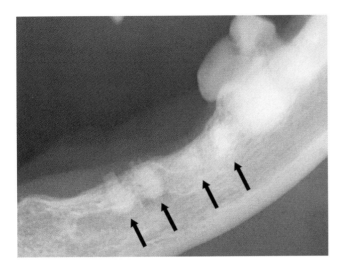

FIGURE 10.5. Root fragments.

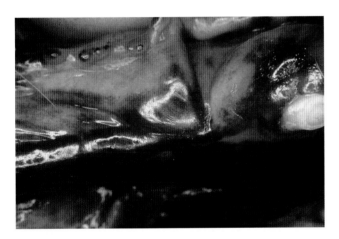

FIGURE 10.6. Clinically missing mandibular first premolar.

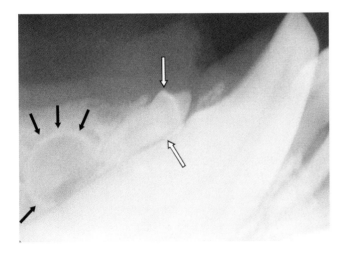

FIGURE 10.7. Radiograph revealing a cyst (closed arrows) affecting the non-erupted mandibular first premolar (open arrows).

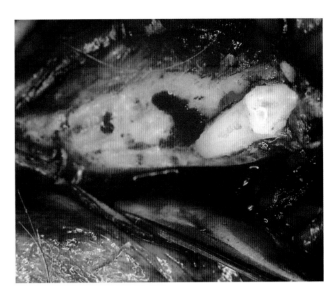

FIGURE 10.8. Exposed non-erupted mandibular first premolar and radicular cyst.

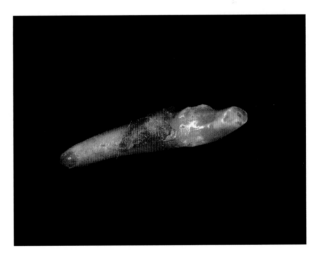

FIGURE 10.9. Extracted mandibular first premolar.

- Fractured teeth where the tooth cannot be saved, or where the owner will not consent to endodontic care (Figure 10.10).
- Class 2, 3, and 4 feline odontoclastic resorptive lesions (FORLs).
- Nonresponsive feline lymphocytic plasmacytic stomatitis syndrome cases.
- Extensive internal or external root resorptions resulting in a nonrestorable tooth (Figure 10.11).

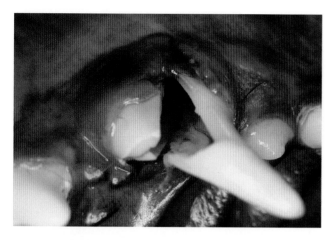

FIGURE 10.10. Class 3b fracture of an immature maxillary canine tooth.

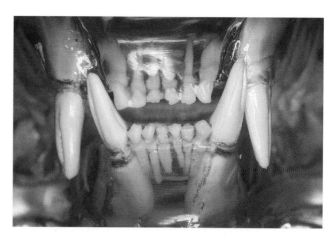

FIGURE 10.12. Single-rooted canines and incisors (feline model).

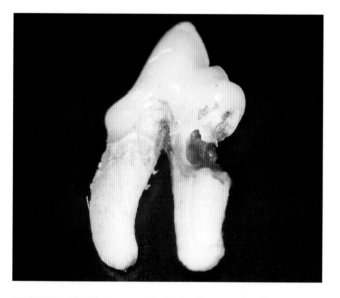

FIGURE 10.11. Large subgingival resorptive lesion.

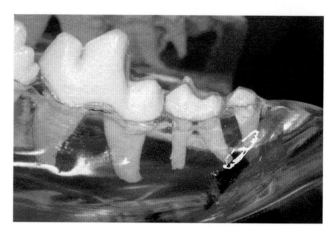

FIGURE 10.13. Canine mandibular molars (model).

ANATOMY

In the *dog*, the following generally occur:

- The incisors, canines, and first premolars have one root (Figure 10.12).
- The mandibular teeth distal to the first premolar have two roots (in most cases the mandibular third molar has one root) (Figure 10.13).
- The maxillary second and third premolars have two roots; the fourth premolar and the two molars have three roots (Figure 10.14).

In the *cat*, the following generally occur:

- The premolars and mandibular molars have two roots, except for the maxillary fourth premolar,

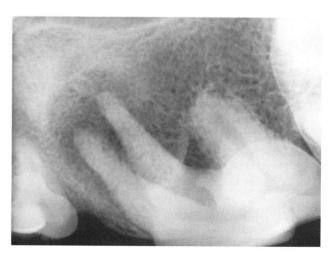

FIGURE 10.14. Radiograph of a triple-rooted maxillary fourth premolar in a dog.

which has three. The maxillary molar may have 1–3 roots. Bone overlying the maxillary teeth is thinner compared to bone around the mandibular teeth (Figure 10.15).

- There are variations concerning the number of roots each premolar and molar has (Table 10.1). Ten percent of cats have three rooted maxillary third premolars. A pre-operative radiograph should be evaluated before extraction (Figure 10.16).

Types of extraction include:

- *Simple (closed)* extraction may be indicated where teeth are markedly mobile due to support loss from advanced periodontal disease or trauma. Multirooted teeth require *sectioning* into single-rooted units before extraction.
- *Surgical* extraction entails incisions for flap exposure. This allows access to the root to remove the buccal and/or lingual alveolar plate to ease extraction of teeth. Surgical extraction is indicated for

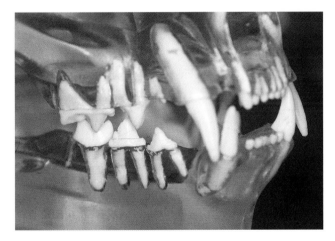

FIGURE 10.15. Feline incisors, canines, premolars, and molars (feline model).

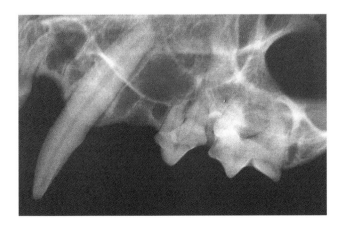

FIGURE 10.16. Radiograph showing feline maxillary canine and third and fourth premolars.

Table 10.1. Root variation among teeth.

Type of Tooth		Number of Roots
Dogs	Incisor	1
	Canine	1
	Maxillary first premolar	1
	Maxillary second and third premolar	2
	Maxillary fourth premolar	3
	Maxillary first and second molar	3
	Mandibular first premolar and third molar	1
	Remaining mandibular premolars and molars	2
Cats	Incisor	1
	Canine	1
	Maxillary second premolar	1
	Maxillary third premolar	2
	Maxillary fourth premolar	3
	Maxillary molar	1–2
	Mandibular premolars and molar	2

teeth with large roots, such as canine teeth and those teeth that are well anchored within the alveolus.

PRE-EXTRACTION RADIOGRAPHS

Dental radiographs obtained before extraction provide information regarding shape, number, position of roots, and degree of bony anchorage. Radiographs also supply documentation for the medical record and can be used as an education tool to gain consent from the client to perform needed care.

ORAL SURGICAL INSTRUMENTS

Tray setup for simple extractions includes the following (Figure 10.17):

- Gauze sponges
- Thumb forceps (Burns 700-5020; Cislak, Adson tissue pliers 1x2 serrated; Schein 101-4803)
- 4-0 and 5-0 absorbable suture with curved cutting needle-chromic cat gut (Burns 271-2646, Schein 568-1601)

- Dental elevators/luxators (Burns 271-9080, Schein 888-3220, Cislak)
- Small-breed extraction forceps (Burns 271-9045, Schein 100-2617, Cislak EX 27)
- Needle holder
- Suture scissors
- Mouth props designed to keep the patient's mouth open while dental extractions are being performed—mechanical (Burns 951-7150, Schein 100-3041) and wedge (Burns 606-4183; Schein 568-6710 large; Burns 060-4183, 568-6101 small) (Figure 10.18)

Tray setup for surgical extractions includes the following:

- Suction tip if suction is available (Burns 950-1570, Schein 100-0944)
- Gauze sponges
- Thumb forceps
- Elevators:

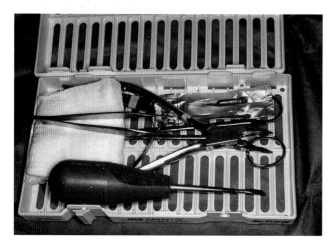

FIGURE 10.17. Sterile extraction pack.

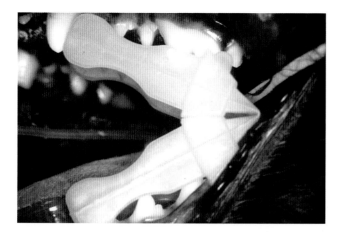

FIGURE 10.18. Mouth prop (Apex orthodontics).

- Freer periosteal (Burns 700-5740, Schein 600-6125) (Figure 10.19)
- Molt periosteal (Burns 271-9008, Schein 600-9526) (Figure 10.20)
- Nos. 301 (Figure 10.21), 301s, 301ss (301: Burns 951-1600, Schein 100-7934, Cislak EX 4—301, EX 5—301s canine)
- Wing-tipped (Burns 606-3204, Cislak Winged 4 sizes EX-103) (Figures 10.22, 10.23)
- Luxators (Burns 271-9080, Schein 888-3220) (Figure 10.24)
- Root tip picks (Heidbrink, Miltex B11, Cislak RT1) (Figure 10.25)
  Bone curette 5-0 (Cislak EX 2)
  Needle holder (Burns 700-8650, Schein 100-2146)
  Scissors (Schein 102-5420)
  Nos. 11, 15 scalpel blades (Schein 100-0249)
- Extraction forceps (Cislak EX 7 small breed, EX 23 large breed) (Figure 10.26)
  Sutures (4-0, 5-0), chromic gut on cutting needle
- Round burs numbers 2 and 4 (Burns #2 952-5110, #4 952-5116; Schein #2 100-0288, #4 100-4535)
- Tapered cross-cut fissure No.701L (Burns 952-5236, Schein 100-7228) burs

Elevators

Dental elevators are placed between the tooth's root and alveolar bone to wedge the tooth from the alveolus. Basic components of an elevator are the handle, shank, and blade or tip. Some elevators also have serrated ridges on the cutting edge to decrease slipping during extraction.

An elevator is used to engage the tooth through a purchase point (a groove or hole between the tooth and alveolus caused by periodontal disease or created with a bur). The elevator is grasped with a tennis racquet grip, with one finger extending along the blade to act as a stop, should the instrument slip while elevating. The handle is slightly twisted and held for 10–30 seconds to help fatigue the periodontal ligament and cause bleeding that aids tooth displacement. The surgeon must be sure the root has a clear unobstructed path of exit. Use of excessive force to bypass an obstruction will fracture the alveolus, the jaw, and/or the tooth.

Elevators include:

- Apexo No. 81 used to luxate large root segments (Burns 951-1667, 81 ELE Cislak, Schein 600-0069).
- 77R elevator used essentially the same as the No. 81 Apexo. Slight curvature of the shank makes it more efficient for posterior regions of the mouth (Burns 951-1560, Schein 600-9432, Cislak No. 77R) (Figure 10.27).

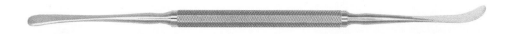

FIGURE 10.19. Freer elevator.

FIGURE 10.20. Molt elevator.

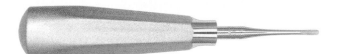

FIGURE 10.21. 301 elevator.

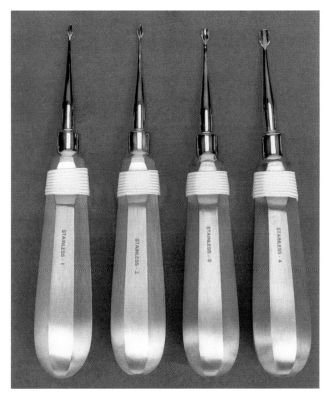

FIGURE 10.23. Winged elevator set.

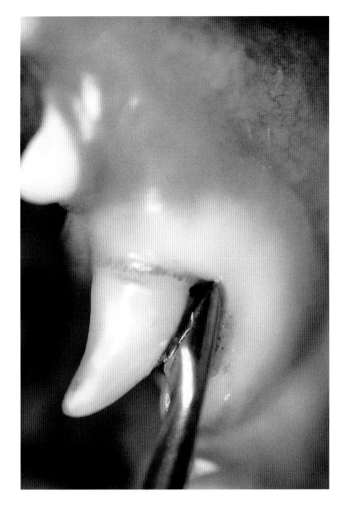

FIGURE 10.22. Winged elevator.

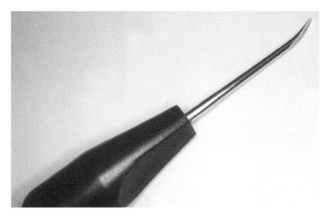

FIGURE 10.24. Luxator.

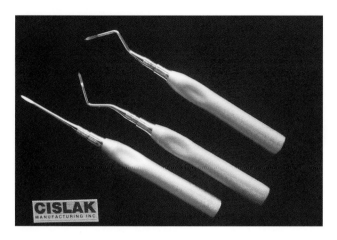

FIGURE 10.25. Root tip pick set.

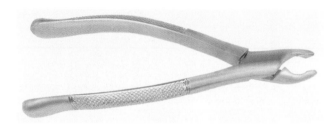

FIGURE 10.26. Extraction forceps.

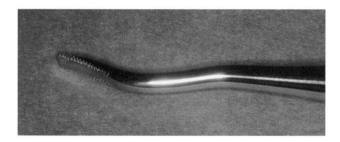

FIGURE 10.27. 77R elevator.

- Heidbrink No.1 elevator has a blade approximately twice as large as the Apexo No. 81 (Burns 951-1618, Schein 600-1429, Cislak #1 ELE) (Figure 10.28).
- Cryer Root Elevators Nos. 44 and 45 are a paired set of instruments used to elevate large root segments. The triangular working tip helps prevent driving maxillary root fragments into the nasal cavity during the extraction process (44: Burns 951-1761, Cislak EX-17, Schein 189-4332) (45: Burns 951-1763, Schein 189-1740, Cislak EX 18) (Figure 10.29).
- Crane pick No. 8 has a pointed blade that extends from the axis of the shank at approximately 45° (Figure 10.30) (Burns 843-0796, Schein 600-6511, Cislak #8 ELE).
- The No. 301 dental elevator is an all-purpose instrument that is available in small, medium, notched,

and bent styles. The 302 and 303 elevators are also commonly used in small animal dental practice. Their thin tips are especially suited for removing small roots (301: Burns 951-1600, Schein 100-7934, Cislak EX 4) (302: Burns 951-1602, Schein 100-5293, Cislak ELE 302) (303: Burns 951-1604 Schein 100-6873, Cislak ELE 303).
- Wing-tipped elevators (Burns 606-3204, Cislak kit #EX-103).
- Periosteal elevators (Molt and Freer) are used to elevate the periosteum from the underlying bone.

Luxators

Luxators have tips with wide, thin slicing edges for easy insertion into the sulcular space used to sever the gingival attachment. The luxator is considered an advanced oral surgical instrument for use only by the experienced dental surgeon. Luxators are not elevators and should

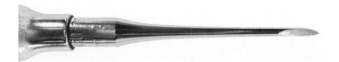

FIGURE 10.28. Heidbrink No. 1 root tip pick.

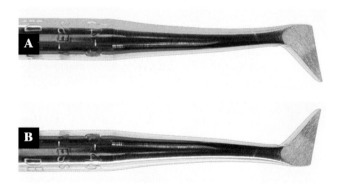

FIGURE 10.29. Cryer root elevators.

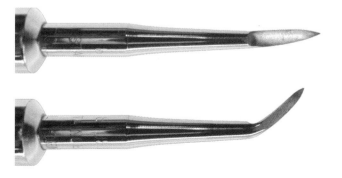

FIGURE 10.30. Crane pick No. 8.

not be used as a lever because this might cause bending or blade breakage.

A luxator kit is available with four instruments and a sharpening stone (black handle—3 mm curved blade for general use; grey handle—3 mm straight blade for interproximal use; brown handle—5 mm curved blade, larger roots; tan handle—5 mm straight blade, interproximal). (Burns 271-9070, Schein 888-3220, Standard handle eight-piece Cislak) (Figure 10.31).

To use the luxator:

1. Place two-thirds of the tip into the periodontal space on the mesial side of the root. Sever the periodontal ligament by directing the handle side to side (Figure 10.32).
2. If root remains firm, repeat the procedure on the distal side. Maintain contact with the root surface at all times.
3. Use an elevator after the luxator to place torque on the tooth and to stretch the periodontal ligament. After mesial and distal elevation, the tooth should dislodge. If the tooth does not elevate, flap expo-

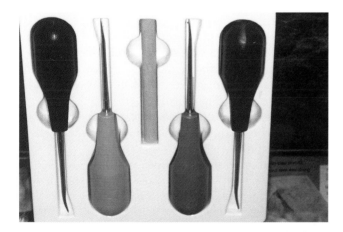

FIGURE 10.31. Luxator kit.

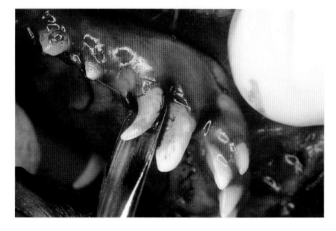

FIGURE 10.32. Luxator blade placed in the periodontal space of a persistent primary tooth.

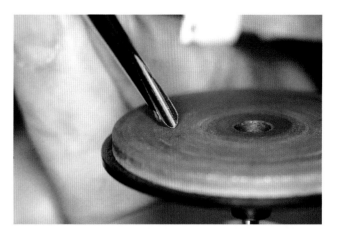

FIGURE 10.33. Mechanically sharpening a luxator blade.

sure and removal of the facial alveolar plate is indicated for extraction.

Luxators can be sharpened by hand by holding an oiled sharpening stone in the one hand and the luxator in the other. The concave surface of the tip is placed on the sharpening stone and stroked away. The blade is lifted after each stroke and replaced at the original site. The process is repeated until the blade is sharpened. Luxators also may be sharpened by using a motorized sharpening stone (Figure 10.33).

Extraction Forceps

Extraction forceps are used to remove mobile teeth from the alveolus. Forceps are composed of three parts: handle, hinge, and beak. The handle enables the forceps to be grasped to deliver adequate leverage through the hinge to the beak. Pressure should be applied in an apical direction followed by a coronal direction to help tear the periodontal fibers. Care must be taken not to apply excessive pressure or torque when using extraction forceps to extract a tooth.

EXTRACTION TECHNIQUE

The veterinarian should obtain informed consent from the pet owner before any dental extraction procedure is performed.

The type, amount, and direction of force applied during the extraction process depends upon characteristics of the tooth:

- Shape
- Size
- Number and anatomy of root(s)
- Thickness and anatomic relationships of the alveolar plate

- Proximity to vital anatomical structures, sinus and neurovascular structures

Extraction of Persistent Primary Teeth

Extraction should take place as soon as a persistent primary tooth is identified, to avoid orthodontic displacement of the erupting permanent tooth and subsequent malocclusion. The maxillary secondary (permanent) canines normally erupt rostral to persistent primary canine teeth. The mandibular secondary canines normally erupt lingual to persistent primary teeth. Careful removal of a primary tooth is necessary to prevent root fracture and trauma to the secondary tooth.

Use the following steps for a non-flap surgical extraction:

1. After appropriate application of local anesthetic and irrigation with 0.12% chlorhexidine solution, sever the gingival attachment with a #15 scalpel blade applied apically 360° around the tooth through the sulcus (Figure 10.34).
2. Place the blade end of an elevator or luxator between the root and alveolar bone. Place 10–60

seconds of minimal-to-moderate axial elevator torque against the tooth and alveolus (Figure 10.35).

3. Persistent torque will eventually stretch and fatigue the periodontal ligament, creating bleeding into the periodontal space. Bleeding and fatigue of the ligament enables the operator to gently lift the tooth from its alveolar socket. Initially, these pressures may be strongly resisted with little or no progress, but as torque time is increased, the tooth eventually becomes mobile. As the procedure continues, depress the elevator handle to elevate the root from its socket. Caution must be taken not to move the tooth in a lingual/palatal to facial or mesial to distal direction, because this might cause root, alveolar, or jaw fracture. If the tooth is not mobile enough for gentle lifting, more time is necessary for luxation or elevation to fatigue periodontal support. If the tooth does not become mobile with the above process, elevate a gingival flap for removal of the coronal aspect of the buccal alveolar plate, making extraction easier.
4. Use veterinary extraction forceps to gently rotate the mobile tooth on its long axis, tearing the remaining connective tissue fibers. The forcep beaks should be in full contact with the tooth's long axis. Most human extraction forceps do not grasp dog and cat's teeth adequately. The improper use of or the use of improperly sized forceps can lead to tooth fracture (Figure 10.36).
5. After the tooth is extracted, remove granulation tissue from the apex of the alveolar socket with a bone curette.
6. An extraction site is an open wound with alveolar bone exposed. All extraction sites greater than 2 mm should be sutured without tension. If such a

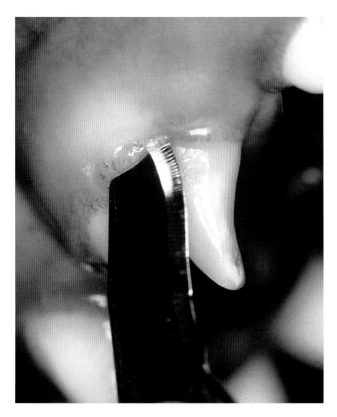

FIGURE 10.34. No. 15 blade used to incise the periodontal ligament around the primary maxillary canine.

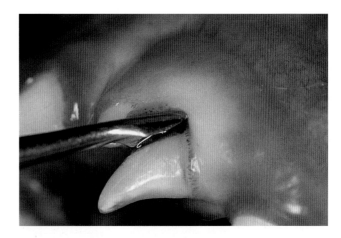

FIGURE 10.35. A winged elevator blade is inserted between the root and alveolus.

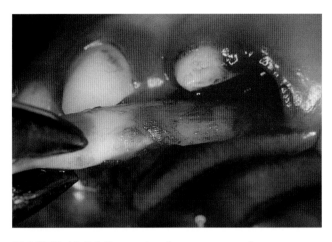

FIGURE 10.36. Extraction forceps are used to remove the tooth.

wound is left open in which to granulate, food and debris can enter, causing delayed healing and increased patient discomfort. In some cases, a gingival flap may need to be elevated to oppose the defect without tension.

7. Pain relief medication is prescribed for all extraction cases.

Surgical Extraction—Flap Exposure

Surgical extraction with flap exposure is the preferred method to remove nonmobile canines, maxillary fourth premolars, mandibular first molars, fractured roots, and other teeth where nonsurgical extraction is not possible. Proper design of the flap facilitates extraction and permits accurate closure of the gingiva without tension. Arterial blood usually flows from distal to mesial. When possible, either an envelope flap, which does not entail vertical releasing incisions, or mesial (versus distal) incisions are made at the tooth corner (line angle) to expose the buccal alveolar bone. Flap incisions should extend apical to the mucogingival line to include the elastic alveolar mucosa.

Absorbable suture material should be used to close exposure flaps. Monocryl (Ethicon, Inc.) is a synthetic, monofilament suture material that combines absorption with the strength and smoothness of nylon suture. A swaged-on 3/8-circle, reverse-cutting needle (FS-2 or P-3, Ethicon, Inc.) is preferred by the author.

Use the following general surgical extraction technique for single- or multi-rooted teeth after infusing local anesthesia:

1. Incise the gingival attachment circumferentially at the base of the sulcus with a #11 or #15 scalpel blade (Figure 10.37).

2. Reflect the gingiva apically, using a Molt or Freer periosteal elevator (Figure 10.38).
3. Remove buccal alveolar bone overlying the root or remove a trough of bone along an outline approximately one-third to one-half of the root's length using a round dental bur in a water-cooled handpiece (Figure 10.39). To allow adequate placement of the elevator tip, cut shallow grooves using a dental bur at the mesial and distal aspects of the tooth. After placing the elevator, rotational torque can be applied until the tooth is loosened. Take care not to rotate the maxillary canine or corner incisor roots palatally, forcing the root apex into the nasal cavity.
4. If the tooth is double- or triple-rooted, use a round or cross-cut fissure bur on a water-cooled high-speed dental handpiece to section the tooth into single-rooted units, starting at the furcation and cutting coronally (Figure 10.40). The fourth maxillary

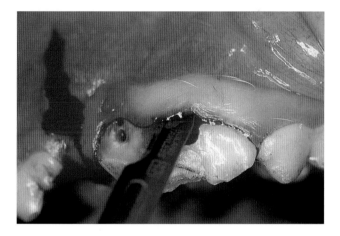

FIGURE 10.37. Incision into the gingival sulcus.

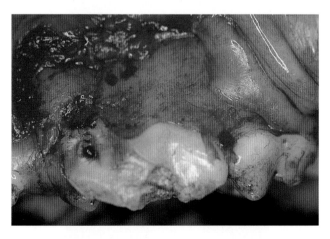

FIGURE 10.38. Flap exposing the underlying buccal bone.

premolar has a mesiopalatal root that may be sectioned at a 30–45° angle to the long axis of the tooth to reach the furcation (Figures 10.41).

5. Place an elevator tip in the kerf (the space created by the sectioning cut) between segments. Rotate the elevator on its long axis like a screwdriver with the concave edge engaging and elevating while the convex surface rests against the fulcrum segment (Figures 10.42, 10.43). Light-to-moderate torque is placed in one direction for 10–60 seconds before reversing torque in the opposite direction, to further stretch and break down the periodontal ligament. The root segment will loosen when the periodontal ligament is stretched sufficiently. Take care

not to engage an adjacent tooth, which might become dislodged due to excessive force.

6. Use dental extraction forceps to remove the mobile tooth from the alveolus. Extraction forceps should only be applied to lift the tooth from the alveolus after the tooth is sufficiently loosened with an elevator, not as a tooth-loosening device. Often, fractured roots or alveoli result if extraction forceps are used with excessive rotational torque on teeth that have not been elevated enough.

7. If granulation tissue or debris is present, perform gentle curettage and debridement of the extraction site with a bone curette.

8. Closely inspect each extracted tooth root to ensure complete extraction (Figure 10.44). Unless the apex

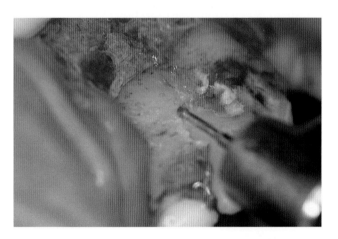

FIGURE 10.39. Round bur in a high-speed drill used to remove part of the lateral alveolus to expose the buccal roots.

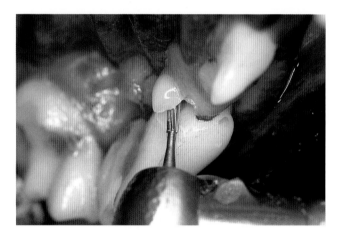

FIGURE 10.41. Fissure bur used to section the mesiopalatal root of the maxillary fourth premolar.

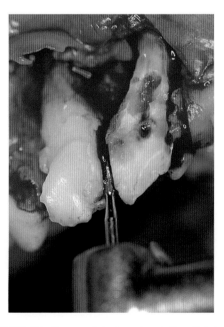

FIGURE 10.40. Bur used to hemisect the distal and mesiobuccal roots of the maxillary fourth premolar.

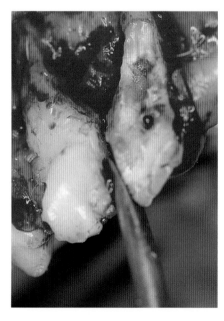

FIGURE 10.42. An elevator tip placed between the distal and mesiobuccal roots of a dog's maxillary fourth premolar.

is affected by resorption, the extracted root tip should be round and smooth upon extraction. Always take a post-operative radiograph.

9. Alveolar bone shaping (alveoloplasty) and smoothing is often indicated following extraction. Alveoloplasty eliminates existing and surgically induced abnormalities—e.g., sharp, protruding alveolar edges, loose and detached bony spicules, bulging tuberosities, and other irregularities—with a small round bur on a high-speed water-cooled handpiece to provide a smooth bony base for suturing the gingiva (Figure 10.45).

10. Optionally, place synthetic bone graft material (Consil Nutramax Laboratories) to aid in maintaining the alveolar ridge and jaw strength while providing a frame for new bone growth.

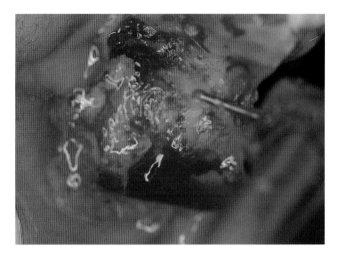

FIGURE 10.45. Alveoloplasty to remove sharp edges.

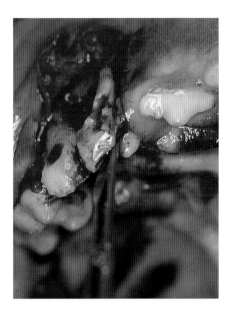

FIGURE 10.43. The elevator tip placed between the mesiobuccal and mesiopalatal roots of a dog's maxillary fourth premolar.

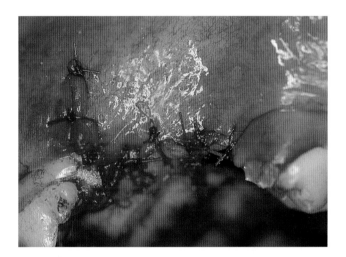

FIGURE 10.46. Sutured mucoperiosteal flap.

11. 3-0 to 5-0 absorbable sutures are used to close the mucoperiosteal flap (Figure 10.46).

Extraction of Incisor Teeth

Incisors are normally single-rooted. The first (central) incisors have the smallest crown:root height ratio (Figure 10.47). Third (corner) incisors have the longest roots. Maxillary incisor roots curve palatally with apices within a few millimeters of the nasal cavity. The mandibular incisors have long slender roots that are relatively straight with flattened sides (Figure 10.48).

Follow this technique for incisor extraction:

1. After local anesthesia infusion, incise the gingival attachment 360° around the tooth with a #11 or #15 scalpel blade or a sharp dental luxator inserted into gingival sulcus.

2. Insert an elevator between the incised gingiva and the tooth, applying pressure apically while rotating

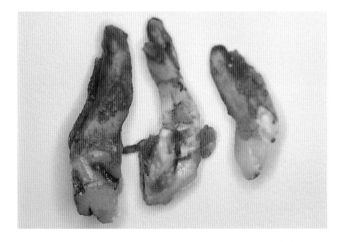

FIGURE 10.44. All root fragments are inspected for complete extraction.

the handle. The instrument is held in this rotated position for a period up to 60 seconds.

3. Repeat step 2 in multiple locations around the tooth, stretching the periodontal ligament creating mobility.

4. When the tooth is sufficiently loosened, use a small breed extraction forceps to grasp the crown near the gingival margin. Rotate the incisor and gently remove it from the alveolus.

5. Suture the defect without tension (a releasing flap incision may be necessary for closure).

Extraction of Maxillary Canine Teeth

The maxillary canine root lies within millimeters of the nasal cavity's lateral wall. Care must be taken during extraction not to apply force in a direction causing the apex to move palatally resulting in penetration of the nasal cavity (Figure 10.49).

Use the following steps for maxillary canine tooth extraction:

1. After infusion of local anesthesia, insert a #11 or #15 scalpel blade into the sulcus to incise the gingival attachment circumferentially around the tooth.

2. Make an incision at the line angle (corner) of the maxillary canine and carry it distally to follow the

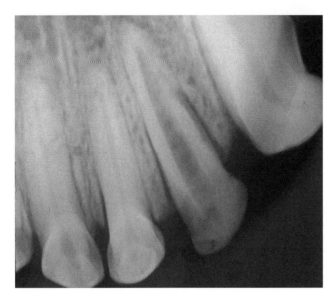

FIGURE 10.47. Radiograph for comparison of the maxillary incisor crown:root ratio.

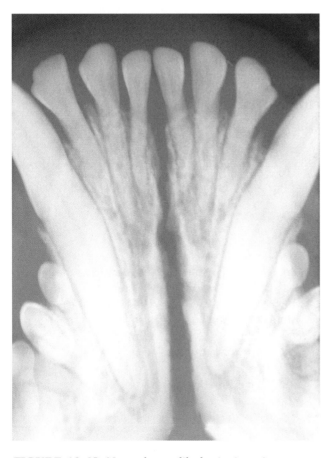

FIGURE 10.48. Normal mandibular incisors in a pug.

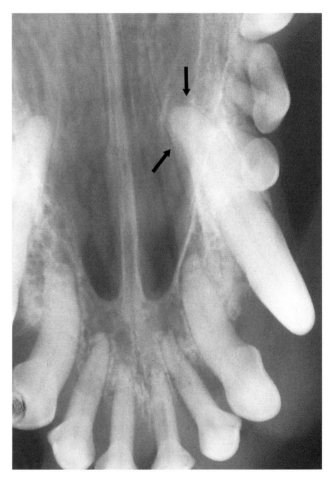

FIGURE 10.49. Radiograph of the maxillary canine, demonstrating close proximity of the apex to the nasal cavity.

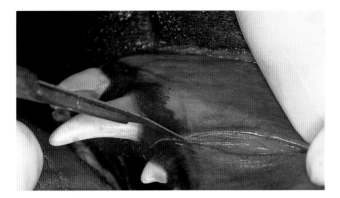

FIGURE 10.50. Full-thickness line angle incision following the root anatomy.

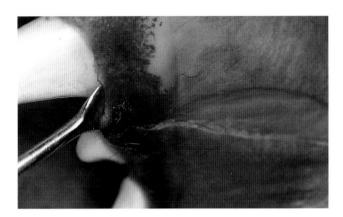

FIGURE 10.51. A periosteal elevator inserted in the gingival sulcus to dislodge the attached gingiva from the alveolus.

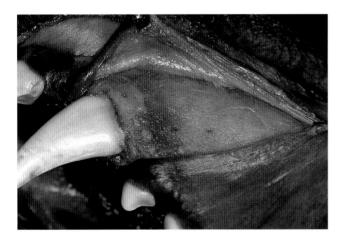

FIGURE 10.52. Exposed lateral alveolus overlying the maxillary canine.

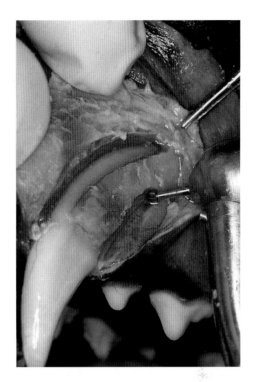

FIGURE 10.53. Root outline using a round bur on a water-cooled high-speed drill.

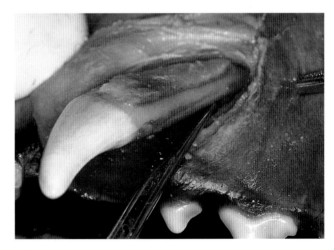

FIGURE 10.54. Torque applied to elevator to dislodge canine.

juga. The length of the incision should be 1/2–3/4 of the root length. Take care to avoid the infraorbital blood vessels and nerves, especially in brachycephalic breeds (Figure 10.50).

3. Create a full-thickness mucoperiosteal flap with the help of periosteal elevators. Angle the elevator toward the periosteum, exposing the buccal cortical bone (Figures 10.51,10.52).

4. Use a round bur on a high-speed water-cooled handpiece to remove the labial cortical bone overlying the root. Alternatively, outline the root with a round bur (Figure 10.53).

5. Place an elevator or luxator in the periodontal space between the canine and alveolus. Apply rotational torque (with an elevator, not a luxator) to gently lift the tooth away from the alveolus (Figure 10.54). If there is not sufficient space for the luxa-

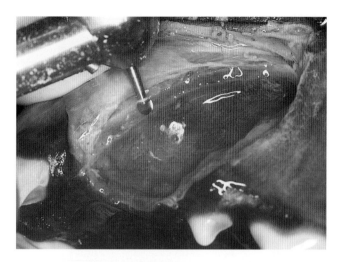

FIGURE 10.55. Alveoloplasty to remove sharp bony projections.

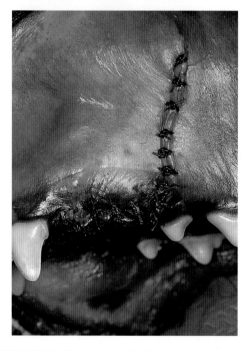

FIGURE 10.56. Flap sutured without tension.

tor or elevator to be placed, make slots in the alveolar bone both mesially and distally.

6. Elevate the canine bucally.
7. After the tooth is extracted, the surgical site should be radiographed to confirm complete extraction. Perform alveoloplasty with a large round bur on a water-cooled high-speed handpiece to remove rough or sharp bony projections in the extraction site (Figure 10.55). The alveoloplasty is complete when the extraction site is smooth to the touch.
8. Use an osseoconductive material (Consil, Nutramax Laboratories) to fill before suturing.

9. Close the mucoperiosteal flap (Figure 10.56) without tension. If more gingiva is needed to decrease tension, use a #15 scalpel blade to partially incise the periosteal fibers perpendicularly on the palatal side of the flap.

With *mandibular canine extraction*, the tooth roots occupy a majority of the rostral mandible. One technique uses a facial approach:

1. After infusion of local anesthesia, insert a #11 or #15 scalpel blade into the sulcus to incise the gingival attachment circumferentially around the tooth.
2. Create a mucoperiosteal flap by making an incision outlining the distal part of the mandibular canine root through the frenulum. The length of the incision should be 1/2—3/4 of the root length. Take care to avoid the mental blood vessels and nerves.
3. Raise the flap with periosteal elevators. Angle the elevator toward the bone to include the periosteum, exposing the labial cortical bone.
4. Use a round bur on a water-cooled high-speed handpiece to remove part of the labial cortical bone overlying the root. Place an elevator in the periodontal space. To avoid symphyseal separation, hold both mandibular arches with one hand as a single unit while using the elevator with the other hand. Apply rotational torque to gently lift the tooth away from the alveolus.
5. Elevate the canine labially.
6. After the tooth is extracted, the surgical site should be radiographed to confirm complete extraction. Alveoloplasty is performed to remove rough or sharp bony projections in the extraction site with a large round bur on a high-speed water-cooled handpiece. The alveoloplasty is complete when the extraction site is smooth to the touch.
7. Use an osseoconductive material (Consil, Nutramax Laboratories) to fill before suturing.
8. Close the mucoperiosteal flap without tension. If more gingiva is needed to decrease tension, use a#15 scalpel blade to partially incise the periosteal fibers perpendicularly on the underside of the flap.

The *lingual approach for mandibular canine extraction* avoids disruption of the lip attachment and the mental neurovascular structures:

1. After infusion of local anesthesia, use a #15 scalpel blade and periosteal elevator to create a lingual-based, full-thickness, mucoperiosteal flap overlying the canine to be extracted. The flap base located next to the mandibular symphysis should be twice the width of the apex (Figure 10.57).
2. Use a periosteal elevator to separate the gingiva from the lingual alveolus (Figure 10.58).

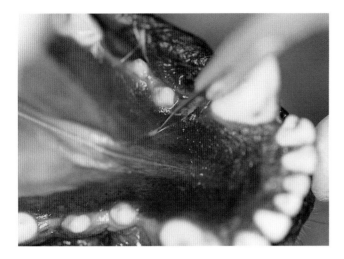

FIGURE 10.57. Flap to lingually expose the mandibular canine.

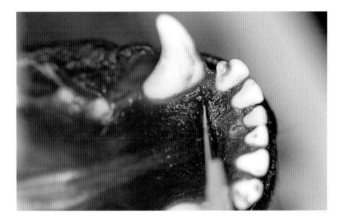

FIGURE 10.58. Flap exposure.

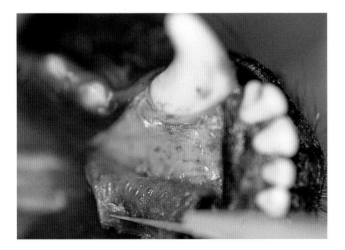

FIGURE 10.59. Lingual alveoloplasty.

3. Perform a lingual alveoloplasty, using a round bur in a water-cooled high-speed handpiece between half and three quarters of the tooth length (Figure 10.59).
4. Use an elevator to loosen the tooth from the alveolus.

5. When it becomes markedly mobile, extract the canine with extraction forceps.
6. Work through steps 6–9 from the buccal approach given previously.

Extraction of Premolar Teeth

In the dog, the following occur:

- The maxillary and mandibular first premolars have a single, straight, conical root permitting easy rotation with extraction forceps after elevation.
- The second and third premolars have two roots, which require sectioning into single-rooted components before extraction. The maxillary third premolar lies in close proximity to the infraorbital foramen, which should be palpated and avoided during extraction (Figures 10.60–64).

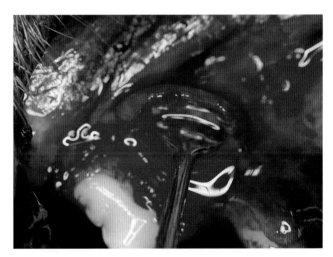

FIGURE 10.60. Flap exposure of a dog's maxillary second premolar using a periosteal elevator.

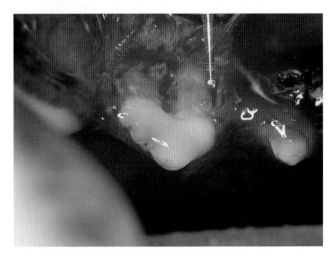

FIGURE 10.61. Removal of the buccal alveolar bone overlying the roots, if ankylosis is present.

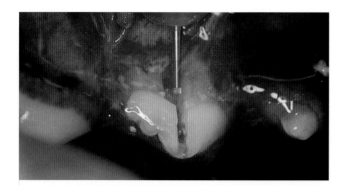

FIGURE 10.62. Hemisection of the two roots.

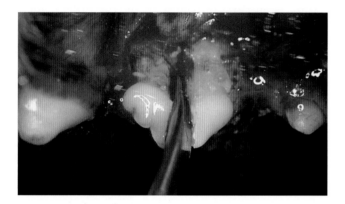

FIGURE 10.63. An elevator inserted to loosen the roots.

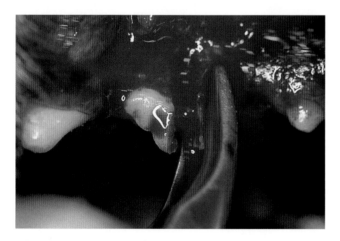

FIGURE 10.64. Extraction forceps, used to remove the hemisected and elevated crowns and roots.

• The maxillary fourth premolar (carnassial) has three roots (distal, mesiobuccal, and mesiopalatal). Sectioning this tooth into three single-rooted segments facilitates removal.

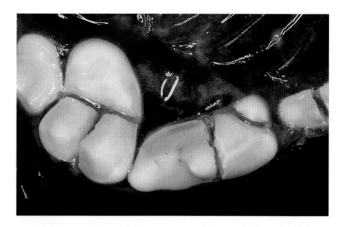

FIGURE 10.65. Sectioned maxillary third and fourth premolars and first molar of a dog.

In the cat, the maxillary second premolar has one or two fused roots; the maxillary third premolar has two roots. In addition:

• The maxillary fourth premolar has three roots located similarly to the dog.
• The maxillary molar has one to two roots either separate or fused.
• All mandibular teeth distal to the canines normally have two roots.

Use this technique for extraction of the maxillary fourth premolar:

1. After local anesthesia infusion, use a #15 scalpel blade and Freer or Molt elevator to create a full-thickness mucogingival flap (described in chapter 6) exposing the buccal alveolar bone.
2. Using a round bur on a water-cooled high-speed handpiece, remove the buccal alveolar plate around the exposed buccal roots. Section the crown using a #701L long tapered transverse cross-cut fissure bur or a water-cooled high-speed handpiece.
3. Section the mesiopalatal root with a diagonal cut from distopalatal to mesiobuccal through the furcation (Figure 10.65).
4. Elevate each section, as if it were a single-rooted tooth. Examine all apices for complete extraction. In cases of ankylosis, remove the buccal alveolar bone over the root surface for exposure. Use a round bur on a water-cooled high-speed handpiece to remove as much of the remaining ankylosed tooth substance as possible.
5. After extraction and post-operative radiograph, use a #2–4 round bur on a water-cooled high-speed handpiece to smooth sharp pieces of the alveolar ridge. Suture the mucoperiosteal flap without tension.

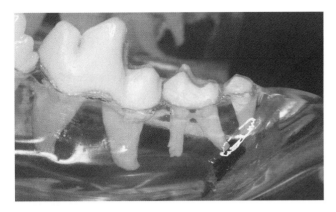

FIGURE 10.66. Mandibular first, second, and third molars in the dog (model).

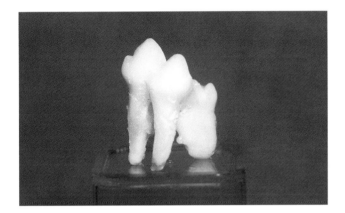

FIGURE 10.67. Canine maxillary first molar.

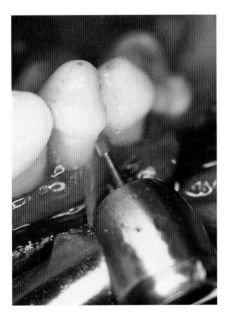

FIGURE 10.68. High-speed water-cooled handpiece using a bur to section the buccal roots of the maxillary first molar of a dog.

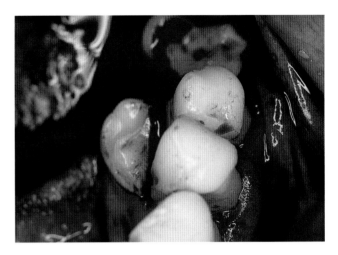

FIGURE 10.69. Sectioned palatal root of the maxillary first molar in a dog.

Molar Extraction

In the dog, the first and second maxillary molars have three diverging roots arranged in a tripod configuration. The mandibular molars have two roots except for the most distal which usually has one root. The gingiva overlying the molar to be extracted is flapped, and the tooth is sectioned in a similar manner as other multi-rooted teeth for extraction (Figures 10.66–10.69).

Feline mandibular molars have two roots. Radiographs help visualize mesial and distal roots before extraction.

Hemisection for Partial Tooth Extraction

Occasionally one or more roots and parts of the crown can be saved when the diseased root has been removed, preserving tooth function. The decision to save part of the tooth is based on tooth importance, periodontal support of the remaining root(s), and client consent. Contraindications to hemisection procedures include reduced periodontal support and/or inability to provide an endodontic seal of the saved root(s).

Use the following steps for hemisection technique:

1. Perform conventional endodontics, if planned, before hemisection; partial coronal pulpectomy (vital pulp therapy), if planned, is performed *after* the hemisection.
2. Use a cross-cut fissure or round bur to section the tooth, starting at the furcation entrance and continuing coronally until the tooth is sectioned.
3. Elevate and extract the diseased root(s) and associated portion of the crown.
4. Restore the exposed pulp chamber access resulting from the hemisection with a bonded composite restorative material after endodontic treatment.

Surgical Exposure for Root Fragment Retrieval

Teeth occasionally fracture from trauma or during dental procedures. Leaving a root fragment behind, after elevating or using extraction forceps, invites future infection and patient discomfort.

Fractured roots usually occur in the apical third of the tooth. Intraoral radiographs are helpful to determine the size and shape of the root fragment. The technique used for root fragment removal varies according to the location, shape of the root, character of the surrounding bone, and access. To give sufficient exposure for removal, an envelope flap (or releasing interdental incisions) is made over the alveolus housing the fractured root (Figure 10.70):

1. When creating a full-thickness flap, keep the sharp edge of a Molt elevator against the bone, with the convex side of the blade held against the soft tissue.
2. Use a round bur on a high-speed handpiece to remove part of the alveolar bone bucally, overlying the root fragment. The root fragment will appear to be harder than the surrounding bone. Use the bur to outline the fragment (Figure 10.71).
3. Use a root tip pick or elevator to remove the exposed root fragment from the alveolus (Cislak root forceps #4658, Peets forceps #5217) (Figure 10.72).
4. Suture the flap without tension.

Some practitioners atomize the fractured root by using a large (#4–6) round bur on a water-cooled high-speed handpiece to "bur out" the root fragment without performing a flap. This is not a recommended procedure, because it either removes too much surrounding bone or not enough tooth. Blind burring of the root also places nearby neurovascular structures open to injury.

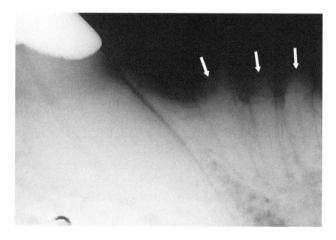

FIGURE 10.70. Radiograph revealing three fractured mandibular root fragments.

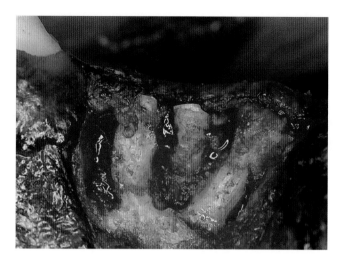

FIGURE 10.71. Root fragments exposed.

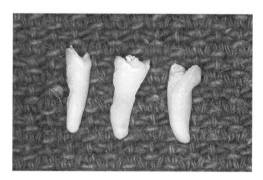

FIGURE 10.72. Extracted root fragments.

UNERUPTED, UNDER-ERUPTED, IMPACTED, EMBEDDED TEETH

An *unerupted* tooth is present subgingivally but has failed to perforate the oral mucosa. An *under-erupted* tooth occurs when the tooth erupts far enough to break through the gingiva but most of the crown is subgingival. An *impacted* tooth is prevented from erupting by a physical barrier, such as thickened gingiva (Figures 10.73, 10.74), adjacent crowded teeth, or horizontal alignment in the alveolus (Figures 10.75–10.80). An *embedded* tooth is covered with bone.

The surgical removal of the mucosal flap covering an unerupted tooth (operculectomy) is likely to be effective in the young animal with a tooth that has an open apex and has eruptive potential. After 9 months of age, the tooth is less likely to erupt even if the impediment is removed. Extraction is recommended in the under-erupted tooth, because a periodontal pocket will form where debris can collect, leading to inflammation (pericornonitis).

Radiographs are necessary to evaluate areas of missing or partially erupted teeth and to show whether the tooth:

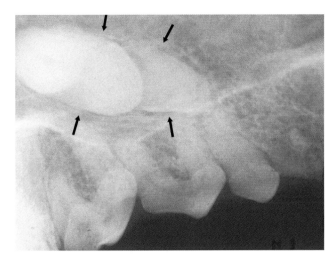

FIGURE 10.73. Radiograph of embedded maxillary canine tooth.

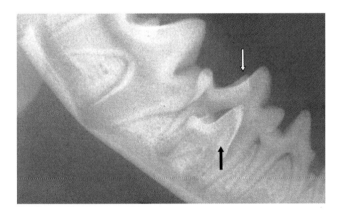

FIGURE 10.74. Partially erupted mandibular fourth premolar (black arrow), caused by failure of primary tooth (white arrow) exfoliation.

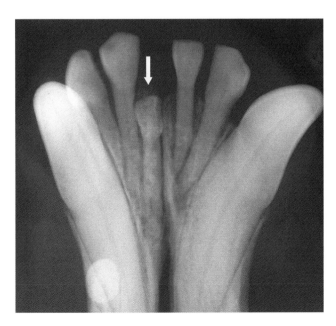

FIGURE 10.75. Radiograph of an unerupted incisor.

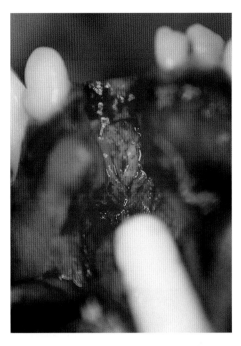

FIGURE 10.76. Flap-exposed alveolus overlying the unerupted incisor shown in fig. 10.75.

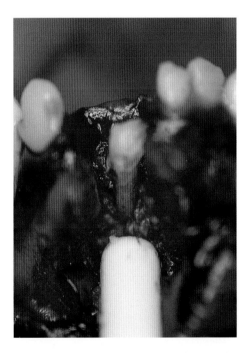

FIGURE 10.77. Exposure of unerupted central incisor before extraction.

- Is absent, therefore no treatment is necessary.
- Is present in a vertical or near vertical nonerupted position. If the animal is younger than 9 months, an operculectomy can be performed to remove the overlying fibrous gingiva covering the crown. If the patient is older than 9 months, the tooth lacks eruptive force and should be extracted or radiographically

and clinically monitored every 3–6 months for at least one year.

- Is partially erupted. If a cyst is not present around the root, an orthodontic device may be fabricated to help extrude the tooth. If a cyst exists, the tooth should be extracted and the cyst lining thoroughly curetted. If a cyst does not exist and orthodontic care is not an option, the tooth can be followed clinically and radiographically every 3–6 months for several years (Figures 10.81–10.83).
- Is misdirected in a horizontal position. If the tooth is impacted, extraction is the treatment of choice to eliminate the possibility of future cyst development (Figure 10.84).

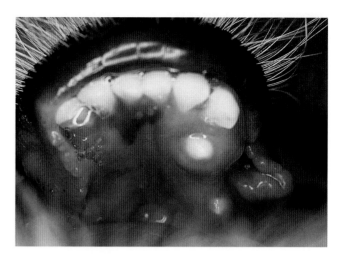

FIGURE 10.80. Partially erupted mandibular canine tooth in a dog after operculum barrier removed.

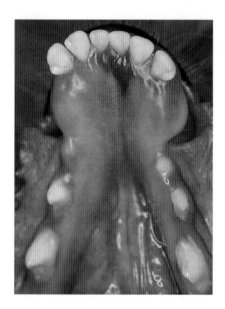

FIGURE 10.78. Clinically missing mandibular canines in a dog.

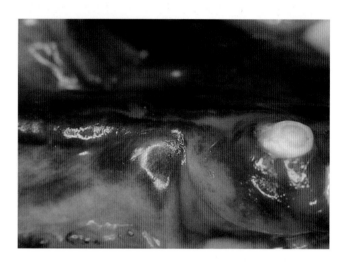

FIGURE 10.81. Clinically missing mandibular first premolar.

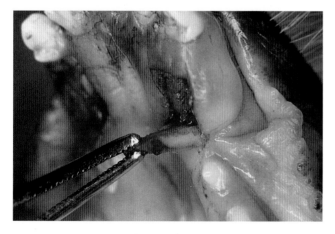

FIGURE 10.79. Surgery to remove thickened gingiva (operculum) overlying the impacted mandibular canine.

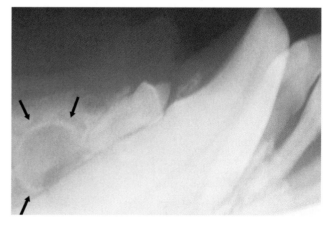

FIGURE 10.82. Radiograph of periapical cyst involving the first mandibular premolar in a dog.

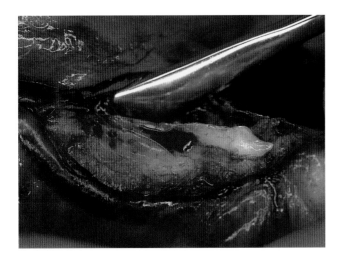

FIGURE 10.83. Flap exposure of horizontally positioned mandibular first premolar in a dog.

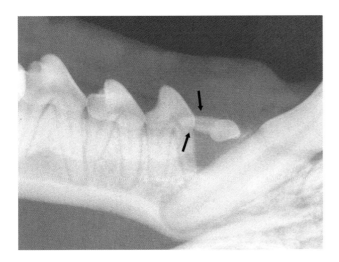

FIGURE 10.84. Radiograph of horizontal orientation of first mandibular premolar in a dog causing bone loss.

Feline Odontoclastic Resorptive Lesions (FORLs)

Approximately half of all cats older than 6 years old will have at least one FORL. FORL lesions have also been called:

- Caries, an inaccurate term because these lesions are not the result of demineralization and loss of the tooth structure, as are human caries (cavities)
- Neck or cervical line lesions, which describe where most of the clinical pathology exists, in the neck or cervical region where the crown and root meet
- External or internal root resorptive lesions
- External odontoclastic resorptions (EORs)

FORLs are usually clinically apparent at the labial or buccal surface near the cementoenamel junction (CEJ). FORLs can be found on any tooth, although the teeth most commonly affected are the mandibular third premolars, molars, and maxillary third and fourth premolars. Some FORLs affecting the canines occur apical to the CEJ and often are not clinically apparent. Purebred cats, especially Siamese and Persians, appear to be more susceptible than other cats.

The etiology of FORLs is unknown. Theories supporting autoimmune mediating cellular and humoral factors, calici virus, and metabolic imbalances relating to calcium regulation, as well as excess vitamin D in commercial cat foods, have been proposed. Histologically, FORLs are filled with multinucleated odontoclasts, which resorb dentin.

Clinically, resorptions appear as areas where the tooth substance is resorbed, often filled with hyperplasic gingiva. Patients affected with FORLs may show hypersalivation, head shaking, sneezing, anorexia, oral bleeding, or have difficulty apprehending food. The lesion may erode into sensitive dentin, causing the cat to show pain with jaw spasms (chatter) when touched with a shepherd's hook explorer. Even so, most affected cats do not show clinical signs and many suffer in silence.

FORL CLASSES AND TREATMENT OPTIONS

There are five classes and two types of FORLs. The resorptive lesions should be staged 1–5, and then the roots classified as type I or II.

FORL types:

- *Type I* lesions arise in the cervical area of the tooth and extend inward and/or up and down the root. Type I leasions are inflammatory in nature, arising from periodontal inflammation. Radiographically, Type I lesions have relatively normal root structure.
- The more common *Type II* lesion begins subgingivally and may be caused by vitamin D toxicity. Radiographically, the roots appear to be resorbing. The periodontal ligament will not be readily recognizable due to ankylosis.

FORL classes:

- *Class 1 FORLs* involve cementum without entering dentin (Figure 10.85) and are not clinically sensitive when probed. Radiographs are used to confirm that the lesion does not extend into the dentin or pulp. Research indicates that class 1 FORLs may not exist as enamel only lesions, but occur as all FORL lesions secondary from an undermining as a result of dentin destruction. Preliminary studies support the use of Alendronate for controlling the progression of FORLs (significant side effects in humans). Follow-

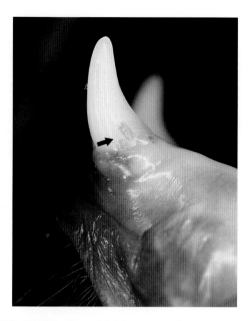

FIGURE 10.85. Class 1 FORL: enamel lesion in a mandibular canine.

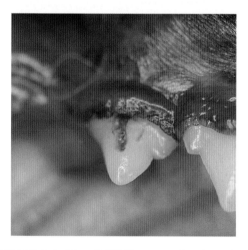

FIGURE 10.86. Class 2 FORL: resorption into the dentin of the maxillary third premolar in a cat.

up examinations are recommended, including intra-oral radiographs when the cat is anesthetized.

- *Class 2 FORLs* penetrate cementum into dentin (Figure 10.86). Due to dentinal communication with the pulp, these lesions can be painful. Treatment options include extraction or glass ionomer restoration. At one time, application of glass ionomer restorative was the preferred treatment for class 2 FORLs. Follow-up has shown a poor long-term success rate, (80% failure rate after 2 years). The current treatment of choice is extraction.
- *Class 3 FORLs* enter the pulp (Figure 10.87), and the current recommended treatment is extraction. Restoration with glass ionomer restoratives or root canal therapy does not yield long-term successful results in the majority of cases.

- *Class 4 FORLs* have extensive root and crown damage (Figure 10.88). Often, gingiva grows over the resorbed crown fragment, leaving a sensitive lesion upon probing. Treatment is flap surgery to remove the crown and extraction of the root fragments.
- *Class 5 FORLs* lack a clinical crown (Figure 10.89), but root fragments remain on radiographs. The decision to perform surgery to extract the remaining root(s) is based on the patient's pain and the lesion's appearance. If the cat feels discomfort when the lesion is probed, the overlying gingiva is inflamed or fistulated, or there is radiographic evidence of pathology around the root remnant, the root(s) should be extracted after a surgical exposure.

CROWN AMPUTATION   *Crown amputation* is preferred by some as an alternative to flap exposure and full tooth extraction in the therapy of FORLs. This is a controversial practice because it leaves the root with hopes of eventual resorption (Figures 10.90,10.91).

Cases proposed for crown amputation are those that have at least class 3 involvement, without evidence of periodontal disease on radiographs or probing, mobili-

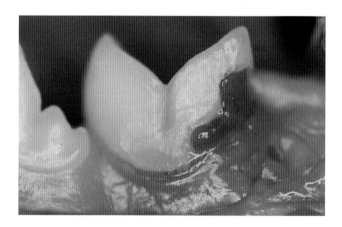

FIGURE 10.87. Class 3 FORL: pulpal exposure of the mandibular molar.

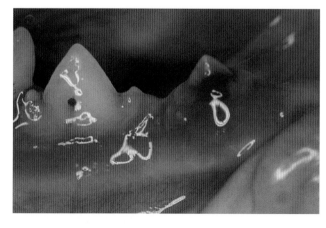

FIGURE 10.88. Class 4 FORL: partial crown resorption of a mandibular third premolar.

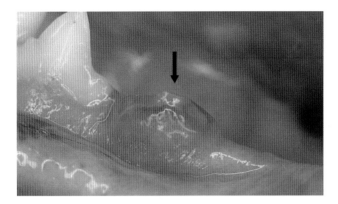

FIGURE 10.89. Class 5 FORL: a mandibular third premolar clinical crown not visible.

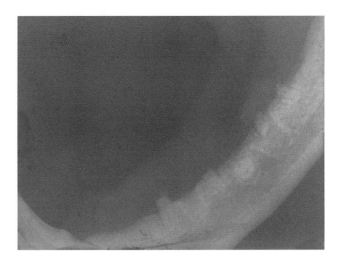

FIGURE 10.90. Radiograph of multiple root fragments after crown amputation.

ty, or apical pathology.

Use the following technique for crown amputation:

1. Make an envelope flap that extends mesial and distal to the affected tooth, exposing the CEJ and alveolar ridge.
2. Using a #2 or #3 sterile round bur on a high-speed water-cooled handpiece, remove the crown 1–2 mm below the alveolar ridge.
3. Smooth any sharp bony projections and close the gingiva with 5-0 absorbable sutures.

LYMPHOCYTIC PLASMACYTIC GINGIVOSTOMATITIS SYNDROME (LPGS)

Cats can also be affected by lymphocytic plasmacytic gingivostomatitis syndrome (LPGS). The etiology of LPGS has not been determined. An immune-mediated hypersensitivity to bacteria (plaque) and viruses is suspected due to histopathology findings of plasma cells.

Clinical signs of advanced LPGS include:

- Dysphagia
- Weight loss
- Ptyalism
- Bruxism—grinding teeth
- Scratching the face due to pain
- Apparent oral pain
- Unkempt hair coat

Oral examination findings with LPGS include the following:

- Marked gingivitis and periodontitis evident 360° around the incisors, premolars, and/or molars (Figure 10.92).
- Caudal stomatitis "faucitis" is present in approximately 50% of the cases. Faucitis clinically appears

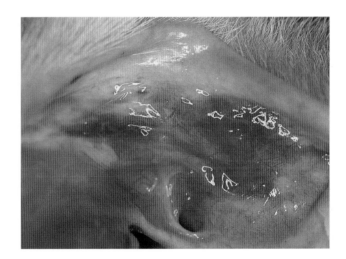

FIGURE 10.91. Clinical appearance of inflamed gingiva with retained roots.

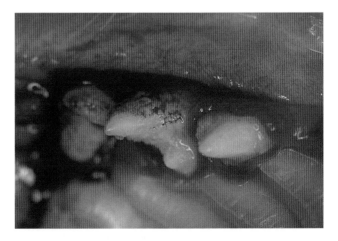

FIGURE 10.92. Generalized inflammation around the attached and alveolar gingiva of the maxillary third and fourth premolars of the cat.

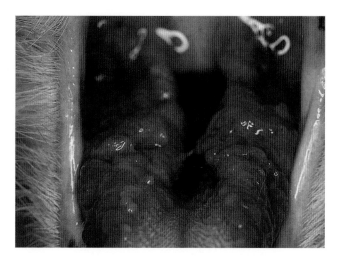

FIGURE 10.93. Marked faucitis in a cat affected with LPGS.

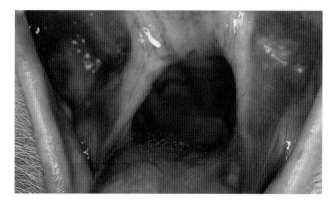

FIGURE 10.94. Resolution of faucitis (in Figure 10.93) 2 months after extraction of all teeth distal to the canines.

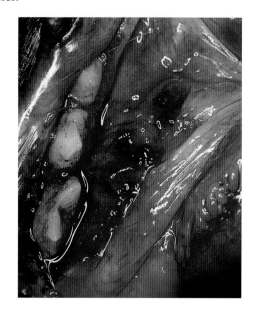

FIGURE 10.95. Marked stomatitis around the mandibular teeth before therapy.

as cobblestone-like hyperemic lesions lateral to the palatoglossal folds, soft palate, and oropharynx. In some cases, faucitis persists despite treatment efforts (Figure 10.93).

Radiograph Findings with LPGS

Intraoral radiographs often reveal moderate-to-severe periodontal disease, with bone loss and retained or fractured roots. All stages of FORLs can also be apparent clinically and radiographically.

LPGS Therapy

Therapy for LPGS can be frustrating. Strict home care aimed to control plaque usually does not lead to long-term success. Corticosteroids, gold salts, coenzyme Q-10, metronidiazole, megestrol acetate, laser surgery, antibiotics, bovine lactoferrin, azithromycin, alpha-interferon, cyclosporin, and omega 3 and 6 fatty acid supplements have been used to treat the disease, with mixed long-term results. Repeated reposital corticosteroid injections usually provide clinical improvement initially but eventually decrease the body's ability to resist the inflammatory process and predispose the patient to diabetes mellitus. Surgical extraction of the plaque-retentive cheek teeth appears to yield the most positive results (Figure 10.94–10.97).

The following is a sample approach to the LPGS patient:

1. Evaluate pre-operatively, including testing for feline leukemia, feline immunodeficiency virus, organ function, and urinalysis. A majority of the cases will have elevated globulin levels and be negative for FeLV as well as FIV.
2. Obtain intraoral radiographs of the oral cavity, including the subgingival areas of missing teeth.
3. Chart the mouth, including probing depths.
4. If a tooth is affected by moderate to severe periodontitis typified by greater than 25% support loss, it should be extracted. Additionally, remove root fragments observed clinically or radiographically. Repeat radiographic examination of the surgical area after extraction to ensure complete tooth removal. Alternatively, extract all teeth distal to the canines after the diagnosis of LPGS is made, to decrease the need for multiple surgical appointments.
5. If a CO_2 laser is available, partially vaporize inflamed palatoglossal lesions to decrease the inflammatory mass and patient discomfort. In partially responsive cases, repeat laser vaporization treatment monthly until the inflammation is under control.
6. Give antibiotics approved to treat dental infections for 2 weeks post-operatively.
7. Dispense pain relief medication.

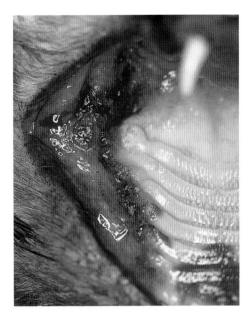

FIGURE 10.96. Extraction of multiple teeth followed by laser rastering.

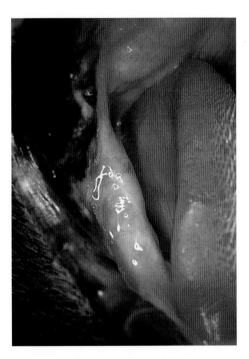

FIGURE 10.97. Resolution of LPGS after extractions in the patient shown in fig. 10.95.

8. Give prednisone (1–2 mg/kg) daily and taper over a 10-day period if the cat is anorexic.
9. Starting 2 weeks after surgery, advise and show the client how to brush the cat's remaining teeth daily and follow with 0.12% chorhexidine irrigation.
10. Re-evaluate the patient every other week. Within 3 months, the faucitis should disappear. In persistent cases, if not already done, extract all teeth distal to the canines unless the canines and incisors are clin-

ically or radiographically diseased, in which case, the affected canines and incisors are also removed.
11. If lesions persist, radiograph the mouth for evidence of tooth fragments, which, if found, should be surgically extracted.
12. If lesions persist, remove all remaining teeth.

NOTE: Approximately 20% of the cases will not be controlled with surgical, laser, and medical care.

SPECIAL CONSIDERATIONS FOR EXTRACTING FELINE TEETH

Extracting feline teeth requires exacting technique. Presurgical radiographs are important to evaluate root anatomy and pathology. Teeth with dental resorptive lesions can be ankylosed (type II), making extraction very difficult. Pulverizing or atomizing the root within the alveolus with a water-cooled high-speed handpiece and dental bur may result in removing excess supporting bone, removing too little tooth, or trauma to adjacent anatomy, and should be avoided. Removal of part or all of the facial or buccal/labial alveolar plate around a root fragment with a round or 701L long cross-cut taper fissure bur aids with exposure and can help the extraction process.

Use the following technique for extracting single feline teeth:

1. After infusion of local anesthesia, make interdental incisions on either side of the tooth to be extracted, using a #11 or #15 scalpel blade (Figure 10.98).

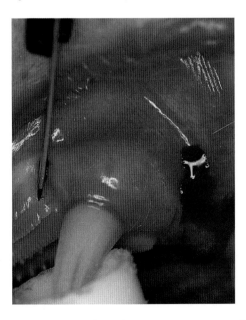

FIGURE 10.98. Interdental incisions to create a full-thickness mucoperiosteal flap for a maxillary canine tooth.

2. Insert the scalpel blade tip or sharp luxator into the gingival sulcus. Incise the soft tissue attachments 360° (Figure 10.99).

3. Raise the full-thickness mucoperiosteal flap with a Molt or Freer periosteal elevator to provide root access (Figures 10.100, 10.101).

4. Use a #2 round bur on a high-speed water-cooled handpiece to remove the coronal aspect of the facial or buccal/labial alveolar plate from the tooth root (Figures 10.102–10.105). Occasionally, radiographs reveal a bulbous root apex, which requires additional widening of the overlying alveolus.

5. Section multirooted teeth into single-rooted segments (Figures 10.106–108).

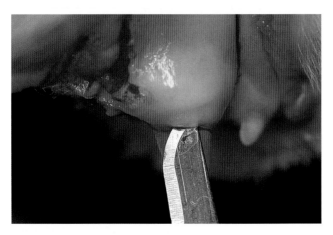

FIGURE 10.99. Intersulcular incision.

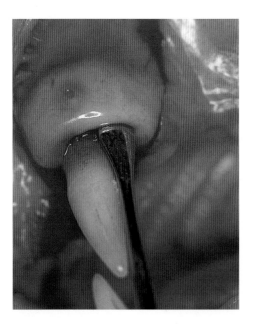

FIGURE 10.100. Attached gingiva separated with a Molt elevator.

6. Use a winged elevator to elevate the tooth root (Figure 10.109) from the alveolus before using the extraction forceps for tooth removal:

- Feline teeth are small and brittle, and sometimes fracture if the elevator is used with excessive

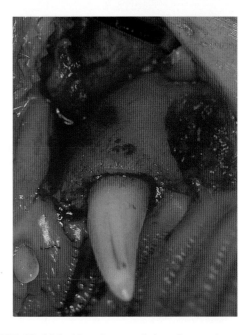

FIGURE 10.101. Alveolus overlying the canine root exposed by flap elevation.

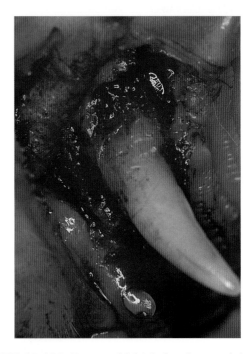

FIGURE 10.102. Removed labial alveolus overlying the root.

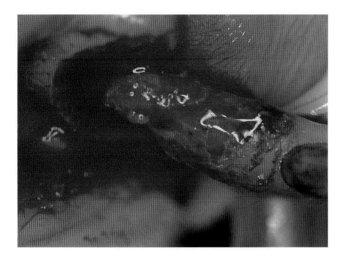

FIGURE 10.103. Extraction forceps used to deliver the canine from the alveolus.

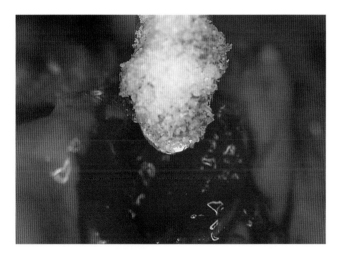

FIGURE 10.104. Consil, an osseoconductive material (alloplast), placed in the defect.

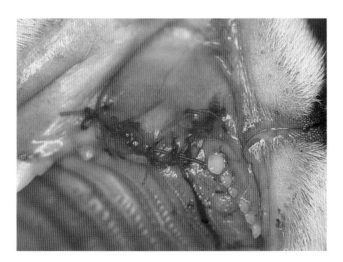

FIGURE 10.105. Flap closure.

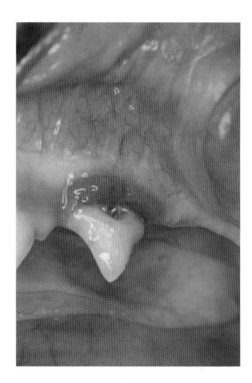

FIGURE 10.106. Inflamed gingiva around the mandibular third premolar.

force. In the event of a root fracture, every attempt should be made to retrieve the fragment. A small root elevator or root tip pick can be used after the removal of the overlying alveolar plate to expose the root.

- When operating on mandibular teeth, be aware that the mandibular canal lies immediately beneath the cheek teeth apices. Marked hemorrhage and damage to the inferior nerve may occur when the mandibular canal is entered. Excessive hemorrhage may be controlled by digital pressure and closure of the mucoperiosteal flap.

- The mandibular canines occupy a large area of the rostral mandible. Extraction must be performed carefully to avoid iatrogenic injury (Figures 10.110–10.116).

- Maxillary canine teeth affected by *chronic alveolar osteitis* clinically present with unilateral or bilateral buccal swellings. Oral probing and radiographic examination reveal marked periodontal disease. The affected teeth should be extracted after the bulging alveolus is exposed via a full-thickness mucoperiosteal flap, and alveoloplasty is performed to decrease the bulge before closure.

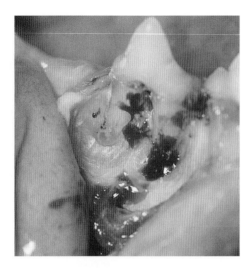

FIGURE 10.107. Exposure of the buccal alveolus.

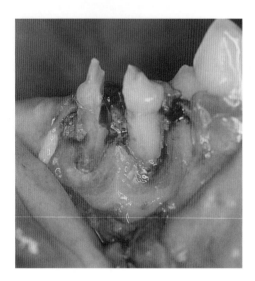

FIGURE 10.108. Two roots sectioned.

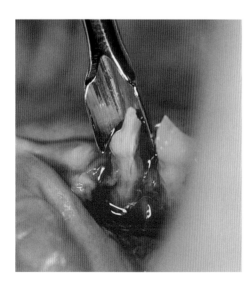

FIGURE 10.109. Winged elevator used to loosen the roots in the alveolus.

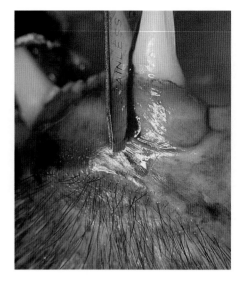

FIGURE 10.110. Line-angle incison as the mesial extent of the gingival flap of a mandibular canine tooth.

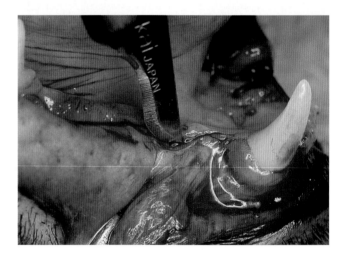

FIGURE 10.111. Number 15 blade used to incise the frenula for flap exposure of the mandibular canine.

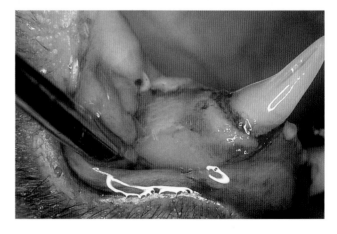

FIGURE 10.112. Labia alveolus exposed.

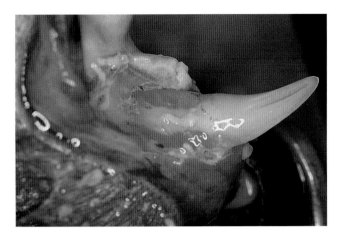

FIGURE 10.113. Labial alveolus removed to aid extraction.

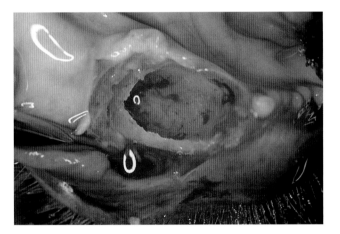

FIGURE 10.114. Mandibular alveolus after canine was extracted (note the sharp edges).

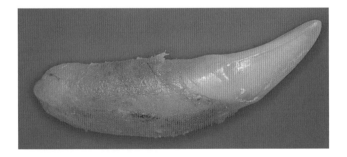

FIGURE 10.115. Extracted mandibular canine.

7. After extraction, re-contour the remaining rough edges of bone (alveoloplasty) with a round bur placed in a high-speed water-cooled handpiece. If the defect is large, place bone graft or osseoconductive material to promote osseous integration.
8. Suture the full-thickness mucoperiosteal flap without tension. In some cases, it is necessary to cut the periosteum for a tension-free closure.

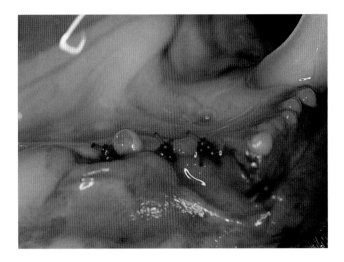

FIGURE 10.116. Sutured flap.

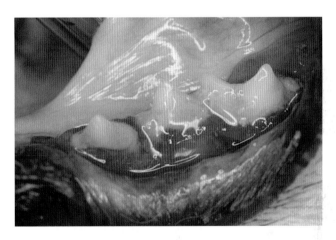

FIGURE 10.117. Example of a cat affected by stomatitis.

9. Administer appropriate pain control medication and send medication home with the client to administer for 2 weeks.

Use this technique for extracting multiple adjacent feline teeth (Figure 10.117):

1. Intraorbital and/or inferior alveolar nerve blocks are performed to provide local anesthesia. Incise the sulcular gingival attachment 360° with a #15 scalpel blade around all teeth to be extracted. Make horizontal incisions at the coronal interproximal areas between the affected teeth. Carry vertical interdental incisions just past the mucogingival line at the mesial and distal extent of the flap.
2. Elevate the gingiva bucally and lingually/palatally, using a periosteal elevator (Figures 10.118, 10.119).
3. Use a round bur on a high-speed water-cooled handpiece to remove at least half of the buccal alveolar plate, exposing the roots.

4. Section multiple-rooted teeth into single-rooted segments with a round or taper fissure bur. Sectioning normally should begin at the furcation and extend through the crown (Figure 10.120).
5. Gently stretch the periodontal ligament and extract the single-rooted segments with a #1 or #2 winged elevator used between the roots.
6. Perform alveoloplasty after extraction to remove diseased bone and sharp bone fragments.
7. Apply implant material (Consil, Nutramax Laboratories) to the defect to promote osseous growth and maintain alveolar ridge height and jaw strength.
8. Close the full-thickness mucoperiosteal flap over the extraction sites without tension, using 4-0, 5-0 absorbable suture.
9. Administer an antibiotic approved for dental disease and pain control medication daily for 2 weeks.

Post-Operative Recommendations

Post-operative recommendations after surgical extraction include the following:

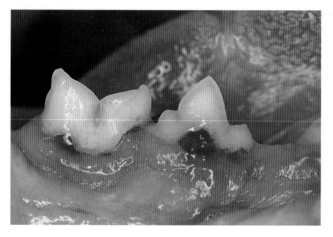

FIGURE 10.118. Mandibular third and fourth premolars and first molar affected by FORLs.

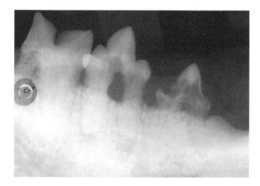

FIGURE 10.119. Radiograph revealing multiple FORLs.

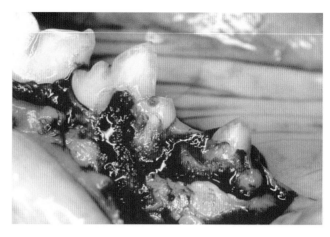

FIGURE 10.120. Flap exposure of mandibular cheek teeth.

- The diet should be softened for at least 1 week after surgery. This can be accomplished by instructing the client to pre-wet the animal's food with warm water for about 20 minutes before feeding.
- A 0.12% chlorhexidine solution can be sent home with the owner to apply twice daily for a week, as an oral rinse.

DENTAL AVULSION, LUXATION, AND SUBLUXATION

Avulsion is the complete displacement of a tooth out of the alveolar socket, with or without a concomitant alveolar fracture. The most commonly affected teeth are the canines followed by the incisors. The etiology includes trauma from fights with other dogs or car accidents. Time is of the essence when managing tooth luxation and avulsion. These are true dental emergencies (Figure 10.121).

Successful tooth reimplantation depends on the viability of the periodontal ligament. The tooth should be handled only by the crown. Examination of the tooth will usually reveal part of the periodontal ligament attached. If the avulsed tooth is exposed to air for greater than 2 hours, the prognosis is poor. If the tooth is completely avulsed, the pet owner should be advised to place it in milk as a transport medium until the owner can get the patient to the animal hospital. The owner should not attempt to clean or debride the tooth root, which could damage the cementum. Chilled low-fat milk is superior to saliva or water as a temporary storage medium for the survival of periodontal fibroblasts.

After the tooth and patient have been examined, the

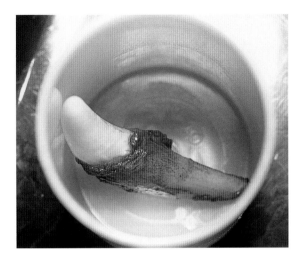

FIGURE 10.121. Avulsed canine.

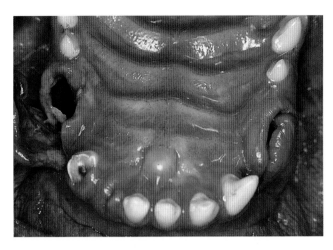

FIGURE 10.122. Right and left maxillary canine alveolar defects remaining after bilateral avulsions.

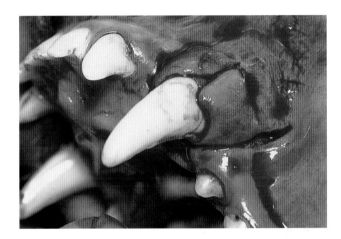

FIGURE 10.123. Avulsed canine teeth replaced into alveoli.

veterinarian should gently remove gross debris with saline and, under anesthesia, replace the tooth into the socket with digital pressure. The alveolus should not be debrided or the clot removed before reimplantation. After the tooth is replaced in the alveolus, it is splinted with 22G orthopedic wire, acrylic (Pro-temp Garant–ESPE), or orthodontic buttons and elastics. The goal of fixation is to hold the tooth in place so the periodontal ligament can heal. The splint should be loose enough to allow physiologic movement. Rigid stabilization of the tooth may result in a portion of the root being held too tightly against the alveolar process causing ankylosis and root resorption. Short-term non-rigid fixation for 2–3 weeks is usually sufficient for healing. During the stabilization period, a soft diet is recommended. The client is also advised to irrigate the mouth with 0.12% chorhexidine after each meal (Figure 10.122–10.126).

There is an absolute need for endodontic attention in the mature avulsed tooth (patient older than 9 months), because pulpal contents with compromised or no blood supply will necrose, leading to periapical disease and potential reimplantation failure. Conventional endodontics should be performed in the mature patient after the tooth is firmly anchored in the alveolus (2–3 weeks after avulsion). Some practitioners prefer using calcium hydroxide as obturation material initially, followed by replacement with gutta percha 1 year later; others use gutta percha initially, precluding a second procedure.

In cases of immature teeth with open apices, revascularization of the pulp tissue after immediate reimplantation is possible. Clinical and monthly radiographic re-examinations are advised to follow tooth vitality. Conventional endodontic procedures should be performed after the apex closes. If the apex does not close, apexification procedures can be performed to stimulate hard tissue formation at the apex.

Luxation is the partial or complete displacement of a tooth: into the alveolar socket (intrusive luxation), out of the alveolar socket (extrusive luxation), or laterally (lateral luxation). The alveolar bone is often fractured during the luxation. Radiographically, a wider than normal periodontal ligament space is usually evident. The vascular supply to the periodontal ligament and the root canal is usually compromised in cases of luxation. Treatment involves replacing the tooth into as normal a position as possible, followed by splinting for 2–3 weeks (Figures 10.127, 10.128). Endodontics is required after the tooth is stabilized, usually 2–3 weeks post-operatively.

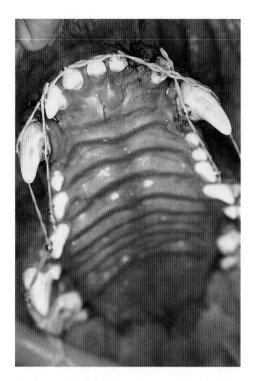

FIGURE 10.124. Replaced canines stabilized with orthodontic buttons and elastics.

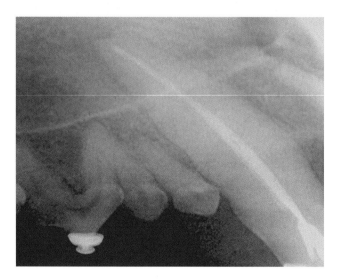

FIGURE 10.125. Radiograph showing conventional endodontics of the maxillary canine tooth after stabilization.

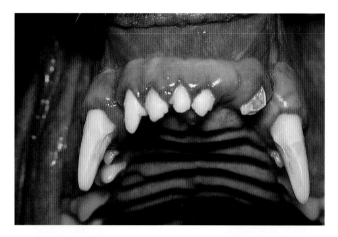

FIGURE 10.126. Six months after stabilization period and endodontic care.

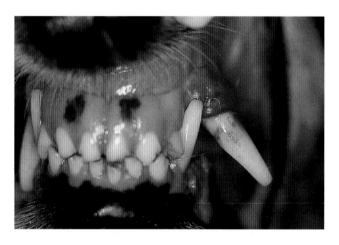

FIGURE 10.127. Luxated left maxillary canine.

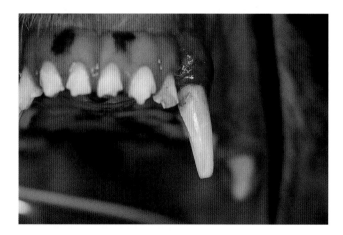

FIGURE 10.128. Luxated canine replaced to functional position before stabilization procedure.

Subluxation occurs when there is an injury of the periodontal ligament with loosening of the tooth, but without displacement. Clinically, the tooth will display abnormal mobility. Radiographic changes will not usually be apparent. The amount of mobility dictates the necessity for stabilization. Endodontic care may have to be performed after the tooth is stabilized, depending on the degree of subluxation and disruption of pulpal nourishment. Progression of periapical pathology on follow-up radiographs is an indication of the need for endodontics.

In all cases of avulsion, luxation, and subluxation, post-operative pain relief medication and antibiotics are recommended.

BONE SEQUESTRA

Bone sequestra may develop when a piece of alveolar or cancellous bone is separated from its blood supply. Clinically, the gingiva around the sequestra usually appears denuded and inflamed. Diagnostic intraoral radiographs reveal an island of bone partially or totally surrounded with a radiolucent halo. Treatment involves identifying and removing the sequestered bone. (Figures 10.129–131).

ODONTOGENIC CYST SURGERY

As a tooth develops within the jaw, the crown is surrounded by a sac of epithelial tissue.

When the tooth breaks through gingiva, the epithelium over the crown is lost. If the tooth never breaks

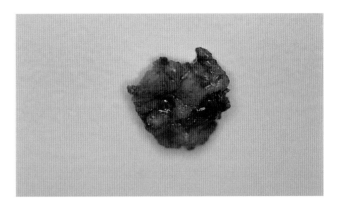

FIGURE 10.130. Sequestrum surgically removed.

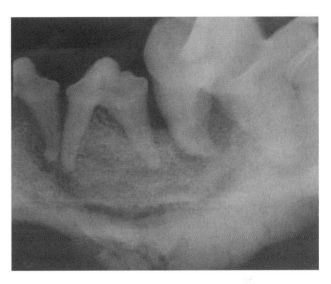

FIGURE 10.131. Radiographic appearance of mandibular sequestra secondary to osteomyelitis.

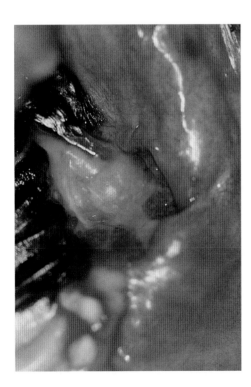

FIGURE 10.129. Clinical appearance of eroded gingiva above a bony sequestra.

through, epithelium remains around the unerupted crown. In time, the epithelium may start to produce fluid, causing the development of a dentigerous cyst.

A cyst is composed of three structures: a central cavity (lumen), an epithelial lining, and an outer wall (capsule). The cystic cavity usually contains fluid or semisolid material, such as cellular debris, keratin, or mucus. There are two broad categories of odontogenic cysts that occur in the oral cavity: developmental (dentigerous) and inflammatory (periapical).

A *dentigerous cyst* surrounds the crown of an impacted or unerupted, vital tooth. The cyst is usually attached at the cementoenamel junction. The crown is inside the cyst, the root outside. Dentigerous cysts may expand into adjacent bone, move adjacent teeth, and/or resorb roots in the area. Neoplastic transformation to ameloblastoma and epidermoid carcinoma is possible.

Types of Otontogenic Cysts

An *eruption cyst* is a dilation of the normal follicular space surrounding the crown during eruption. An eruption cyst presents as a fluctuant soft-tissue swelling of the alveolar ridge. Treatment is generally not needed. However, if necessary, it involves surgically excising the cyst around the clinical crown.

A *dentigerous cyst* is a dilation of the normal space around the crown of a tooth that is unerupted or impacted. Radiographic findings show the crown of an unerupted tooth contained in the radiolucent area while the root(s) is anchored in alveolar bone. Clinically, the enamel will be completely developed in a dentigerous cyst. Treatment involves the thorough surgical removal of the unerupted tooth and curettage of the cystic wall. The defect can then be filled with an osseoconductive material (Figures 10.132–10.134).

A *periapical (radicular) cyst,* also referred to as an apical periodontal cyst, develops at the apex of an erupted tooth whose pulp has been devitalized. The etiology of a periapical cyst usually begins with trauma, causing pulpal necrosis, apical granuloma, and cyst formation. Radiographically, a defined radiolucent area associated with the apex is noted. Treatment options include extraction, root canal therapy, hemisection and root canal therapy in multirooted teeth, and root canal therapy in association with an apicoectomy for persistent cases to permit curettage of the cystic lesion (Figures 10.135, 10.136).

ORAL TUMOR SURGERY

Benign and malignant oral tumors affect dogs and cats. Oral tumors may be classified as odontogenic or non-odontogenic, depending on their origin; as inductive or

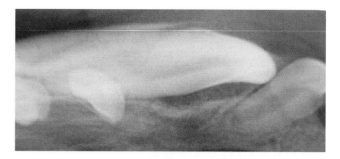

FIGURE 10.133. Radiograph of the dentigerous cyst around the canine in the patient in fig. 10.132.

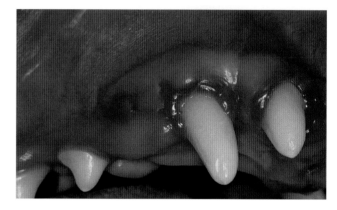

FIGURE 10.134. Clinically functional canine tooth four months post-operatively.

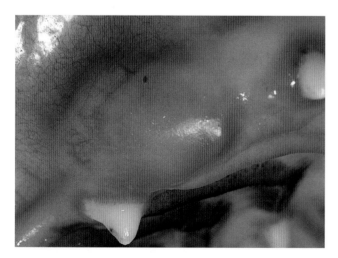

FIGURE 10.132. Swelling present around the aveolar ridge in a dentigerous cyst.

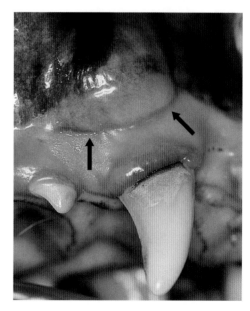

FIGURE 10.135. Marked swelling apical to the canine and maxillary first premolar.

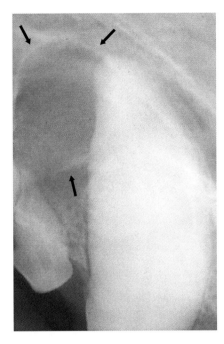

FIGURE 10.136. Radiograph of a radicular cyst of the mandibular first premolar.

non-inductive, depending on the interaction of epithelial and mesenchymal tissues; or by the epithelial, mesenchymal, or mixed epithelial-mesenchymal origin of the neoplastic cells.

Before surgery, the mass should be staged per the World Heath Organization (WHO) primary tumor-regional nodes-metastasis (TNM) system.

The tumor is:

- Inspected and palpated for presence of ulceration or necrosis.
- Examined for adjacent tooth mobility not related to fracture or periodontal disease.
- Evaluated for regional lymph node involvement. Regional nodes are checked for size, shape, pain on palpation, and lack of mobility.
- Radiographed for areas of bone resorption or new bone production. Thoracic radiographs are taken for metastatic evaluation.

Then the following TMN chart is used:

- T—Primary tumor
  - T-1 tumor less than 2 cm
  - T-2 tumor between 2 and 4 cm
  - T-3 tumor greater than 4 cm
- N—Regional lymph nodes
  - N-0 non-palpable nodes—no metastasis expected
  - N-1 palpable ipsilateral non-fixed node—metastasis suspected
  - N-2 palpable contralateral non-fixed node—metastasis suspected
  - N-3 fixed nodes—metastasis suspected
- M—Distant metastasis
  - M-0 no distant metastasis
  - M-1 Evidence of metastasis to other than cervical nodes

Tissue sampling can be accomplished by:

- *Fine needle aspiration*, which is also helpful for lymph node sampling.
- *Exfoliative cytology* is used to examine tumor cells on the mass periphery. *Note:* some oral tumors do not exfoliate cells. Aspiration or cut tissue evaluation generally yields results that are more reliable.
- *Incisional biopsy*, which is indicated for large lesions and those with a more ominous malignant appearance not conducive to initial total removal. Incisional biopsies can be performed with a scalpel blade, disposable biopsy punch, or a Tru-cut needle (Schein 568-4604, Burns 697-5622). A Michelle trephine (Schein 568-2090), or Yamshidi needle (Burns 599-4650, Schein 568-7310) can be used to biopsy masses that have bone involvement.

A pie-shaped or *elliptical wedge* of soft tissue is removed for incisional biopsy. Incisions on either side of the ellipse should converge in a V shape to join in deeper sublesion tissues. The ellipse length should be three times the width. Lesions from fixed alveolar or palatal tissue do not require the 3:1 ellipse shape because of the inability to close the surgical defect. Normal tissue is not purposely incised to prevent opening previously unexposed tissue planes.

Once the cytologic or histopathologic diagnosis has been rendered, additional surgical excision, chemotherapy, and/or radiation therapy can be performed. Ideally, the surgeon should provide clean surgical margins of at least 1 cm for benign lesions and at least 2 cm for malignant lesions.

The optimum goal is to render the patient tumor-free. When this goal is not possible because of the extent of disease or type of tumor, palliative surgery can be performed to achieve temporary local control.

Surrounding the tumor is a pseudocapsule composed of normal, neoplastic cells, and a reactive zone composed of inflammatory cells. Surgical options for oral tumor management include the following:

- *Intracapsular* excision, which removes the tumor from inside the capsule. Intracapsular excision is indicated to treat well-differentiated odontomas, which can be curetted from the maxilla or mandible.
- *Marginal* excision, which removes the lesion visually (Figure 10.137), but is poorly suited for benign

odontogenic tumors such as epuli. Marginal excision may leave remnants of the tumor in place, resulting in regrowth.

- *En bloc* excision removes the tumor, pseudocapsule, reactive zone, and a wide margin of normal tissue. En bloc excision is indicated in the treatment of malignant and infiltrating tumors (Figures 10.138, 10.139).
- *Radical* resection removes major parts of the maxilla and/or mandible. Radical resection is indicated in the treatment of aggressive benign and malignant tumors that invade the mandible or maxilla (Figure 10.140).

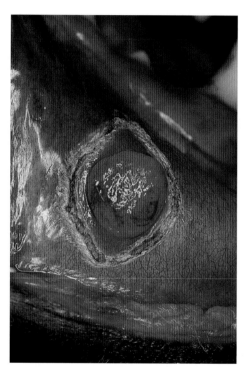

FIGURE 10.137. Marginal excision.

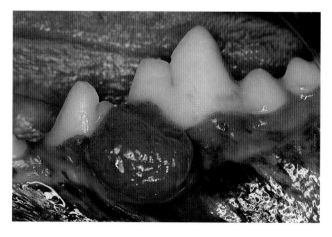

FIGURE 10.138. Mandibular mass in a dog.

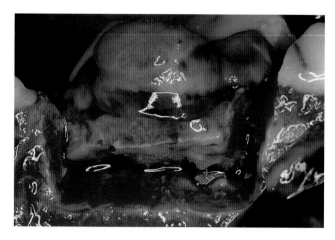

FIGURE 10.139. En bloc excision of the mandibular mass from fig. 10.138.

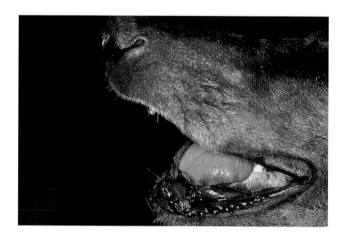

FIGURE 10.140. Radical resection of the rostral mandible.

Common Canine Oral Tumors

Epulides arise from the epithelial rest cells of Malassez which are remnants of Herwig's epithelial root sheath residing with the periodontal ligament. Epuli are the most common benign oral tumors in dogs. The most common epuli in small animal patients are classified as:

- *Fibromatous epuli* (Figure 10.141) occur in both dogs and cats. Ages of affected animals range 1–17 years (mean = 7.5 years). Both pedunculated and sessile forms exist. Fibromatous epuli usually have a smooth, pink surface. Marginal excision is usually not sufficient to treat fibromatous epuli. Removal of the tumor, tooth, and periodontal ligament is the treatment of choice.
- *Ossifying epulis* (Figure 10.142) is similar to the fibromatous epulis, but contains an osteoid matrix. Both fibromatous and ossifying epuli are often clas-

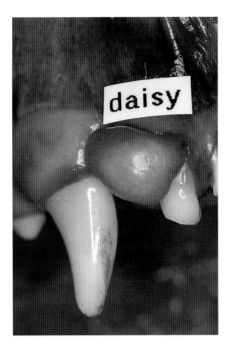

FIGURE 10.141. Fibromatous epulis between the maxillary corner incisor and canine tooth in a dog.

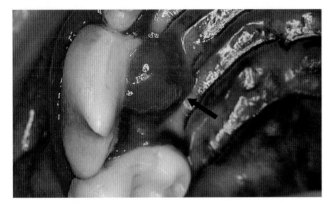

FIGURE 10.142. Ossifying epulis on the palatal aspect of the maxillary fourth premolar in a dog.

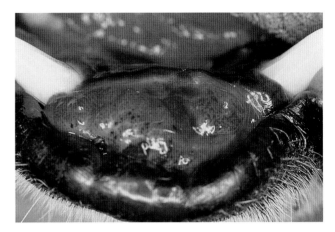

FIGURE 10.143. Acanthomatous epulis of the rostral mandible.

sified as *peripheral odontogenic fibromas*. Most ossifying epuli occur around the maxillary premolars. Treatment involves en bloc removal of the tumor, tooth, and alveolus from which it is growing.

- *Peripheral ameloblastoma (acanthomatous epulis)* (Figure 10.143) is classified as benign, but has the tendency to invade adjacent bone. Acanthomatous epuli can occur around any tooth but most commonly affects the mandibular canines. Surgery must be radical with at least 1 cm clean margins. Extraction of any teeth that may impede incisional healing is indicated. Radiation has also been used

successfully, but may cause the benign tumor to transform to a malignant tumor and/or produce osseoradionecrosis. Although the combination of surgery and radiation may be most effective (requiring less aggressive surgery), radiation sometimes is not readily available, so surgery may be the only option. Multiple (10) weekly injections of Bleomycin (5 mg) injected intralesionally has also been shown to be effective in a small number of reported cases.

Malignant melanoma (Figure 10.144) is the most common oral malignancy in dogs. Malignant melanoma most fequently occurs in older males, especially cocker spaniels, German shepherds, chow chows, and dogs with heavily pigmented mucous membranes. Oral melanomas behave aggressively.

Affected patients often present with oral bleeding, ptyalism, and halitosis. Tumor size on presentation is an important predictor of patient survival. In the dog, melanomas <2 cm carry a better survival rate (median 511 days) than those >2 cm (164 days). Tumors located rostrally also have better prognosis than those located distally, probably because they are discovered earlier and are more amenable to wide surgical excision.

The lip or mucocutaneous junction is another site for melanoma in the dog's oral cavity. Lip melanomas do not commonly invade bone, allowing more aggressive resection of surrounding tissue and overall favorable prognosis.

By the time the tumor is clinically diagnosed, it often has invaded bone and metastasized to the lymph nodes and lungs. Unfortunately, oral melanomas respond poorly to surgical excision unless treated early and aggressively by mandibulectomy or partial maxillectomy.

Melanomas are somewhat radioresponsive. One study showed a median survival time of 14 months after radiation therapy alone. In the study, 800 cGy was administered on days 0, 7, and 21 for a total dose of 2,400 cGy in 3 weeks.

In another study, intralesional cisplatin and/or carmustine or methothrexate implants injected at 1–2 week intervals were used with varied success of >50% decrease in tumor volume (70% of cases).

Squamous cell carcinoma (SCC) (Figure 10.145) is the second most common malignant tumor in the dog, originating from the gingival epithelium; it appears red and ulcerated, and may have cauliflower projections. Older large-breed dogs are predisposed. The prognosis depends on location in the oral cavity. Those located rostrally carry a better prognosis than those located at the base of the tongue or in the tonsilar region, which are locally aggressive and tend to metastasize. In a 1960 study, tonsilar SCC was found to occur 10 times more commonly in dogs from urban settings compared to rural dogs. SCC carries a better long-term prognosis than malignant melanoma or fibrosarcoma in the dog.

SCC in the dog may be widely surgically excised or irradiated, especially if the lesion is located rostrally. Surgically, a maxillectomy or partial mandibulectomy can be performed with a goal of a clean surgical margin of 2 cm. Radiation alone delivers a median survival rate of 15–17 months. Medically, piroxicam (orally 0.3 mg/kg/every other day), a nonsteroidal anti-inflammatory agent, can be used for palliation.

The prognosis for survival following treatment of lingual SCC is poor. In one study, only 25% of treated dogs survived a year or more. Dogs tolerate partial glossectomy involving 40–60% of the tongue. Aggressive excision of the tongue in order to get clean surgical margins may result in patient morbidity due to inability to eat.

Fibrosarcoma (Figure 10.146) has the predilection for the maxilla of large, male, middle-aged, dogs—especially retrievers. The gingiva around the maxillary fourth premolar is commonly affected. Oral fibrosarcomas carry a poor prognosis because of localized destruction.

In published studies, partial maxillectomy or mandibulectomy with at least 2 cm margins have resulted in a 12-month median survival rate. Conservative excision results in rapid recurrence. Oral fibrosarcomas are generally radioresponsive. In one study, radiation was shown to provide a median progression-free survival rate of 23 months. Radiation and aggressive surgery together resulted in mean survival times of 32 months in another study. Palatal fibrosarcomas carry a poor prognosis because of the inability to adequately resect the tumor.

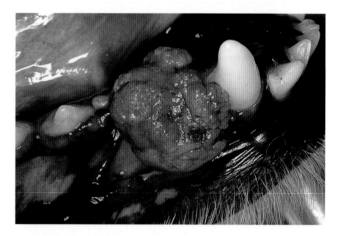

FIGURE 10.145. Squamous cell carcinoma in the mandible of a dog.

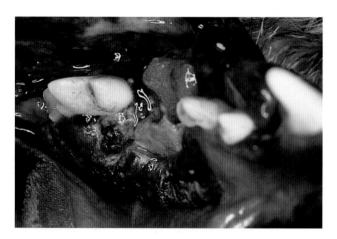

FIGURE 10.144. Malignant melanoma infiltrating the mandible of a dog.

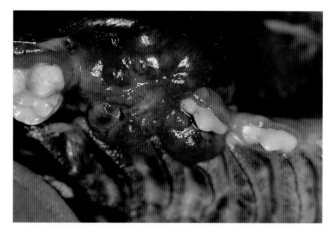

FIGURE 10.146. Fibrosarcoma infiltrating the maxilla of a dog.

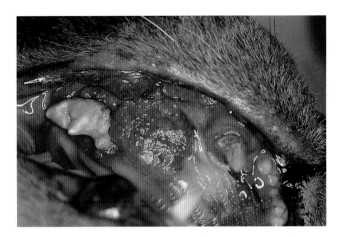

FIGURE 10.147. Squamous cell carcinoma in the maxilla of a cat.

Feline Oral Tumors

In one study, 50% of feline oral swellings presented to the dental department of a veterinary university were nonmalignant, and were mostly from osteomyelitis secondary to retained roots of teeth affected by FORLs.

Squamous cell carcinoma is the most common oral malignancy in the cat. Feline oral squamous cell carcinoma carries a poor prognosis. Rostral involvement provides a slightly more favorable prognosis with wide excision than does tonsilar or sublingual tumors. Surgery, chemotherapy, and/or radiation will usually not cure the disease. Median survival time of cats with oral squamous cell carcinoma, even with treatment, is less than 6 months once diagnosed. One-year survival rarely exceeds 10% of those treated (Figure 10.147).

Fibrosarcoma is locally invasive and slow to metastasize in the cat. Wide excision is the treatment of choice.

MAXILLECTOMY AND MANDIBULECTOMY

Partial maxillectomy and mandibulectomy are considered advanced oral surgical procedures. The most common reason to remove part of the maxilla or mandible is for wide excision of oral tumors. The extent of excision should be based on many factors, including the following:

- Clinical and radiographic extent of the lesion
- Pre-operative cytological and/or previous histopathological diagnosis

- The ability to achieve at least a 2 cm surgical margin if the lesion is malignant, 1 cm if the lesion is benign
- The ability to close without tension
- Anatomical structures

Before surgery, the patient is treated with appropriate antibiotics and pain relief medication. When anesthetized, the oral mucosa is irrigated with 0.12% chlorhexidine. Regional anesthetic nerve blocks are also performed. Use the following steps for tumor excision:

1. Lightly trace an initial incision to provide at least a 1 cm margin for benign lesions and a 2 cm margin for malignant lesions.
2. Excise soft tissue to the bone, ligating large blood vessels as encountered. Plan the soft tissue incision and bone removal so that the suture line is supported by bone.
3. Elevate tissues subperiosteally. Take care to leave soft tissue attached to the underlying bone where the soft tissue comes within 1 cm of the tumor.
4. Make mucosal flaps larger than the defect to assure tension-free closure.
5. Before closure, smooth sharp edges with a round bur inserted in a water-cooled hig-speed handpiece.
6. Place 4-0 to 5-0 absorbable sutures, using a reverse cutting needle in a simple interrupted pattern. Place sutures 3–4 mm apart and 3–4 mm from the opposing margins.
7. Extract any teeth that occlude on the mucosal flap, or crown reduction, vital pulpotomy, and crown restoration.

After surgery, the patient is maintained on a soft gruel diet or fed through a pharyngostomy tube until it can apprehend and swallow. Antibiotic and pain relief medication is administered for 2 weeks post-operatively.

Maxillectomy

Rostral unilateral or bilateral premaxillectomy is performed to remove tumors or repair rostral maxillary trauma. Caudal and hemimaxillectomy are used to remove tumors of the caudal maxilla. The infraorbital artery is located apical to the distal root of the second premolar and preserved if in the surgical site. The major palatine artery emerges from the palatine foramen at the level of the carnassial tooth, midway between the midline and dental arcade. It should be ligated if the palate is incised. Removal of the excised portion of the maxilla often exposes the nasal cavity, which needs to be covered with a labial mucosal-submucosal flap.

Mandibulectomy

Mandibulectomies are classified according to the part excised: unilateral or bilateral; rostral hemimandibulectomy, central or caudal hemimandibulectomy; three-quarter or total hemimandibulectomy. After the soft tissue attachments are incised to the bone, osteotomies are performed, avoiding the tooth roots. The first osteotomy is at the mandibular symphysis followed by the pre-planned area between the premolar teeth. A curved mosquito hemostat can be used to locate the mandibular alveolar artery for ligation. If the artery retracts into the mandibular canal, the canal can be packed with bone wax to control hemorrhage. After tumor removal, the labial mucosa is sutured to the sublingual and contralateral mandibular mucosa without tension. When the chin has been included in the resection, skin is sutured to the mucosa of the floor of the mouth rostrally to reconstruct a lip margin (Figures 10.148–10.158).

Total unilateral mandibulectomy may lead to a drift of the remaining mandible toward the mandibulectomy side, although this rarely produces a functional problem other than the mandibular canine tooth traumatizing the palate. Crown amputation and direct pulp capping should be considered to relieve palatal trauma, if present.

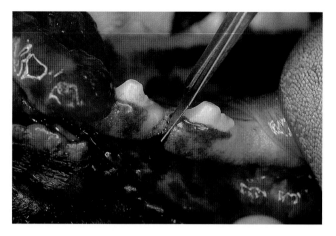

FIGURE 10.149. Incision between third and fourth mandibular premolars.

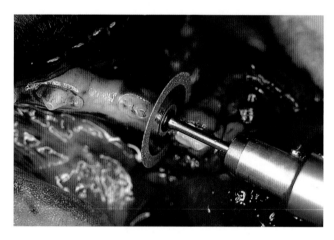

FIGURE 10.150. Diamond disk used for mandibulectomy (advanced procedure).

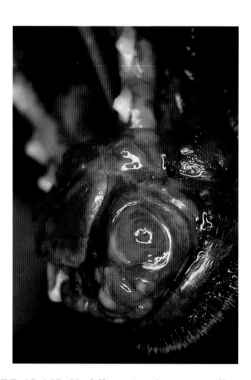

FIGURE 10.148. Undifferentiated sarcoma affecting the rostral mandible.

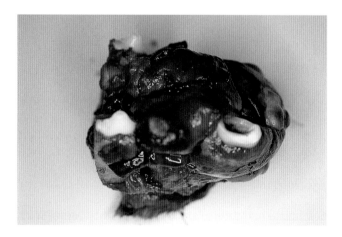

FIGURE 10.151. Excised rostral mandible.

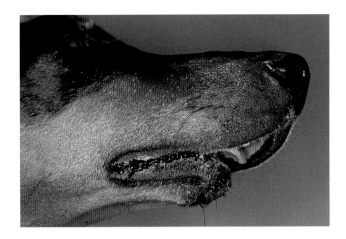

FIGURE 10.152. Patient shown in fig. 10.148 two months after rostral mandibulectumy.

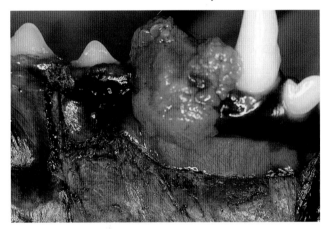

FIGURE 10.153. Incision outline for rostral hemi-mandibulectomy for excision of squamous cell carcinoma lesion in a dog.

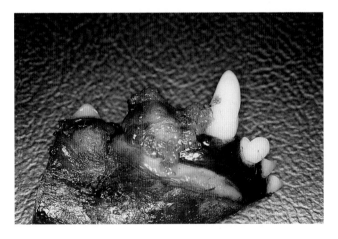

FIGURE 10.154. Rostral hemimandibulectomy segment.

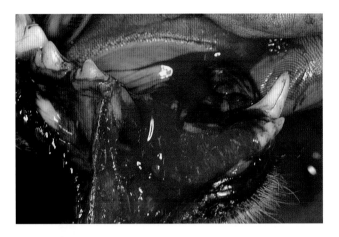

FIGURE 10.155. Surgical site after rostral hemi-mandibulectomy in a dog.

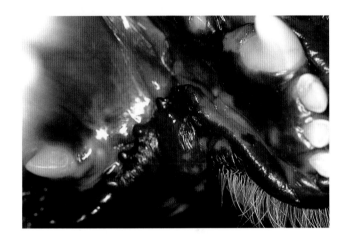

FIGURE 10.156. Sutured defect two months after a rostral hemimandibulectomy.

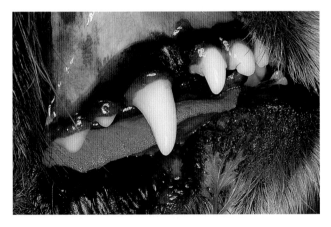

FIGURE 10.157. Functional post-operative result following a rostral hemimandibulectomy.

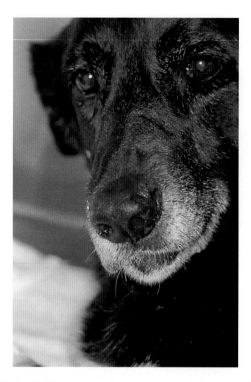

FIGURE 10.158. Clinical appearance after a rostral hemimandibulectomy.

JAW LUXATION/FRACTURE

Maxillary and mandibular fractures occur secondary to trauma or preexisting pathology (periodontal, metabolic, and neoplastic). In the cat, mandibular symphyseal separations are most common. Dogs most often fracture the mandible between the first premolar and second molar. Before the fracture can be fully evaluated under deep sedation or general anesthesia, the patient must be stabilized. Both jaws as well as the temporomandibular joint should be thoroughly examined manually and radiographically.

A traumatic rostral or caudal temporomandibular dislocation may be responsible for a patient that acutely cannot close its mouth or closes in a non-occlusal position. Usually, the condyloid process displaces rostrodorsally. The luxation may be unilateral or bilateral. If unilateral, the mandible deviates to the side opposite the luxated joint. Diagnosis of luxation alone or luxation with fracture can be confirmed with lateral oblique radiographs. Treatment involves placing the animal under general anesthesia, inserting a fulcrum (a pencil or tubular device) across the second molars, and closing the jaws to insert the luxated condyle(s) into the temporomandibular joint.

Jaw fracture repair concepts include the following:

- Rapid return to function and anatomic reduction are the most critical concerns.

- Intact teeth in the fracture line are not extracted if they do not interfere with fracture reduction.
- Malpositoned teeth created by the fracture are extracted or repositioned and splinted in functional positions.
- Grades 3 and 4 periodontally affected teeth are extracted or hemisected and the viable roots restored if they are within the fracture line. Follow-up clinical and radiographic evaluation is recommended.
- Esophagostomy tube placement may be necessary in cases of multiple or severe jaw fractures.
- Temporary tape muzzles can be used to stabilize minimally displaced favorable fractures. The patient must be monitored to ensure that the muzzle does not interfere with normal breathing (Figures 10.159, 10.160).
- Bone plates are not commonly used in fracture repair because of iatrogenic root trauma and the difficulty in achieving functional occlusion.
- External fixation using pins and acrylic sidebars can be used for fracture stabilization. External pin fixa-

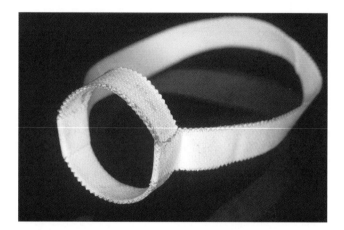

FIGURE 10.159. Support muzzle made from waterproof tape.

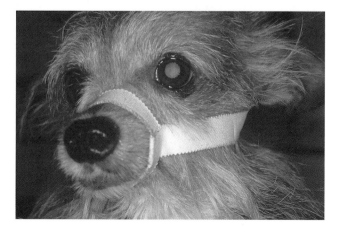

FIGURE 10.160. Tape muzzle applied to patient.

tion causes significant iatrogenic trauma to tooth roots and/or the mandibular canal.

- Interdental fixation with wire, acrylic splints, and/or orthodontic buttons and elastics is the preferred method to repair most small-animal jaw fractures.
- Functional occlusion is more important than cosmetics.

Maxillary Fractures

Maxillary fractures occur from trauma or preexisting pathology. Fractures resulting in minimal displacement without a malocclusion may be treated using a tape muzzle. Fractures resulting in instability should be stabilized. General surgical and orthopedic principles apply after physical and radiographic examination: apposition of fracture components as close to normal and functional anatomy as possible. Stability can be provided using nonmobile teeth as anchors for splinting material, interdental wiring, acrylic, or orthodontic buttons and elastics. Dental acrylic can be used to provide support across the hard palate. Six to eight weeks are generally recommended for healing (Figures 10.161–10.163).

Trauma may also result in palatal fracture. Physical examination usually reveals palatal separation without displacement. Suturing the separation leads to healing within 2 months (Figure 10.164).

Mandibular Fractures

Pathological fractures occur most commonly in the region of the first molars and canine teeth, caused by marked bone loss from periodontal or neoplastic disease. Traumatic mandibular fractures commonly affect the middle third of the mandible. Radiographic and

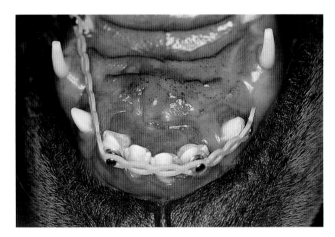

FIGURE 10.162. One month after application of orthodontic buttons and elastics used to stabilize maxillary fracture.

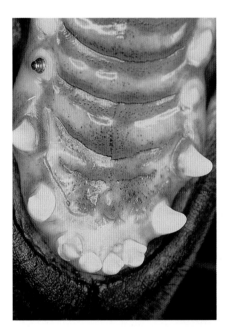

FIGURE 10.163. Healed fracture site 4 months postoperatively.

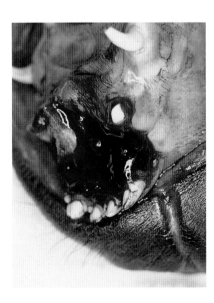

FIGURE 10.161. Maxillary fracture in dog caused by a horse kick.

clinical evaluation is critical to formulate appropriate therapeutic options.

Fractures occurring in a rostroventral direction are relatively stable (favorable). Caudoventral mandibular fractures are generally unstable (unfavorable), because of digastric muscle distraction of the fracture segments. Interdental orthopedic wire placed on either side of the fracture segment and stabilization using Protemp Garant (3M ESPE) can be used to repair mandibular body fractures.

Multiple mandibular fractures can also occur. Management of a comminuted mandibular fracture involves advanced dental procedures not within the scope of this text.

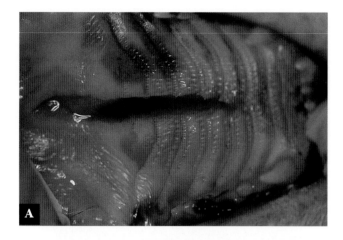

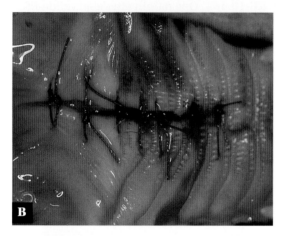

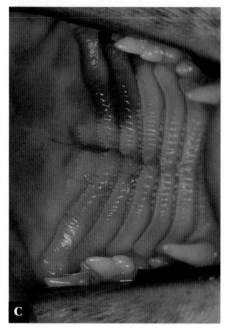

FIGURE 10.164. (A) Feline palatal separation from trauma; (B) defect sutured; (C) healing palatal separation.

Fractures of the mandibular ramus and condyloid process are uncommon. The surrounding muscle mass usually stabilizes the fracture segments. If unstable and grossly displaced, mandibular ramus fractures can be wired. Condylar fractures will usually functionally heal without surgery.

Dental acrylic helps to immobilize the fractured segments. Acrylic splints are indicated for fractures rostral to the first mandibular molar and the maxillary fourth premolar.

Use this technique for the intraoral splint fabrication:

1. Align the fracture segments into a functional anatomic position. Occlusal evaluation is difficult in the intubated animal. To properly evaluate occlusion, the animal is either intubated through a pharangostomy or the animal can be intravenously anesthetized and closely monitored. Suture open lesions if possible.
2. Apply 24 gauge stainless steel orthopedic wire in a Stout's multiple loop fashion to stabilize the fracture before application of the acrylic splint (Figure 10.165).
3. Clean, polish (using a non-fluoride polish), and acid-etch the affected teeth in the fracture area.
4. Apply petroleum jelly to the maxillary dentition.
5. Use ProTemp Garant to fabricate the splint. Add most of the composite resin to the lingual surface of the mandibular teeth, so as not to interfere with occlusion (Figure 10.166).
6. While the acrylic is still soft, close the maxilla to full occlusion with the mandible.

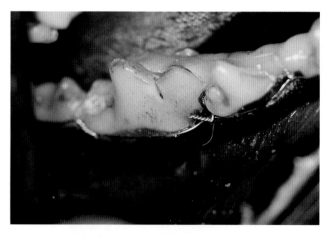

FIGURE 10.165. Interdental wiring using an Ivy loop wiring technique to stabilize a mandibular body fracture.

7. After the splint is hardened, open the mouth for fine adjustments and smoothing with a dental bur.

8. Send the owner home with 0.12% chlorhexidine rinse to apply twice daily to the splint area. Place the patient on a soft food diet.

9. Allow the splint to remain for 3 weeks or until rigid stabilization has occurred, evidenced both clinically and radiographically.

Use this technique for extraoral splint fabrication; the skin surface over the fracture site is prepared surgically:

1. Externally place Kirschner wires and/or threaded Steinman pins perpendicular to the edges of the mandibular fracture segments. Incise oral mucosa to the bone in the area before the pins are placed. Confirm functional occlusion. Introduce pins into the bone, using a low-speed drill operated at less than 300 rpm. Take care to avoid roots and the mandibular canal. Ideally, at least 6 cortices should be engaged in each major fracture segment. Pin placement should be at least 1 cm from the fracture lines.

2. Embed exposed cut pin ends into an acrylic bridge or a padded external fixation apparatus for stability while maintaining a functional occlusion.

3. Take post-operative radiographs to access fracture reduction.

4. Clinically evaluate the surgical site weekly and radiograph every 3–4 weeks.

5. Allow the external fixature to remain until there is radiographic evidence of healing. External fixature removal may be staged.

6. While the external fixation is in place, the patient should be fed a gruel diet.

Symphyseal Separations

Mandibular symphyseal separations occur secondary to automobile or high-rise fall injuries, especially in the cat. Stabilization can be obtained through circumferential or figure-eight wiring of the segments in as near normal anatomic position as possible, coupled with ProTemp Garant (Figures 10.167, 10.168).

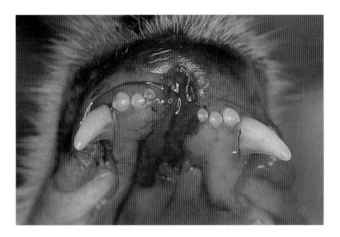

FIGURE 10.167. Feline symphyseal separation.

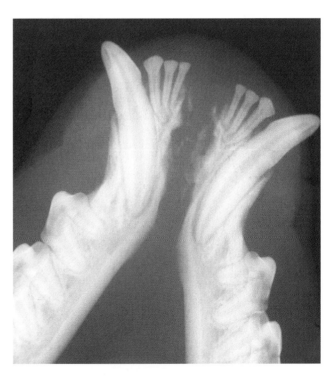

FIGURE 10.168. Radiograph of symphyseal separation.

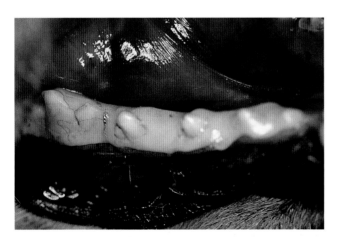

FIGURE 10.166. ProTemp Garant placed over wired mandibular body fracture for additional stabilization.

Use the following circumferential wiring technique for stabilization of mandibular symphyseal fractures:

1. Place an 18 gauge needle behind the mandibular canines ventrally through the skin into the labial mucosa (Figure 10.169).
2. Thread 22 gauge stainless steel orthopedic wire through the needle.
3. Remove the needle and reinsert on the opposite side.
4. Direct the wire toward the skin (Figure 10.170).
5. With needle holders or wire twisters, tighten the wire, which is cut 3–4 mm from the exit point and bent parallel to the skin. Do not over-tighten, which may lead to labioversion of the mandibular canine teeth (Figures 10.171, 10.172).
6. The wire is removed in 3 weeks.

Use the following *figure-eight wiring technique* with caution, because this procedure may induce localized periodontitis and cause lingual canine displacement:

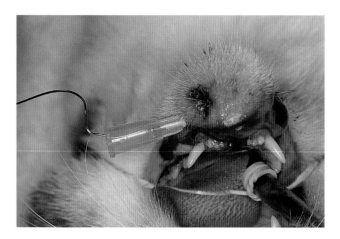

FIGURE 10.169. Wire threaded through the 18 guage needle placed ventral to the canines.

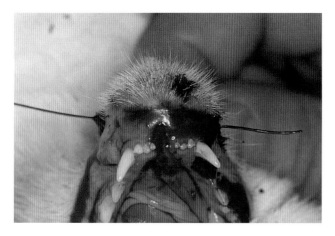

FIGURE 10.170. Wire ventral to the canines.

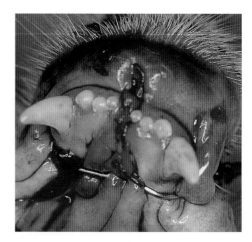

FIGURE 10.171. Clinical post-operative appearance.

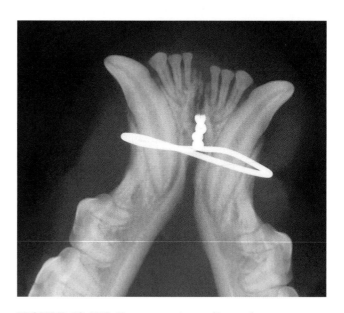

FIGURE 10.172. Post-operative radiograph.

1. Clean and polish the mandibular canines with a non-fluoride paste.
2. Loop 22 guage orthopedic wire from the mesial surface of one mandibular canine to the distal surface of the other. Pass additional loops until stability occurs.
3. Twist the wire on the distolabial surface where the procedure began.
4. Apply composite material over the wire to protect the tongue from trauma.

Temporomandibular Joint Instability

Clinical instability of the temporomandibular joint may cause clicking or catching of the condylar process on the zygomatic arch. When this occurs, the animal may be unable to close its mouth. The jaw can be manually reduced to allow normal closure of the mouth, but a wide excursion such as a yawn may result in a locked open mouth. Surgical correction of the problem entails removing the part of the zygomatic arch that is interfered with and/or removing part of the coronoid process of the mandible.

Shar-Pei Tight Lip Syndrome— Vestibular Deepening Surgery

Shar-Pei dogs can be affected by a condition where the mandibular lip is attached higher than normal pulling the lip over the anterior mandibular teeth (tight lip syndrome). The mucosal surface of the lip may cover only the incisors or extend past the incisors to the premolars (Figure 10.173).

Follow these steps for surgical repair:

1. Place the animal in ventral recumbency with the head suspended by a tie around the maxilla to an overhead support. The surgical area is disinfected with 0.12% chlorhexidine and infiltrated with local anesthesia containing epinephrine.
2. Make incisions to the depth of the anterior mandibular vestibule. In severe cases, incising the frenula is necessary (Figure 10.174).
3. Peel away the periosteum with a Molt No. 2 and/or No. 4 periosteal elevator (Figure 10.175).
4. Harvest a full-thickness buccal alveolar mucosal graft from the maxillary facial mucosa apical to the premolars (Figure 10.176).
5. Suture the graft to the lower-lip defect with 4-0 absorbable suture material (Figures 10.177, 10.178).

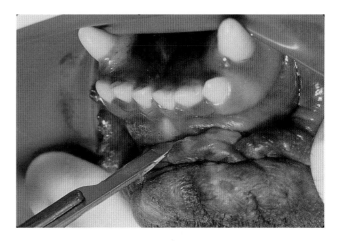

FIGURE 10.174. Incision into the anterior mandibular vestibule.

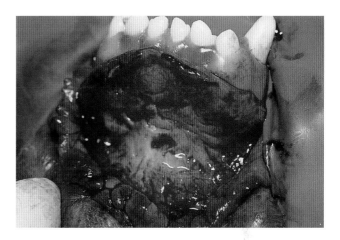

FIGURE 10.175. Periosteal elevator used to enlarge host site.

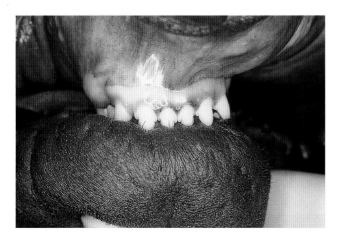

FIGURE 10.173. Shar-Pei tight lip.

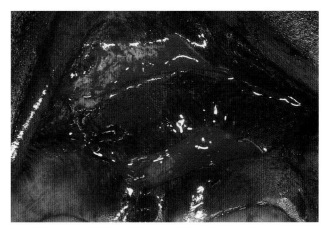

FIGURE 10.176. Graft being harvested.

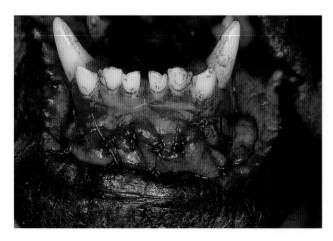

FIGURE 10.177. Sutured graft.

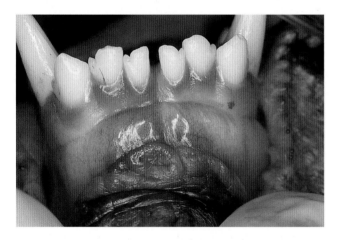

FIGURE 10.178. Two-month post-operative result resolving tight lip.

6. Instruct the client to rinse the surgical area twice daily with 0.12% chlorhexidine rinse.
7. Dispense antibiotic and pain control medication. Generally, healing is complete in 3 weeks.

LASER USE IN VETERINARY DENTISTRY

The term *laser* is an acronym for light amplification by stimulated emission of radiation. The laser is a highly concentrated light focused into an extremely small spot delivering a large amount of energy. When the laser light hits an object, it reflects, transmits, scatters, or is absorbed. Power can be adjusted to incise, excise, vaporize (ablate), or cauterize.

As photons are absorbed, they are converted into thermal energy. When tissue temperature is elevated to 60–65° C, protein denaturation occurs. When tissue temperatures reach 100° C, water undergoes a phase transformation from liquid to steam. As soon as the pressure of the steam overcomes the strength of tissue confinement, vaporization occurs. The classic laser ablation crater consists of an area where tissue has been vaporized (temperatures above 100° C), surrounded by an area of thermal necrosis (temperatures between 60–90° C), encircled by an area of inflammation and edema (temperatures up to 60° C).

Heat generated in tissue seeks equilibrium and diffuses from an area of high heat concentration to an area of low heat concentration. Heat distribution in tissue generated by laser irradiation is dependent on the wavelength of the beam, the optical properties of tissue, the concentration of energy deposited, and the length of time taken to deposit that energy into tissue. Differences in tissue content of substances—such as water, protein, hemoglobin, and melanin—can substantially influence the affect of a specific wavelength.

Although the influence on tissue can differ substantially between different wavelengths, the influence of a single wavelength on tissue varies, depending upon the amount of time that is taken to deposit a specific amount of energy into the tissue.

Lasers can be used to resect, dissect, excise, incise, or amputate oral tissues as one would use a scalpel. One important difference compared to scalpel surgery is that hemostasis can be provided while the tissue is being incised.

The cutting action depends on the type of laser and the tissue on which you are operating. Generally, lasers operated in continuous mode cut comparably to a scalpel, while those in lower-pulsed modes (10–20 pulses/second) incise slower or rougher. Diode lasers used in contact mode often drag when making oral incisions.

Types of Lasers Used in Oral Procedures

Lasers are named by the lasing medium they contain. Popular lasers include carbon dioxide, neodymium yttrium aluminum garnet (Nd:YAG), argon, ruby, diode, holmium:YAG, Erbium:YAG, and pulsed dye. The carbon dioxide and diode lasers are most frequently used in small animal practice.

ARGON LASER (488-514 NM) The argon laser's wavelengths, operating in the visible blue-green region (488.0 and 514.5 NM), are absorbed strongly by hemoglobin, which lets the laser energy cut, vaporize, or coagulate most oral tissues. Dental argon lasers are low-power devices (5 watts or less). Fibers must be used in a contact mode or near-contact mode to cut or vaporize oral tissue. Argon lasers are used in either continuous-

Glossary of Dental Laser Terms

Continuous wave laser beams emit an uninterrupted shaft of light at the output power setting for as long as the switch is turned on.

Energy is the capacity to do work (to vaporize tissue). Laser energy is measured in joules (J). Energy is a product of power (watts, W) and time of application (seconds). It takes 2.4 J of energy to vaporize 1 mm of soft tissue at a fluence of approximately 4 J/cm.

Fluence or **energy density (ED)** is the total amount of energy delivered per unit area. Fluence is the product of irradiance and time of laser application. The concentration of energy and irradiance are functions of the power output of the laser, the spot diameter over which the power is distributed, and the duration of the laser exposure. Change in spot diameter by a factor of 2 changes the power concentration (watts/πr^2) by a factor of 4. Thus, 10 watts delivered in a spot diameter of 1.0 mm delivers power at 1,270 W/cm^2, and the same 10 watts delivered in a spot diameter of 0.5 mm delivers power at 5,080 W/cm^2 (Figure 10.179).

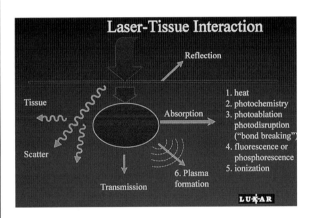

Irradiance or **power density (PD)** is the rate of energy delivery per unit area of target tissue. It is a measure of how intensely the beam is concentrated over a given surface area. The higher the irradiance, the faster a given volume of tissue is vaporized.

Power or **watt (W)** is the rate of energy delivery, or how fast energy flows. A watt is defined as 1 joule per second.

Pulse repetition rate (PRR) is the number of laser pulses per second, measured in Hertz (Hz).

Pulse width (PW) or laser pulse duration is the laser exposure time.

Pulsed operation provides emitted pulses with duration of 1 millisecond or less, and pulse energies of 0.1–1 joule. Pulsed operation results in reduced char and thermal injury to surrounding tissue.

Scanning delivery systems deliver laser energy onto the tissue surface in a highly controlled pattern.

Scanners can be used to treat diffuse oral lesions more uniformly, quickly, and more effectively than manual methods.

Spot size refers to the diameter of the laser beam at the tissue level. Laser delivery may be directed through a lens, or emanate directly from the end of a fiber or hollow waveguide. With lens delivery, the beam is concentrated to a specified spot diameter at a focal point from the lens. The clinician can control laser delivery to the tissue by moving the beam into a focused position (smallest beam diameter) for high power density, or a defocused position (larger spot diameter) for decreased power density. Doubling of the spot size results in a fourfold decrease in power density (Figure 10.180).

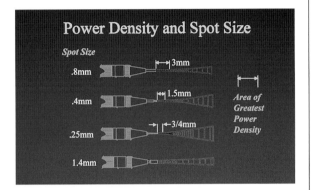

Vaporization is the process of removing solid tissue by converting it into a gaseous vapor in the form of steam or smoke.

Zone of coagulation necrosis is incurably damaged tissue secondary to lateral thermal damage (heat conduction) adjacent to the vaporization crater.

Zone of sublethal injury is located peripherally to the area injured by lateral heat conduction. The zone of sublethal injury has the capacity to recover.

Zone of vaporization is the area occupied by the vaporization crater removed by the explosive laser pulse (Figure 10.181).

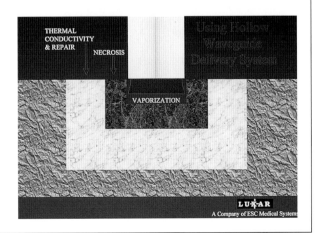

wave or single-pulse mode. Power output of 2.5 W and a spot size of 2.0 mm are used for small (< 2 mm) lesions.

Argon laser wavelengths penetrate into hard dental surfaces up to several millimeters. As a result, there are potential risks of direct laser injury to the tooth pulp. Argon dental lasers can be used for gingival surgery, curing dental composites during tooth restoration, and—in human dentistry—for tooth whitening. Argon lasers may be useful for enamel melting and resolidification to repair small enamel defects.

CARBON DIOXIDE LASERS (10,600 NM)   Carbon dioxide lasers (Figure 10.182) are used in oral surgery for precise cutting or vaporizing soft tissue with hemostasis. Typically, "what you see is what you get" when using the CO_2 laser, compared to the Nd:YAG laser where visible change does not appear in the tissue surrounding the zone of vaporization. The CO_2 wavelength is absorbed by the water content of oral tissues. Shallow thermal necrosis zones of only 100–300 microns at incised tissue edges are typical. Other lasers (Nd:YAG, argon, diode) necrose several millimeters during oral procedures.

Inorganic components of teeth and bone also absorb at the carbon dioxide wavelength. High temperatures

(>100° C) are required to truly vaporize hard tissue. Continuous wave (CW) CO_2 lasers cannot ablate or cut calcified tissue without inducing severe charring and thermal injury to surrounding tissue, and should not be used for that purpose.

Modes used for dental applications include continuous wave and variations of the pulsed mode. For ablation of oral lesions, the superpulse mode is desirable because the pulse width is shorter than the thermal relaxation time of oral soft tissue, decreasing the lateral thermal damage.

For ablation of oral lesions, laser power is set between 10–15 watts in CW mode or 20 watts in a pulsed mode. The spot size used for ablation varies between 2–3 mm in diameter using the 0.4–0.8 mm tip. The lesion is initially outlined with a margin of several millimeters. Using paintbrush strokes (rastering), multiple applications of the laser are placed within the marginal outline. Moist gauze is used to wipe away the treated area of mucosa. Excessive heat conduction appears as charred tissue. Charring results from prolonged contact between the laser beam and the tissue and is usually caused by moving the handpiece too slowly across the lesion. Only minimal charring should be evident (Figure. 10.183).

A pale pink base that does not bleed indicates removal of the epithelium to the level of the basement membrane. The submucosal layer is identified by both the appearance of blood vessels and a yellow granular tissue layer. Within 24 hours after treatment, a fibrin coagulum normally forms on the surface of the surgical wound, which acts as a bandage. The coagulum is replaced by epithelium originating from the wound

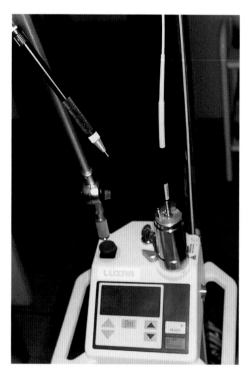

FIGURE 10.182. Carbon dioxide laser.

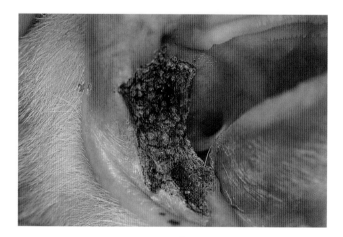

FIGURE 10.183. Temporary char as a result of the CO_2 laser application.

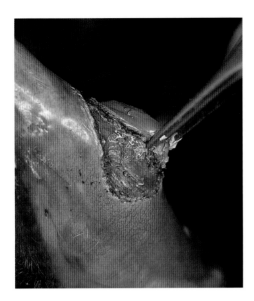

FIGURE 10.184. Traction of tissue during laser excision.

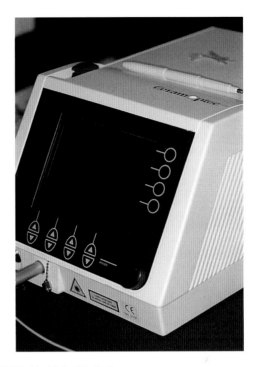

FIGURE 10.185. Diode laser.

edge. Ablation of less than 2.0 cm of mucosa results in complete epithelial resurfacing in less than 3 weeks unless a char layer is left behind, retarding healing.

To use the CO_2 laser as a precise cutting instrument in oral surgery, the laser beam spot size at its focal point should be 0.2–0.3 mm from the tissue. Traction and countertraction of tissue with surgical sponges and tissue forceps facilitate incisional surgical technique (Figure. 10.184).

SEMICONDUCTOR DIODE LASERS (805–980 NM)
Diode lasers (Figure 10.185) in the 800–980 nm range use contact mode optical fibers for cutting and vaporizing oral tissue. Diode units are similar to Nd:YAG lasers. Diode and Nd:YAG laser radiation penetrates deeper (1–2 mm) than either CO_2 or argon wavelengths. Diode lasers can be used for gingivectomy, gingival troughing, subgingival curettage, and other soft tissue procedures.

Frequent water irrigation is used as a heat sink to decrease thermal damage when using the diode laser in the oral cavity. Changes in tissue texture and color are best indicators of the diode's laser effect.

For contact incisional application, mechanical pressure is not necessary; the surgeon needs only sufficient force to guide the handpiece along the incision. When the fiber is in contact mode, it should be kept in contact mode. The fiber can be used first in non-contact (free beam), and then placed in contact mode but not vice versa.

ERBIUM LASERS (2900 NM) The Erbium:YAG laser (Figure. 10.186) has been approved by the FDA for use on human dental hard tissue. This laser can precisely cut or ablate hard dental substances, including enamel with relatively little pulse energy and power, because the 2936 nm wavelength is absorbed by water and hydroxyapatite. Erbium lasers are operated in a Q-switched non-contact mode to generate pulses of about 100 nanoseconds in duration. The handpiece is held approximately 2 cm from the targeted tissue site.

Incisions made in soft tissue with an erbium laser heal almost as quickly as scalpel incisions. Because little collateral thermal injury is produced, only slight hemostasis occurs.

HOLMIUM LASERS (2100 NM) Holmium lasers can cut and vaporize soft tissue similarly to the CO_2 laser, with the added advantage of energy delivery through flexible quartz optical fibers. The holmium laser can also precisely ablate hard materials, such as bone, dentin, and enamel. Pulsed modes with 250–350 msec durations are commonly used. Holmium lasers are used in dental surgery in tissue contact for cutting and vaporization, and in non-contact mode for vaporization and tissue coagulation. Thin flexible fibers allow the holmium laser to be used to debride pulp from pulp cavitiess with or without dentin removal.

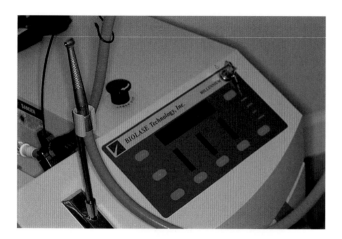

FIGURE 10.186. Erbium laser.

ND:YAG LASERS (1064 NM) The Nd:YAG laser (Figure. 10.187) penetrates deeply (several millimeters) into oral soft tissues. In human dentistry, low-power Nd:YAG lasers are used to provide laser-induced analgesia to teeth without local anesthesia. For oral mass ablation in human dentistry, a large volume of tissue destruction can be accomplished using the Nd:YAG laser. Tissue welding (apposition of incised gingival tissues without sutures) is clinically performed using the Nd:YAG laser in human dentistry using low power settings (0.1–1 W). Nd:YAG laser energy penetrates tissue until it is absorbed by the first heavy pigment it encounters. There is little absorption by water, moderate absorption by hemoglobin, and high absorption by melanin. This highly energetic beam presents potential risk of thermal injury to pulp, periodontal ligament, and bone when working on or near teeth. The Nd:YAG laser may be used in continuous wave, single pulse, repeat pulse, and Q-switched emission modes.

Laser Safety

The veterinarian using a laser in the oral cavity must be concerned with possible damage to sensitive oral structures, including the tooth pulp, periodontal ligament, and bone. The actual zone of damage that can be tolerated depends on the proximity and sensitivity of nearby tissue. The tooth pulp and periodontal ligament are sensitive to thermal injury and tolerable of a rise in temperature of only a few degrees.

Lasers in the dental operating area have the potential to ignite materials on and around the surgical site. Examples of combustible materials include dry cotton swabs, gauze sponges, wooden tongue blades, alcohol wipes, and plastic instruments.

In laser surgery of the oral cavity, the endotracheal

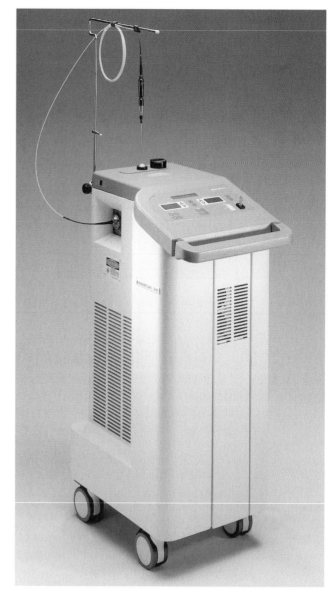

FIGURE 10.187. Nd:YAG laser (Lumenis Inc.) (from Lumenis CD).

tube is a significant fire danger. Special care must be taken to prevent the tube from coming in contact with the laser beam during surgery. Ignition of the endotracheal tube may produce a fire with a blowtorch effect inside the animal's airway. Laser-safe endotracheal tubes are available for use during laser surgery. Additionally, water-moistened gauze should be packed in the pharyngeal area to avoid injury.

The plume or lased smoke is a by-product of laser surgery. The laser plume is primarily composed of vaporized water (steam), toxic substances, such as formaldehyde, hydrogen cyanide, hydrocarbon particles, and cellular products. The smoke can be irritating to those who are exposed to it. A high-volume laser smoke evacuator should be used to remove the plume during oral procedures (Figure 10.188).

Take the following precautions when performing laser surgery:

- When the laser is in use, place a warning sign to alert those who enter the operatory.
- Make sure everyone in the operatory wears shielded eyeglasses. When using the Nd:YAG laser, green safety glasses are used. With CO_2 lasers, clear prescription or plastic glasses can be worn.
- Shield non-target areas. Wet gauze packs—especially around the endotracheal tube and caudal pharynx—are effective shields against the CO_2 laser beam effects. Wet gauze is effective because of the CO_2 laser energy's high absorption into water. Optical backstops consisting of water-moistened gauze may be placed below the target tissue for protection of adjacent tissues from the CO_2 laser beam.
- Remove reflective metal materials from the immediate surgical area. Nonreflective surgical instruments are recommended.
- Use a vacuum evacuation system to draw off the plume cloud created when tissue vaporizes. If inhaled, the smoke plume may be irritating, infectious, or carcinogenic.

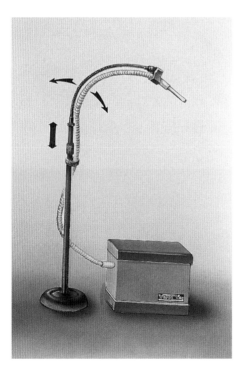

FIGURE 10.188. Smoke evacuator with adjustable stand.

- Remove combustible materials—such as alcohol preps, flammable inhalant agents, oxygen, and drapes—from the immediate laser beam area.

SMALL ANIMAL DENTAL LASER PROCEDURES

Gingivoplasty/Gingivectomy

The CO_2 laser is versatile for precise incising or vaporizing the gingiva. Higher CO_2 laser power (10–15 watts) is used to remove moderate (<2 mm) amounts of hyperplastic gingiva. For thicker areas, the CO_2 laser may be used in a defocused or diverging mode for coagulation to help control bleeding after scalpel blade gingivectomy (Figures 10.189–10.191).

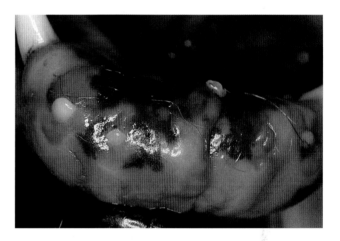

FIGURE 10.189. Gingival hyperplasia in the rostral mandible of a boxer.

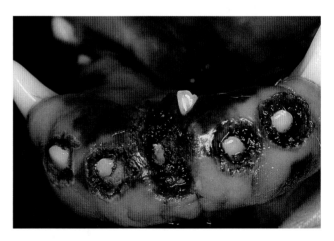

FIGURE 10.190. CO_2 laser removal of hyperplastic gingival.

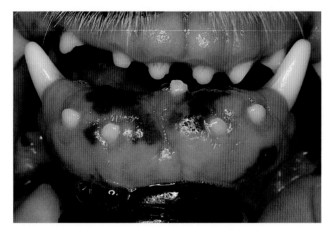

FIGURE 10.191. One-month post-operative gingivo-plasty result.

Oral Biopsy

Lasers can be used for excisional or incisional biopsies with controlled bleeding and improved visualization. Laser excision permits histologic evaluation and establishment of clean margins by a pathologist knowledgeable in laser-tissue interaction.

The CO_2 laser can incise soft tissue in a non-contact mode making it particularly useful for biopsy on buccal and lingual surfaces (Figure 10.192). An excisional outline (Figure 10.193) can be made rapidly, using repeated single pulses (5 watts, 0.3 mm spot size) to circumscribe the desired target tissue. One edge of the incised margin can be elevated with forceps and the lesion undermined at the correct depth of dissection with the laser. With the beam defocused, the surgical wound is briskly "painted" in one pass to seal off small lymphatics, blood vessels, and nerve endings (Figure 10.194). Sutures are not required unless the defect is greater than 3 mm. Argon, Nd:YAG, and diode lasers can also be used for oral biopsies.

Gingival Troughing for Crown Preparation

When preparing a tooth for crown restoration, a trough or space between the free gingiva and crown is created to allow a marginal line for impression material. If prepared with a scalpel blade, the incised gingiva bleeds, generating additional surgical time for hemostasis and potential impression inaccuracy.

The carbon dioxide or diode laser tip held in a near parallel position to the tooth can form a trough. Care should be taken to avoid having the beam contact enamel or dentin. Argon lasers are not recommended for troughing because of the wavelength's strong absorption by blood (Figures 10.195–10.198).

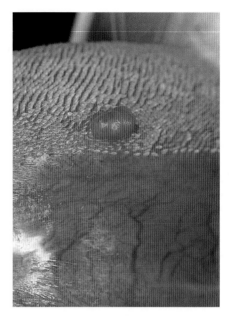

FIGURE 10.192. Solitary tongue lesion.

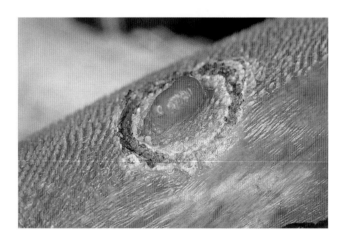

FIGURE 10.193. Laser-outlined surgical margin.

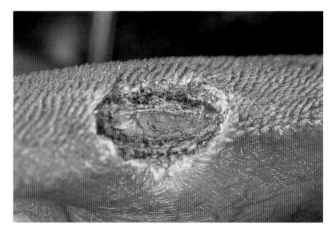

FIGURE 10.194. Tumor ablation.

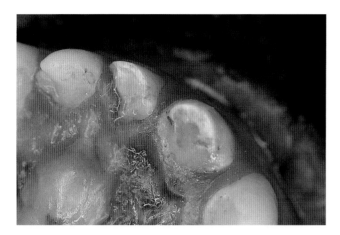

FIGURE 10.195. Fractured maxillary incisors after endodontic therapy and acrylic resin restoration.

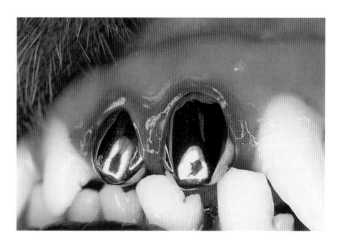

FIGURE 10.198. Cast crown restoration.

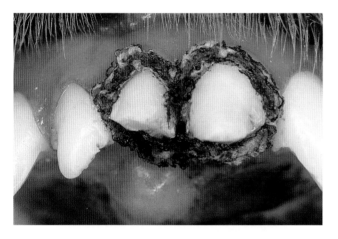

FIGURE 10.196. Laser-created gingival trough to establish a crown finish line.

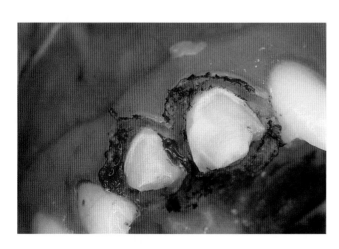

FIGURE 10.197. Trough appearance before crown cementation.

Operculectomy

Operculectomy can be performed with a laser for excision of thick fibrous gingival tissue over an impacted tooth. Ten watts of CO_2 laser energy with 0.3 mm spot size can be used to incise a mucosal flap and expose the underlying crown (Figures 10.199–10.201).

The Nd:YAG laser can also be used at 5–10 watts in contact mode for operculectomy surgery.

Frenectomy

Lasers can be used to perform maxillary and lingual frenectomies with little or no bleeding, and often without the need for sutures. The CO_2 laser used in a non-contact mode vaporizes the frenulum quickly. Either continuous wave mode at 3–5 watts of power with a 0.3 mm spot size for incision, or a pulsed mode at 20 watts and a 1.4 mm spot for ablation can be used. With the frenulum stretched taut, a short vertical incision is made through the mucosa at the mid-portion of the frenulum. Horizontal releasing incisions are then developed through the mucosa on both sides, extending to the periosteum.

Tongue Lesions

Solitary and multiple tongue lesions (Figure 10.202) can be excised using the CO_2 laser (Figure 10.203). Laser parameters of 10 watts with a spot/tip size of 0.4 mm is commonly used. Penetration into the muscularis layer should be avoided. Sutures are generally placed if the post-surgical defect is greater than 3 mm.

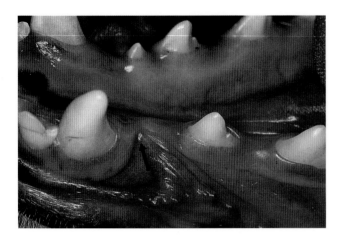

FIGURE 10.199. Clinically absent mandibular first premolar.

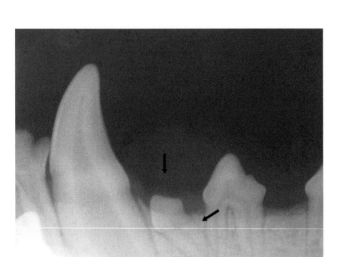

FIGURE 10.200. Radiographic confimation of an impacted mandibular first premolar.

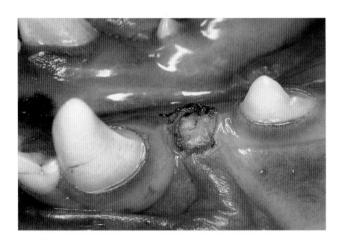

FIGURE 10.201. Operculectomy revealing first premolar crown.

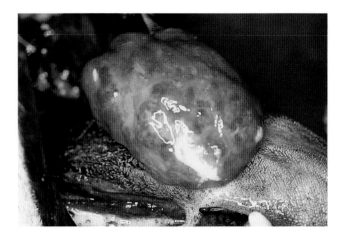

FIGURE 10.202. Large tongue lesion.

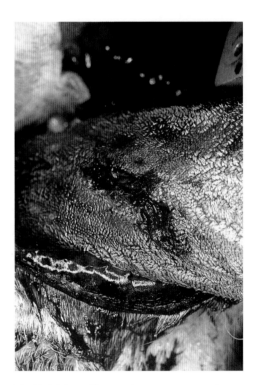

FIGURE 10.203. Palliative laser excision of tongue mass (clean surgical margins not obtained).

Oral Neoplasia

Laser use in oral cancer surgery provides advantages of hemostasis, decreased post-operative edema, and diminished infection. Additionally, because of the laser's ability to seal small blood vessels and lymphatics, there is a reduced likelihood of inducing tumor microemboli during the procedure.

The CO_2, diode, and Nd:YAG lasers can be used for resection of oral cancer. An advantage of using the Nd:YAG laser includes increased hemostasis, compared to the CO_2 laser.

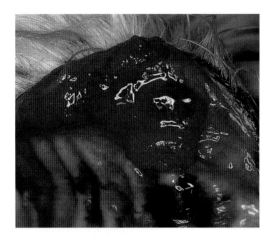

FIGURE 10.204. Squamous cell carcinoma.

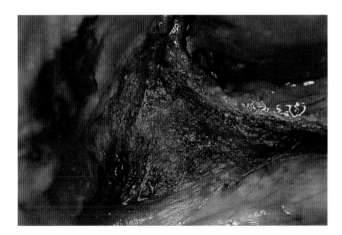

FIGURE 10.205. Palliative tumor debulking.

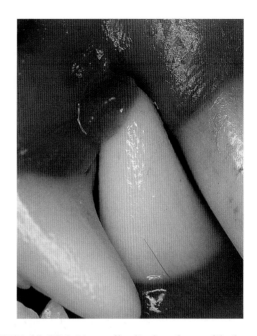

FIGURE 10.206. Lingually displaced mandibular canine impinging on palatal gingiva.

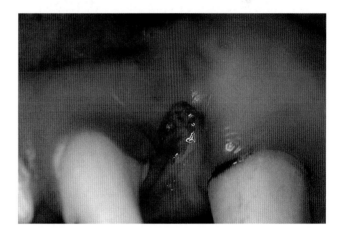

FIGURE 10.207. Laser ablation of the impinged palatal gingiva.

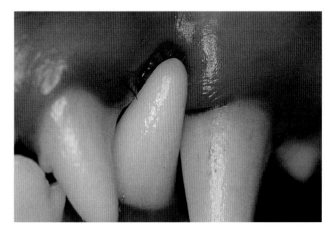

FIGURE 10.208. Post-operative appearance.

Palliative treatment for non-resectable masses can be accomplished using the laser to debulk the mass before radiation therapy or to periodically decrease the tumor size to make the patient more comfortable (Figures 10.204, 10.205).

Gingival Surgery

Gingivoplasty can be performed in cases of minimally lingually displaced mandibular canine teeth to remove gingival areas of palatal impingement. For the gingivoplasty, 8–10 watts of superpulsed CO_2 laser energy in a defocused mode is used to vaporize sequential layers of tissue until the mandibular canine tooth is no longer impinging on the gingiva (Figures 10.206–10.208).

Flap surgery incisions (Figure 10.209) can be performed with the diode or CO_2 laser. Human patients interviewed in one study reported less pain with laser surgery than with scalpel blade flap incisions. Flaps incised with lasers take longer to heal than scalpel incisions.

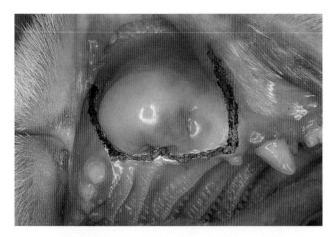

FIGURE 10.209. Laser flap surgical outline around a cat's maxillary canine.

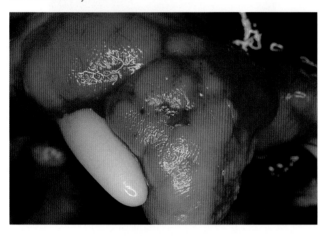

FIGURE 10.210. Marked gingival hyperplasia covering part of a maxillary canine.

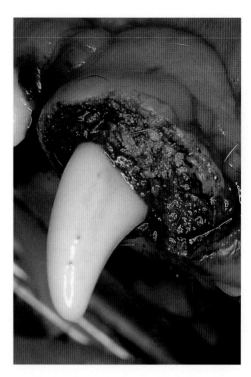

FIGURE 10.211. Majority of gingival tissue excised with scalpel; laser used for fine sculpturing and coagulation.

For the treatment of *gingival hyperplasia*, the CO_2 laser can be set at 4–8 watts in continuous mode and applied over the incised area after blade gingivectomy to shape the gingiva and aid hemostasis (Figures 10.210–10.212).

Removal of traumatic sublingual granulation tissue (gum chewers lesions) can also be accomplished using the CO_2 laser. Following excision, laser power is decreased to 4 watts with a defocused beam to seal small blood vessels. Sutures are not usually needed (Figure 10.213).

Feline Stomatitis Therapy

Feline lymphocytic plasmacytic gingivostomatitis (LPGS) is a multifactorial disease. The CO_2 laser can be used to vaporize areas of palatoglossal inflammation (faucitis), as an adjunct in the treatment of LPGS.

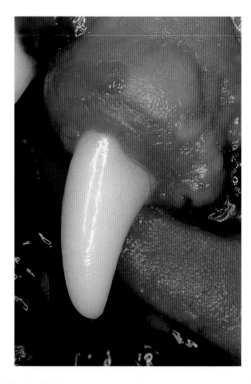

FIGURE 10.212. Appearance 1 month post-operatively.

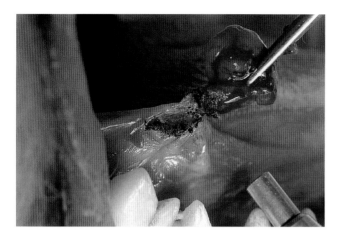

FIGURE 10.213. Excision of traumatic sublingual granulation tissue.

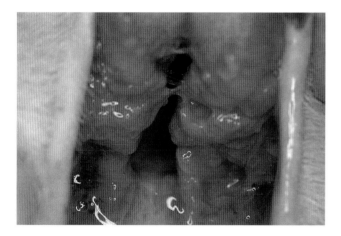

FIGURE 10.214. Marked "faucitis" in a cat affected by feline LPGS.

Post-operatively, an appropriate oral antibiotic and pain relief medication is given for 2 weeks. Monthly rechecks are advised. Depending on response, repeat laser treatments are performed to remove residual inflammation 4–6 weeks apart. Nonresponsive cases should have additional evaluation, dental radiographs, and extractions. Approximately 20% of the stomatitis cases remain resistant to therapy (Figures 10.214–10.216).

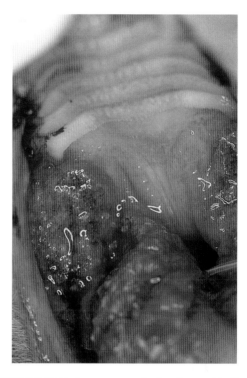

FIGURE 10.215. Appearance during laser ablation of the affected areas.

Pre-operative blood testing (including screens for FIV and Felv), oral examination with charting, and intraoral dental radiographs are evaluated. Initial therapy consists of extraction of those teeth that have feline odontoclastic resorptive lesions and greater than 25% support loss. The CO_2 laser can be used at 2–6 watts of power, with a 0.8–1.4 mm tip in continuous wave mode to vaporize inflamed tissue. The beam is defocused to "paint" (raster) the entire inflamed tissue area. Rastering is repeated until there is minimal bleeding after the char is wiped away. There may be some benefit in using a scanner or a pattern generator for beam delivery. The scanner improves tissue vaporization over a large area and reduces heat buildup in the tissue during ablation. Superpulse mode is not recommended, because the decreased lateral thermal damage decreases the fibrous tissue response.

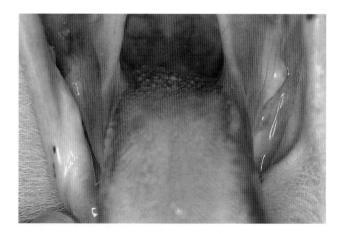

FIGURE 10.216. Resolution of "faucitis" after full mouth tooth extraction and three monthly laser treatments.

Areas of Future Laser Applications

As veterinarians become more comfortable with the use of lasers in the oral cavity, similar applications in human laser dentistry will be employed to help veterinary patients. One use under investigation is etching enamel and dentin for bonding. Preliminary studies show a better etch may be obtained with the laser than with conventional phosphoric acid, leading to improved marginal sealing and decreased microleakage of composite resin restorations.

Human dentists use lasers to remove hard dentin and enamel in cavity preparation and sulcular debridement for the care of periodontal pockets. Lasers may also be used to fuse dentin in the root canal, creating an apical plug of glazed nonporous material, free of organic tissue. Laser use for endodontic disinfection and coagulation for vital pulp therapy may become preferred over the use of calcium hydroxide.

Ongoing research into laser use with FORLs will confirm whether the use of lasers effectively destroys surface odontoclasts to control the progression of stage 1 and 2 lesions and to desensitize and seal exposed dentin (Figure. 10.217).

Lasers may be helpful for periodontal tissue regeneration in furcation areas by vaporizing inflamed tissues and by stimulating wound healing.

RADIOSURGERY

Radiosurgery uses the passage of a high-frequency low-heat radiowave (3.8–4.0 MHz) through tissue to incise or excise and coagulate. Standard electrocautery operates in low frequencies and produces high temperature, causing significant necrosis. Radiosurgery's higher (4.0 MHz, Ellman International, Figure 10.218) frequency

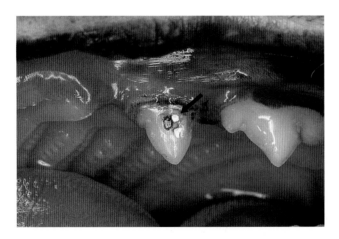

FIGURE 10.217. Experimental use of CO_2 laser to affect surface odontoclasts in Class 2 FORLs.

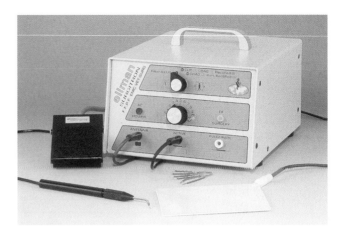

FIGURE 10.218. Ellman radiosurgical unit.

produces a pressureless, smooth incision with hemostasis and minimum tissue alteration (<20 microns).

With radiosurgery, a radiowave is transmitted by two metallic electrodes, one active and the other passive. The passive plate acts as an antenna placed underneath the animal's head close to the surgical site. Direct metal to skin contact is not needed. The radio signal is transmitted from the active electrode through tissue, received by the passive electrode, and returned directly to the radiosurgery unit. The electrode remains cold to the touch.

Soft tissue passing between the electrodes rises in temperature caused by resistance to the radio signal. The radio signal guided through tissue leaves a path of cell destruction, producing an incision. Cell destruction or volatilization creates a smoke plume, which should be removed by a surgical smoke evacuator.

Lateral heat produced during cautery, radiosurgery, or laser procedures, may iatrogenically injure oral tissues. Radiosurgical incisions produce minimal tissue damage due to the low level of lateral heat produced. Lateral heat production is related to:

- Time: Less lateral heat is generated with fast passage of the electrode through tissue.
- Intensity: High intensity carbonizes tissue; insufficient intensity causes sticking of the electrode to tissue.
- Current chosen: Four radiosurgical waveforms are commonly available. Generally, the more pulsatile the waveform (as seen on an oscilloscope), the more lateral heat is generated:
  - The *fully filtered current* produces 90% cutting and 10% coagulation. The fully filtered current is a pure continuous flow of high-frequency energy. The filter provides a continuous nonpulsating current, resembling a scalpel incision. The fully

filtered current can be used for biopsy, frenectomy, mass removal, and surgery near bone.

- The *fully rectified current* produces 50% cutting and 50% coagulation. The fully rectified current can be used for gingivectomy, gingivoplasty, and troughing procedures for crown impressions. The fully rectified current should not be used when operating near bone.
- The *partially rectified current* produces 90% coagulation and 10% cutting with increased lateral heat and tissue shrinkage. Partially rectified currents should not be used near bone. Hemostasis can be accomplished using a unipole ball, broad needle electrode, or bipolar forceps on vessels <2 mm in diameter.
- The *fulgurating* current employs a half-wave current for coagulation and destruction of tissue. The electrode does not actually touch tissue, but coagulates by energy transferred to tissue. The fulguration waveform may be used for hemostasis near bone, removal and destruction of cyst remnants, and destruction of fistulous tracts. The electrode used is in the shape of a pencil or sphere and is positioned about 0.5 mm from the tissue surface.
- Frequency of application: Low frequency generates a less efficient incision and produces more lateral heat. An ideal frequency for use in the oral cavity appears to be 3.8 MHz.

The power setting determines the amount of energy transferred to the tissue. The setting should be high enough to prevent drag of the electrode through the tissue, but not high enough to create sparking.

Electrode Tips

There are many types of electrode tips (Figure 10.219):

- Diamond-shaped tips can be used for removal of tissue that requires suturing. Diamonds are commonly used for small biopsies. Only the bottom third of the electrode should penetrate the tissue, creating a V-shaped incision.
- Small elliptical loop tips can be used for gingival contouring and crown lengthening procedures.
- Larger loop tips can be used for gingivectomy and operculectomy.
- Triangle-shaped tips can be used for gingivoplasty and removal of the interproximal papilla.
- Vari-Tip electrode (Ellman) can be used in many applications (Figure 10.220). The Vari-Tip length is adjustable.
- Ball-shaped tips are used for gross coagulation (Figure 10.221).

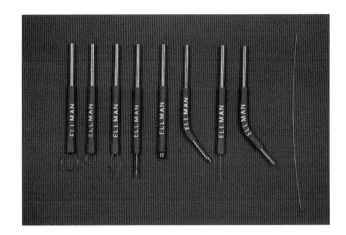

FIGURE 10.219. Ellman electrode tips.

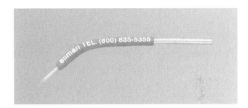

FIGURE 10.220. Vari-Tip electrode.

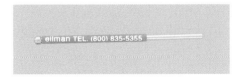

FIGURE 10.221. Ball-shaped tip.

- Pencil-point tips can be used for fine coagulation.
- Fulgurating tips are used for gross superficial destruction of tissue after biopsy and for hemostasis during osseous surgery.

Radiosurgical Techniques

Use the following incision/excision technique; unlike a scalpel blade, no pressure is required:

1. Hold the handpiece like a pen rather than a scalpel handle.
2. Move the electrode as rapidly as possible across the tissue in a brush-like stroke.
3. Keep the electrode perpendicular to the tissue surface.
4. Periodically remove buildup of charred coagulated tissue from the electrode tip.
5. Do not engage power to the electrode until the tip is in contact with the tissue.

6. Allow 8 seconds between cutting strokes in the same site to allow heat to dissipate.
7. Moisten the operative site with gauze soaked in sterile saline to reduce tissue resistance.

GINGIVECTOMY FOR REMOVAL OF HYPER-PLASTIC TISSUE Tissue can be incised with either fully filtered or fully rectified currents. The fully filtered current is used in areas where the tissue is delicate and minimal tissue alteration is desired. The fully rectified current is used where the tissue is thick and fibrotic or in areas of hyperemia that require immediate hemostasis.

1. Use the bendable fine wire electrode (Vari-Tip, Ellman) for gingivectomy. The fully rectified or filtered current can be used. Gingivectomy can also be performed using a loop electrode set to a fully filtered and rectified current.
2. Set the incision angle similar to the physiological angle of the gingiva (30–40°) (Figure 10.222).
3. If necessary, coagulate bleeding vessels, using a ball electrode with the partially rectified current setting.
4. Remove excised tissue with a curette (Figure 10.223).

FLAP SURGERY A reverse bevel incision along the gingival margin can be made using a fine-wire electrode.

1. Make interdental incisions with the electrode.
2. Use a Freer or Molt elevator to raise the mucoperiosteal flap from the underlying bone.
3. Expose the flap and suture similarly to the scalpel blade procedure.

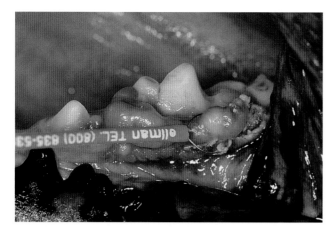

FIGURE 10.222. Marked gingival hyperplasia surrounding the mandibular first molar.

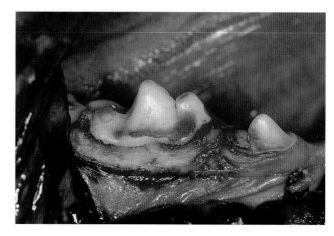

FIGURE 10.223. After radiosurgical removal of hyperplastic tissue.

TROUGHING FOR CROWN IMPRESSIONS A trough is a channel created in the soft tissue around a crown preparation to allow space for placement of impression material. To create a trough, a thin layer of tissue from the sulcus is excised, exposing the crown margin preparation. The length of the Vari-Tip electrode can be adjusted to prevent accidental cutting of the epithelial attachment.

Radiosurgical troughing eliminates the need for retraction cord because of the trough itself and the concurrent hemostasis, which allows the impression to be taken immediately:

1. Prepare the crown with the finish line at the gingival margin.
2. Place the radiosurgical tip parallel to the tooth to prevent removal of excessive tissue height.
3. Move the tip from mesial to distal around the tooth to create the trough.
4. Use a pencil-point electrode tip with a partially rectified current for pinpoint hemostasis.
5. Irrigate the area post-operatively with 0.12% chlorhexidine.

FRENECTOMY A frenectomy is used to loosen tight mandibular lips pressing debris against the gingiva overlying the mandibular canines:

1. Dissect the frenulum toward the mandibular insertion with multiple brushstokes, using the Vari-Tip electrode with a fully rectified current. Make the first incision vertically from the base of the bone where the frenulum attaches between the central incisors to the underside of the lip.

2. Make a third or fourth horizontal releasing incision to remove the frenula from the oral cavity.
3. Coagulate larger bleeding vessels, using a fulgurating current with the pencil-point electrode tip.
4. Suture the resultant defect with 4-0 or 5-0 absorbable suture on a cutting needle.

OPERCULECTOMY An operculectomy removes overgrown dense fibrous gingiva covering an impacted immature tooth to aid eruption. Using a fully rectified current with a Vari-Tip or small loop electrode tip, excise the overlying gingiva.

11
Educating Your Client

Most owners care deeply for their pets and want existing problems treated. For the client to appreciate the degree of disease present, he or she first has to be able to see what the veterinarian considers abnormal. Unfortunately, teeth are hidden behind the lips. Instant or digital photography allows the client "into the pet's mouth."

Dental photography is also an education tool. Images can present the animal's problem and allow the veterinarian to speak about therapy using the pet's pathology to refer to, rather than struggling with a poorly illuminated oral cavity. Gingivitis and periodontal disease show vividly with instant and digital photography. To further educate the dental client, the veterinarian can compare the pet's condition with a textbook representation of disease. This helps confirm that the pet's lesion is a real problem that needs care.

GENERAL PHOTOGRAPHIC TIPS

The final product should be evaluated through the viewfinder or digital screen before the picture is taken. The goal is to get a clear picture of the pathology:

- Extraneous items (fingers, tongue, endotracheal tube, other teeth) which draw the viewer's attention away from the pathology should not be present in the finished image (Figure 11.1).
- The photographed area should be clean of blood and hair.
- The highest magnification available should be chosen to see the lesion and adjacent normal tissue clearly.
- With single lens reflex (SLR) cameras, fine focus can be obtained by moving the camera forward and backward before pressing the shutter.

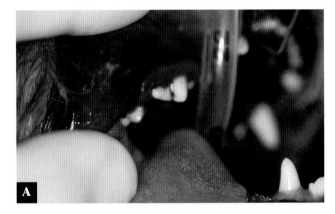

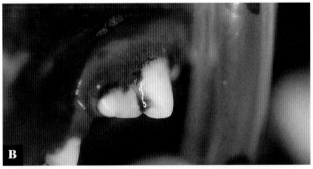

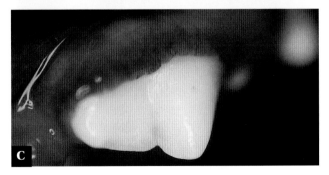

FIGURE 11.1. (A,B) Extraneous items (fingers, endotracheal tube, gauze) to draw viewer's attention away from the subject, and (C) the same subject after teeth cleaning without extraneous items.

363

INTRAORAL INSTANT PHOTOGRAPHY

Intraoral instant cameras are available through the Polaroid Company. They are simple to use, allowing anyone in the office to get an acceptable photo with different levels of magnification. There are two popular models, which focus using infrared beams: the Polaroid Macro 5 SLR (Schein 987-2593) (Figure 11.2) has five built-in enlargement options and a date stamp, and the Polaroid Macro 3 SLR has three built-in enlargement options.

A slide duplicator (Polaroid) (Figure 11.3) can be used to make enlargements of dental radiographs to share with clients or referring veterinarians. To convert the dental film to a photograph, the developed radiograph is placed in a slide holder and inserted into the slide duplicator. A 3X enlargement is developed within one minute.

Providing the client with before and after photographs of pathology when therapy is completed gives readily comprehensible and visually impacting documentation of the case and your skills. One picture set can be inserted in the medical record and the other given to the client to show those at home. A third set of interesting dental cases can be placed in a *Smile Book* to show new clients.

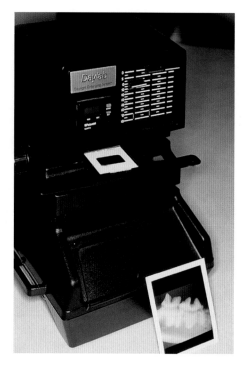

FIGURE 11.3. Polaroid slide duplicator.

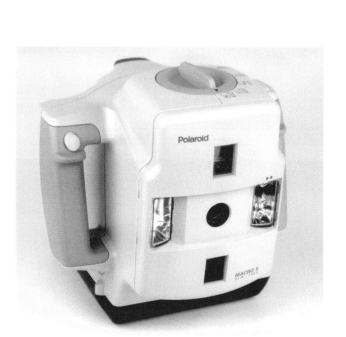

FIGURE 11.2. Polaroid SLR 5.

Unfortunately, sometimes needed dental care is not performed because the owners do not realize the importance or urgency. If the client chooses to decline the recommended therapy in the exam room, the instant photograph can be given to them to share with others at home, or to post on the refrigerator or bathroom mirror until they are ready to accept treatment.

The instant image also allows the veterinarian to show the dental laboratory the condition of the teeth that need repair.

Single Lens Reflex (SLR) Cameras

Single lens reflex (SLR) cameras, once the mainstay of client photographic education, to some extent have been replaced by instant (Polaroid) and digital photography. The main disadvantage of slide or print photography is time of delivery of the final picture compared to other formats. Kodak produces a special dental 35 mm 100 speed film, which has a neutral color base to give true representation of the shades of teeth and gingiva (Figures 11.4, 11.5).

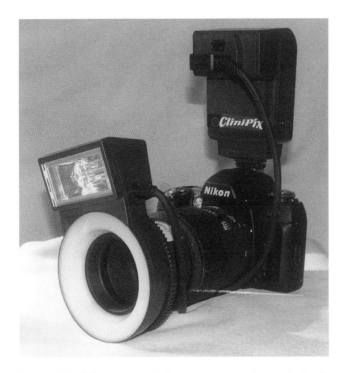

FIGURE 11.4. SLR dental close-up camera (Clinipix Inc.).

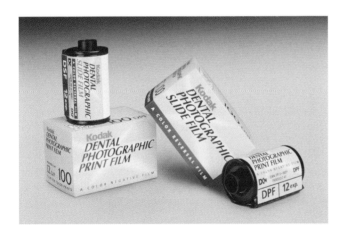

FIGURE 11.5. Kodak dental film.

VIDEOSCOPE

The videoscope system consists of a telescope, digital camera, and monitor. The telescope is shaped like an otoscope (for use in ears as well), and contains rod lenses and optical fibers, which produce a bright, magnified image of high resolution. This allows both practitioner and client to see details that might otherwise be missed or difficult to see. The camera attaches to the eyepiece

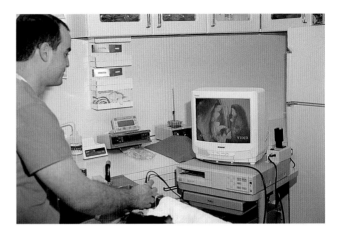

FIGURE 11.6. Technician using the MedRx digital videoscope to image before and after care.

of the telescope, and the image is transmitted to a TV monitor for easy viewing (Figures 11.6). The image can also be transmitted to a documentation device, such as a printer, video recorder, floppy disc drive, or computer for archiving. By placing the system on a mobile cart, the practitioner has the flexibility of performing exams in the exam room or in the treatment area.

The print format may be a photograph or a more detailed report containing multiple images, written diagnoses, and home care instructions. Prints given to clients also help build the practice, when the client shows this print to family or friends.

Digital Photography

The "film" in a digital camera is a computer disk or memory stick. Using the digital camera (depending on make and model), you can:

- Instantly see the area imaged and either accept or delete the image from memory.
- Modify the picture (change contrast, brightness, and hue; crop, enlarge, or decrease image size; add symbols or text).
- Import to a computer application for electronic mail, catalog, or add to the patient record.
- Use images in presentations.
- Print images for a before-and-after series for the client exit discussion to aid the explanation of the procedure performed (Figure 11.7).
- Attach the camera to a television with a video input for client viewing or teaching purposes (Figure 11.8).
- Image radiographs, which can be enlarged and enhanced in the dental operatory to aid interpretation (Figure 11.9).

Yorkie Leroy

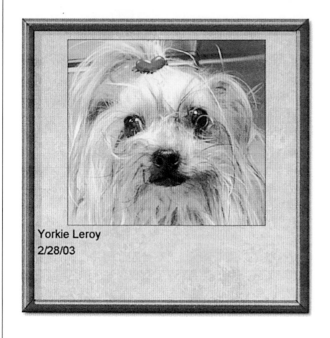

Yorkie Leroy
2/28/03

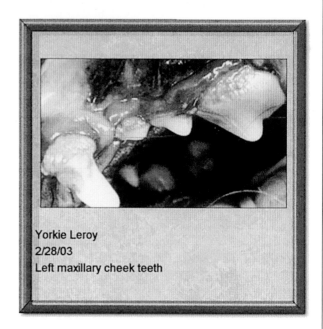

Yorkie Leroy
2/28/03
Left maxillary cheek teeth

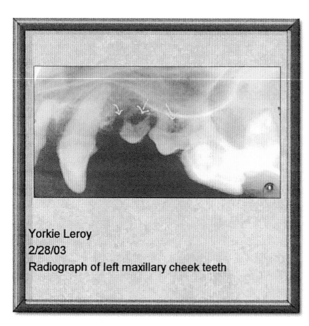

Yorkie Leroy
2/28/03
Radiograph of left maxillary cheek teeth

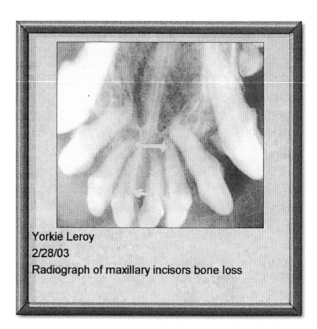

Yorkie Leroy
2/28/03
Radiograph of maxillary incisors bone loss

Hometown Animal Hospital and Dental Clinic

FIGURE 11.7. Printed report for the client showing pathology and therapy.

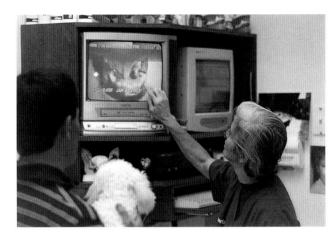

FIGURE 11.8. Digital camera image viewed through television monitor.

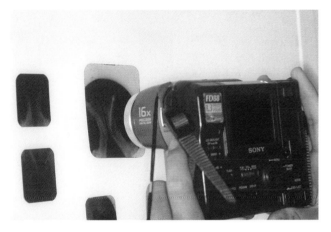

FIGURE 11.9. Camera position for digitized radiographic survey.

Digital Camera Choices

Digital cameras vary by the way they store images:

- Digital cameras use a serial, parallel, or USB cord that connects the camera and computer. Once exposed, the image can automatically download to the computer.
- Other cameras use a detachable disk or memory stick to save the image.
- PC-cards are small matchbox-sized disks that save multiple images. The PC-cards are placed in a cradle attached to the computer for access. The Smart Media format used by Olympus and Toshiba cameras allows the user to insert the card into an adapter that fits into the floppy drive.
- 3 1/2-inch floppy disks are used in some digital cameras to store images and then load them into the computer's A drive for access. Although this format

is convenient, limitations of the image size are imposed by the 1.44 MB floppy disk.
- The resolution of digital cameras has improved to mimic print/slide cameras. Many digital cameras offer a selection of resolution settings. A high resolution increases the quality of the image and markedly increases the picture size (which can be adjusted) (Figure 11.10).
- Kodak DX 4900 has 4.0 megapixel image resolution and uses EasyShare Camera Doc II, a PC interface device that also recharges the digital camera batteries. The dock eliminates USB cables, media cards, or external media card readers (Figure 11.11).
- Image format controls how the picture is stored. Digital cameras store images in many formats. The JPG format has a high level of compression that allows many images to be stored.

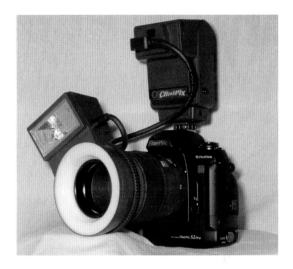

FIGURE 11.10. Clinipix Fujifilm 6 megapixel digital camera with ping flash.

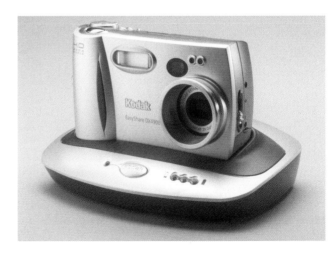

FIGURE 11.11. Kodak DX 4900 dental digital camera kit.

Image Software

The digital camera captures the picture, which is loaded into the computer's software. Most digital cameras are sold with a packaged software program. Advanced software can be purchased separately, which allows you to further enhance and store images in albums.

The following is a step-by-step creation of a digital case report for presentation (Sony Mavica FD-90):

1. Insert labeled disk into camera.
2. Set camera to macro setting for close up if available.
3. Change exposure setting based on ambient light.
4. Take photos before, during, and after procedure.
5. To digitize radiographs, place the developed film on a light box, set camera setting to BW (black and white, or grayscale) and macro, focus with camera lens about 1 inch from the film, and take the picture.
6. Remove disk and load onto the A drive in the computer or flash card adapter, or attach USB cord from the camera to the computer.
7. Load pictures into the application (Figure 11.12).
8. Choose pictures that help display the dental story you want to share with your client or referring veterinarian (Figure 11.13).
9. Arrange pictures in order to be printed.
10. Type explanation under each picture (Figure 11.14).
11. Print with header and footer (Figure 11.15).

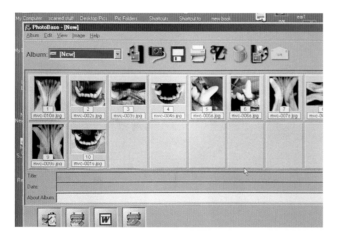

FIGURE 11.12. Images are loaded into the application (ARCSOFT).

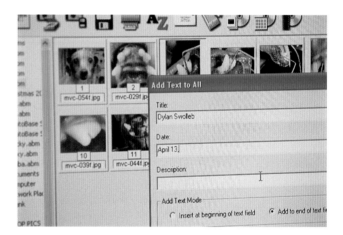

FIGURE 11.14. An explanation is added to appear below each image.

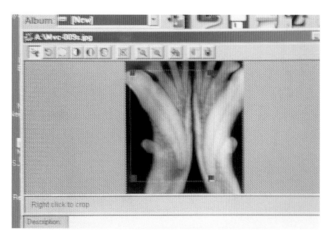

FIGURE 11.13. The best images are chosen.

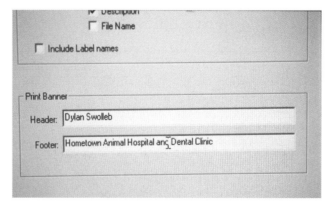

FIGURE 11.15. A header and footer are entered identifying the patient, facility, and date.

Appendix
Vendor Information, Equipment, and Materials

BURNS DENTAL SUPPLIES

High-Speed Handpieces

952-3891	Super Trac Push Button Handpiece
952-7306	Super Trac Swivel Handpiece
952-3865	Replacement Turbine
952-3870	Replacement End Cap
952-0022	True Speed 2 Standard Head High Speed Handpiece 2 Hole
952-0042	True Speed 2 Standard Head High Speed Handpiece 4 Hole
952-0064	Bur Tool
952-1822	Replacement Cartridge
952-0062	Replacement End Cap
864-1915	Quiet-ir L with Power Lever—Midwest
864-1917	Replacement Cartridge
952-3894	Super Trac Mini Handpiece
952-3855	Replacement Cartridge

Fiber-Optic Handpieces

952-3893	Super Trac Fiber-Optic Handpiece
951-8747	w/Straight Tubing
951-8746	w/Coiled Tubing
951-8748	Coiled Replacement Tubing
951-8749	Straight Replacement Tubing
951-8744	Replacement Lamp
894-2231	StarFlex SWL Fiber-Optic Handpiece (swivel not included) Star Dental
894-2198	Swivel Assembly
894-2250	StarBright ISO-C (Six Pin) Swivel Connector w/Lamp
894-2214	Steel Bearing Auto chuck Turbine
894-4043	Swivel and Turbine End Cap Tightening Wrench

Midwest

864-2505	Fiber-Optic Handpiece Less Coupler
864-2510	5-Hole Coupler
864-2512	6-Pin Coupler

Maintenance

952-1940	Lubricant Oil

Low-Speed Handpieces and Accessories
Super Torque Handpieces
952-3750   2-Hole
952-3748   4-Hole
952-3751   Straight Nose Cone
952-3752   Angle Nose Cone w/Latch Angle
952-1136   Latch Type Angle
950-8987   Friction Grip Angle
952-3451   Prophy Angle Snap-On

Contra-Angles
951-4604   10:1 Reduction Gear
951-4615   Contra Angle #200 Latch Style
951-4595   Contra Angle #200 Latch Style Deluxe Sectional

Prophy Cups
951-8500   White Webbed Snap-On
951-8505   White Webbed Screw-On

Dental Burs
Plain Round
952-5100   1/4 FG
952-5102   1/2 FG
952-5106   1 FG
952-5110   2 FG
952-5116   4 FG
952-5122   6 FG
952-5126   8 FG

952-5770   1/2 RA
952-5572   1 RA
952-5574   2 RA
952-5578   4 RA
952-5582   6 RA
952-5586   8 RA

952-5430   1/2 HP
952-5432   1 HP
952-5434   2 HP
952-5438   4 HP
952-5442   6 HP
952-5446   8 HP

Inverted Cone
952-5130   33 1/2 FG
952-5132   34 FG
952-5134   35 FG
952-5138   37 FG

952-5590   33 1/2 RA
952-5592   34 RA
952-5594   35 RA
952-5598   37 RA

952-5450   33 1/2 HP
952-5452   34 HP
952-5454   35 HP
952-5458   37 HP

Cross-cut Taper Fissure

952-5224	699 FG
952-5226	699L FG
952-5234	701 FG
952-5236	701L FG
952-5240	702 FG
952-5246	703 FG
952-5692	701 RA
952-5694	701L RA
952-5698	702 RA
952-5704	703 RA
890-0873	699 HP
890-0876	701 HP
890-0880	702 HP
890-0882	703 HP

Finishing

823-1272	White Pointed Cone FG
823-1278	White Flame FG
823-1256	Dura-White CA

Cross-cut Fissure

952-5204	557 FG
952-5210	558 FG
952-5662	557 RA
952-5668	558 RA
952-5508	557 HP
952-5514	558 HP

Diamonds

Premier Two-Striper Diamonds FG Crown Cut

878-4066	SC5
878-4068	SC8
878-4070	SC10
878-4072	ST6
878-4074	ST8
878-4076	ST11

Diamond Discs

951-1240	Ultraflex Safe Bottom .10 mm HP
951-1242	Ultraflex Double Sided .15 mm HP
951-1235	Flex Discs Single Sided 0.20 mm HP
951-1237	Flex Discs Double Sided 0.30 mm HP

Radiography

699-6709	Vet Image 70 Vet Dental Plus Intraoral X-Ray Unit
606-1412	Vet Image 70 Vet Dental Intraoral X-Ray Unit Mobile Stand

Radiographic Film Superdent D Speed

952-1078	XF-57 #2 Double Film Paper Pack 150/bx
952-1079	XF-57 #2 Double Film Polysoft 150/bx
952-1082	XF-58 #2 1 Film per Packet Polysoft 150/bx
952-1180	XF-58 #2 1 Film per Packet Paper Pack 150/bx
952-1090	XF-54 #0 1 Film per Packet Paper 100/bx

952-1085   XF-42 #3 1 Film per Packet Paper 100/bx

Kodak Ultraspeed Dental X-Ray Film
833-0692   DF-42 #3 1 Film per Packet Paper Pack 100/bx
833-0702   DF-50 #4 1 Film per Packet Paper Pack 25/bx
833-0707   DF-53 #0 2 Films per Packet Polysoft 100/bx
833-0709   DF-53 #0 1 Film per Packet Polysoft 100/bx
833-0713   DF-57 #2 2 Films per Packet Paper Pack 150/bx
833-0714   DF-57 #2 2 Films per Packet Polysoft Pack 150/bx
833-0717   DF-58 #2 1 Film per packet Polysoft Pack 150/bx

Kodak Ektaspeed Plus Film
833-1108   EP-21P #2 1 Film per Packet Polysoft
833-1106   EP-22P #2 2 Films per Packet Polysoft 150/bx
833-0709   EP-01P #0 1 Film per Packet Polysoft 100/bx
833-0692   EB-31P #3 1 Film per Packet Paper 100/bx
833-0702   EO-41P #4 1 Film per packet Paper 25/bx
833-0701   EO-42P #4 2 Films per Packet Paper 25/bx

Film Hangers
885-4400   1 Clip Long
951-2353   2 Clip Long
951-2355   4 Clip Long
951-2357   4 Clip Long
951-2359   10 Clip Short
951-2350   Single Clip 12/bx

Chairside Darkrooms
951-5002   Insta-Developer Portable Darkroom
951-1423   Chairside Darkroom (4 cup)
885-0506   Chairside Mini-Darkroom
951-5005   Insta Mini-Tanx

Processing Solutions
952-1160   Superdent Rapid Process Developer/Fixer (1 qt each)
952-1165   GBX Developer/Fix Set (1 gal each)

Automatic Developer
952-1180   Superdent Developer/Fixer for All Automatic with Rollers (2 gal each)
946-2007   Peri-Pro Film Carriers for #0 Film (Pedo)
946-2008   Peri-Pro Film Carriers for #1 Film (Adult)
946-2060   Peri-Pro Film Carriers for #3 Film (Bite Wing)
946-2058   Peri-Pro Film Carriers for #4 Film (Occlusal)

Mouth Props
606-4182   The Wedge Veterinary Mouth Prop Small Under 20 lb
606-4183   The Wedge Veterinary Mouth Prop Large Over 20 lb

Patient Monitoring Devices
606-5107   VetSpecs ECG, BP, Pulse Oximeter, Temperature
606-0814   Cardell Veterinary Blood Pressure Monitor—Sharn
606-1237   Palco 5340V Pulse Oximeter
606-5002   Pulse Oximeter Hand Held—Nonie 8500V
606-5000   Pulse Oximeter Hand Held w/Alarm—Nonie 8600V

Periodontal Instruments
Explorers, Probes, and Explorer/Probes
271-9105   Cislak Color Coded Explorer/Probe
843-3701   Explorer/Probe 11/23

843-3700   Explorer/Probe 12/23
843-2453   Expro Explorer/Probe #2 handle 23/UNVC15
951-8619   Color Coded Probe Single Ended CP11
843-3693   Color Coded Probe Single Ended CP12
955-0104   Explorer DE #11/12

Scalers
951-9335   Scaler DE #12
951-9374   Scaler Jacquette #2/3
951-9395   Scaler Sickle 23 SE
958-1028   Scaler 204 SD

After Five Curettes—Hu-Friedy
843-2230   Gracey DE #1/2
843-2246   Gracey DE #5/6
843-2233   Gracey DE #7/8
843-2236   Gracey DE #11/12
843-2237   Gracey DE #13/14
843-2238   Gracey DE #15/16

Mini Five Curettes—Hu-Friedy
843-0680   #1/2
843-0683   #7/8
843-0684   #11/12
843-0685   #13/14

Superdent Curettes
950-9546   Gracey DE 13/14
950-9545   Gracey DE 11/12
950-9543   Gracey DE 7/8
950-9522   Columbia DE #13/14
950-9535   McCalls DE #13/14

Sharpening
952-0760   Buffalo Arkansas Sharpening Stone
843-3210   Conical Sharpening Stone #299
843-3204   India Flat Wedge #6
843-3202   Arkansas Flat #4
843-3220   India Stone #309
699-3007   Sharpening Manual
843-3120   Sharpen-EZ Oil
843-2490   Acrylic Test Stick 6/pkg
878-4368   Disc Sharpener

Mechanized Instruments for Calculus Removal and Dental Care
269-0413   iM3 Pro 2000 Starter
269-0515   iM3 Pro 2000 Challenger with suction and flush
269-0517   iM3 Pro 2000 Ultra with suction and fiber optics
263-9603   Vetroson Millenium 25/30 Ultrasonic Scaler
699-9356   Portable Water Tank
606-2935   Vetroson "SS" Insert #3 Insert 25K
606-2945   Vetroson "SS" Insert #10 Insert 25K
697-9874   Vetroson "SS" Insert #3 Insert 30K
695-0188   Vetroson "SS" Insert #10 Insert 30K
606-2942   Universal Perio 30K
906-0300   Biosonic US100 Ultrasonic Scaler
906-0304   Biosonic Insert #10 25K
906-0305   Biosonic Insert #10 30K
906-0307   Biosonic Insert Slim 25K

906-0308	Biosonic Insert Slim 30K
606-2963	Vetroson Powder Polisher/Stain Eraser
829-6000	Bobcat Ultrasonic Scaler
699-5574	ProphyMate Polisher
953-2598	Plastic Disposable Angles
951-8500	Snap-On Prophy Cups
829-0842	Cavitron SPS Ultrasonic Scaler
829-0842	Cavitron Jet SPS Ultrasonic Scaler and Air Polisher
829-1350	Cavitron Prophy Jet Air Polishing System
829-0816	Air Polishing Insert for Cavitron Jet each
829-0818	Air Polishing Insert for Cavitron Jet 3 Pack
829-0820	Air Polishing Insert for Prophy Jet 30 each
829-0819	Air Polishing Insert for Prophy Jet 30 3 Pack

Cavitron Ultrasonic Inserts

829-0554	P10
829-0515	EWPP
829-0530	P3
829-0520	TFI-1 25K
829-0521	TFI-3 25K
829-0766	TFI-9 25K
829-0522	TFI-10 25K
829-0785	TFI-1000 25K
829-0523	TFI-EWPP 25K
829-0792	TFI-3 30K
829-0803	TFI-9 30K
829-0804	TFI-10 30K
829-0797	TFI-EWPP 30K
829-0798	TFI-1000 30K
829-0757	Slimline Assorted 3 PK. 30K
829-0756	Slimline Assorted 3 PK. 25K
829-0758	Slimline Insert SLI-10S Straight 30K
829-0760	Slimline insert SLI-10R Right 30K
829-0759	Slimline Insert SLI-10L Left 30K
829-0752	Slimline Insert SLI-10S Straight 25K
829-0750	Slimline Insert SLI-10R Right 25K
829-0754	Slimline Insert SLI-10L Left 25K

Anesthetics

951-5510	Lidocaine HCL 2% w/Epinephrine 1:100,000 50/bx
951-5500	Lidocaine HCL 2% w/Epinephrine 1:50,000 50/bx
820-0360	Carbocaine HCL 3% 50/can
820-1680	Marcaine HCL 0.5% w/Epinephrine 1:200,000 50/can
950-1743	Benzo-Jel Topical Anesthetic Gel 1 oz Jar Banana
950-1737	Benzo-Jel Topical Anesthetic Gel 1 oz Jar Cherry
950-1738	Benzo-Jel Topical Anesthetic Gel 1 oz Jar Mint
950-1736	Benzo-Jel Topical Anesthetic Gel 1 oz Jar Bubble Gum
805-0100	Aspirating Syringe Astra Type 1.8 cc
887-1410	Monoject Needles 10/bx 27 x 3/4
887-1408	Monoject Needles 10/bx 27 x 1 1/4
887-1416	Monoject Needles 10/bx 30 x 3/4
887-1418	Monoject Needles 10/bx 30 x 1/2

Periodontal Care

843-2422	Freer Elevator
271-9008	EX 20/21 (Molt 2/4)
951-7875	Molt Elevator #9
843-0490	Ochsenbein Chisel #3
843-0491	Ochsenbein Chisel #4

950-2185   Stainless Steel Blades #10 100/bx
950-2186   Stainless Steel Blades #11 100/bx
950-2187   Stainless Steel Blades #12 100/bx
950-2192   Stainless Steel Blades #15 100/bx
990-9015   Stainless Steel Blades #12B 100/bx
990-9016   Stainless Steel Blades #15C 100/bx
950-2150   Surgical Handle #3
950-2151   Surgical Handle #4
990-4284   Needle Holder Crile Wood 6"
843-1824   Needle Holder Crile Wood 6" Grooved
700-8650   Needle Holder Olsen-Hegar 5 1/2
950-6105   Needle Holder Castroviejo 5 1/2
952-1776   Set-Up Trays 13 1/2 x 9 5/8 x 7/8 Blue
952-1793   Set-Up Trays 13 1/2 x 9 5/8 x 7/8 Grey
952-1775   Set-Up Trays 13 1/2 x 9 5/8 x 7/8 White
952-1781   Set-Up Trays 13 1/2 x 9 5/8 x 7/8 Beige
952-1719   Set-Up Trays 13 1/2 x 9 5/8 x 7/8 Mauve
952-1750   Adjustable Tray Rack
952-1752   Zirc Set-Up Tray with Microban 13 1/2 x 9 5/8 x 7/8 Divided Blue
952-1753   Zirc Set-Up Tray with Microban 13 1/2 x 9 5/8 x 7/8 Divided Yellow
952-1754   Zirc Set-Up Tray with Microban 13 1/2 x 9 5/8 x 7/8 Divided Green
952-1751   Zirc Set-Up Tray with Microban 13 1/2 x 9 5/8 x 7/8 Divided White
952-1752   Zirc Set-Up Tray with Microban 13 1/2 x 9 5/8 x 7/8 Divided Mauve
953-8702   Zirc Procedure Tubs with Microban 10 1/4 x 9 1/4 x 2 1/2 Blue
953-8704   Zirc Procedure Tubs with Microban 10 1/4 x 9 1/4 x 2 1/2 Yellow
953-8706   Zirc Procedure Tubs with Microban 10 1/4 x 9 1/4 x 2 1/2 Green
953-8700   Zirc Procedure Tubs with Microban 10 1/4 x 9 1/4 x 2 1/2 White
953-8713   Zirc Procedure Tubs with Microban 10 1/4 x 9 1/4 x 2 1/2 Mauve

Dental Antibiotics
262-5026   Antirobe Aquadrops 12/bx
262-5002   Antirobe Capsules 25 mg 600/bt
262-5004   Antirobe Capsules 75 mg 200/bt
262-5006   Antirobe Capsules 150 mg 100/bt
269-1250   Doxirobe Gel Syringe Kit 3/bx

Teeth Cleaning Products
951-8641   Prophy-1 Prophy Paste 250 gm. Jar
951-8657   Prophy-1 Prophy Paste 200/bx Fruit Coarse
951-8658   Prophy-1 Prophy Paste 200/bx Mint Coarse
951-8655   Prophy-1 Prophy Paste 200/bx Cherry Coarse
951-8652   Prophy-1 Prophy Paste 200/bx Bubble Gum Medium
951-8651   Prophy-1 Prophy Paste 200/bx Mint Medium
850-1670   Nupro Prophy Paste 200/bx Orange Coarse
850-1675   Nupro Prophy Paste 200/bx Mint Coarse
850-1672   Nupro Prophy Paste 200/bx Fruit Coarse
850-1674   Nupro Prophy Paste 200/bx Cherry Coarse
850-1676   Nupro Prophy Paste 200/bx Grape Coarse
850-1660   Nupro Prophy Paste 200/bx Orange Medium
850-1665   Nupro Prophy Paste 200/bx Mint Medium
850-1672   Nupro Prophy Paste 200/bx Fruit Medium
850-1674   Nupro Prophy Paste 200/bx Cherry Medium
850-1676   Nupro Prophy Paste 200/bx Grape Medium
850-1650   Nupro Prophy Paste 200/bx Orange Fine
850-1655   Nupro Prophy Paste 200/bx Mint Fine
850-1652   Nupro Prophy Paste 200/bx Fruit Fine
850-1654   Nupro Prophy Paste 200/bx Cherry Fine
850-1656   Nupro Prophy Paste 200/bx Grape Fine
850-1750   Nupro Prophy Paste 12 oz Jar Orange Coarse

850-1755	Nupro Prophy Paste 12 oz Jar Mint Coarse
850-1752	Nupro Prophy Paste 12 oz Jar Fruit Coarse
850-1754	Nupro Prophy Paste 12 oz Jar Cherry Coarse
850-1772	Nupro Prophy Paste 12 oz Jar Grape Coarse
850-1745	Nupro Prophy Paste 12 oz Jar Mint Medium
850-1742	Nupro Prophy Paste 12 oz Jar Fruit Medium
850-1770	Nupro Prophy Paste 12 oz Jar Grape Fine
952-1626	Topex Prophy Paste 200/bx Cherry Coarse
952-1628	Topex Prophy Paste 200/bx Mint Coarse
952-1638	Topex Prophy Paste 200/bx Pina Colada Coarse
952-1627	Topex Prophy Paste 200/bx Cherry Medium
952-1629	Topex Prophy Paste 200/bx Mint Medium
952-1635	Topex Prophy Paste 200/bx Pina Colada Medium
952-1683	Topex Prophy Paste 200/bx Bubble Gum Fine
952-1687	Topex Prophy Paste 200/bx Mint Fine
270-0380	Prophydent Prophy Paste 1 oz
951-1218	Reveal Disclosing Solution 2 oz
951-1220	Reveal Disclosing Solution 16 oz
999-6883	2-Tone Disclosing Solution 2 oz
998-0233	2-Tone Disclosing Tablets 250/pkg

Topical Fluorides

952-1530	Thixo-Gel APF 32 oz Mint
952-1534	Thixo-Gel APF 32 oz Wild Cherry
952-1532	Thixo-Gel APF 32 oz Bubble Gum
952-9100	Superdent Fluoride 4.4 oz Strawberry
952-9104	Superdent Fluoride 4.4 oz Bubble Gum
952-9102	Superdent Fluoride 4.4 oz Mint
952-9103	Superdent Fluoride 4.4 oz Grape
951-7908	Fluoride Phosphated Topical Solution 16 oz Bubble Gum
951-7905	Fluoride Phosphated Topical Solution 16 oz Cherry
269-0520	FluaFom Topical Fluoride 1.23% 5.5 oz
954-0684	Gel-Tin Home Care 0.4% Stannous Fluoride 12/Bx Mint
954-0680	Gel-Tin Home Care 0.4% Stannous Fluoride 12/Bx Bubble Gum
954-0683	Gel-Tin Home Care 0.4% Stannous Fluoride 12/Bx Berry
954-0682	Gel-Tin Home Care 0.4% Stannous Fluoride 12/Bx Grape
953-2016	Stannous Fluoride Gel Mint 3.8 oz
953-2017	Stannous Fluoride Gel Berry 3.8 oz
953-2018	Stannous Fluoride Gel Bubble Gum 3.8 oz

Rinses

269-0564	CHX Guard Oral Rinsing Solution 8.1 oz w/Applicator & Finger brush
269-0531	CHX Guard Refill Bottle 8.1 oz
269-0531	CHX 12% Chlorhexidine Oral Cleansing Solution 8 oz
269-0533	Maxi-Guard Oral Cleansing Spray 4 oz Canine/Feline
264-2215	Novaldent Chlorhexidine Rinse 4 oz
264-2210	Novaldent Chlorhexidine Rinse 8 oz
270-0375	Hexarinse Oral Rinse Solution 8 oz
269-2185	Vetus Hexoral Rinse Chlorhexidine 0.12% 8 oz
269-2186	Vetus Hexoral Zn Rinse Chlorhexidine 0.12% and Zinc Chloride 0.12% 8 oz

Gels

269-0566	CHX-Guard LS Long Acting Gel 1.1 oz Syringe
269-0529	CHX Gel .12% w/Finger brush 32 gm
269-0552	Maxi-Guard Oral Gel Taste Free 4 oz

Toothbrushes

269-0527	CET Finger Toothbrush
269-0501	CET Canine Toothbrush

269-0502	CET Cat Toothbrush
269-0518	CET Dual-Ended Toothbrush
271-0800	Dentivet Finger brush
952-1604	Toothbrushes Child

Dentifrices

270-0365	Dentivet Toothpaste
271-0800	Dentivet Toothpaste Kit w/Finger brush and Toothbrush
269-0542	CET Chews Small/Medium 5 oz
269-0548	CET Chews Small/Medium 16 oz
269-0543	CET Chews Large 5 oz
269-0549	CET Chews Large 16 oz
269-0555	CET Chews X-Large 8 oz
695-0490	CET Dental Center
269-0562	CET Finger brush Kit 44 gm Toothpaste and Finger brush Malt
269-0560	CET Finger brush Kit 44 gm Toothpaste and Finger brush Poultry
269-0509	CET Puppy/Kitten Dental Kit
269-0417	CET Forte Tartar Control Kit (Beef Flavor) for Dogs
269-0415	CET Forte Tartar Control Kit (Seafood Flavor) for Cats
269-0434	CET Forte Chews Poultry 24/bx
269-0436	CET Forte Chews Poultry 96/cannister
269-0430	CET Forte Chews Fish 24/bx
269-0432	CET Forte Chews Fish 96/cannister
269-0550	CET Forte Petite Chews for Dogs 24/bx
269-0539	CET Trial Size Dentifrice Dispenser 36/bx Poultry w/Fluoride
269-0514	CET Dentifrice for Pets 70 gm Malt
269-0512	CET Dentifrice for Pets 70 gm Mint
269-0506	CET Dentifrice for Pets 70 gm Poultry w/Fluoride
269-0513	CET Toothbrush and Enzymatic Dentifrice Kit Malt
269-0516	CET Toothbrush and Enzymatic Dentifrice Kit Mint
269-0510	CET Toothbrush and Enzymatic Dentifrice Kit Poultry w/Fluoride
269-0510	CET Dental Kit for Cats

Endodontics

951-1350	Gates Glidden Drills RA 6/Vial #1
951-1352	Gates Glidden Drills RA 6/Vial #2
951-1354	Gates Glidden Drills RA 6/Vial #3
951-1356	Gates Glidden Drills RA 6/Vial #4
951-1358	Gates Glidden Drills RA 6/Vial #5
951-1360	Gates Glidden Drills RA 6/Vial #6
951-1370	Gates Glidden Drills RA 6/Vial Asst 1-6
264-9480	Barbed Broaches 47 mm Asst 1-5
950-1785	Barbed Broaches 22 mm 10/bx XXXXF Purple 0
950-1783	Barbed Broaches 22 mm 10/bx XXXF White 1
950-1781	Barbed Broaches 22 mm 10/bx XXF Yellow 2
950-1779	Barbed Broaches 22 mm 10/bx XF Red 3
950-1777	Barbed Broaches 22 mm 10/bx Fine Blue 4
950-1787	Barbed Broaches 22 mm 10/bx Medium Green 5
950-1789	Barbed Broaches 22 mm 10/bx Coarse Black 6
951-2421	H-Files 21 mm 6/bx #15
951-2423	H-Files 21 mm 6/bx #20
951-2425	H-Files 21 mm 6/bx #25
951-2427	H-Files 21 mm 6/bx #30
951-2429	H-Files 21 mm 6/bx #35
951-2431	H-Files 21 mm 6/bx #40
951-2445	H-Files 21 mm 6/bx #15-40
951-2447	H-Files 21 mm 6/bx #45-80
951-2451	H-Files 21 mm 6/bx #15
951-2453	H-Files 21 mm 6/bx #20

951-2455   H-Files 21 mm 6/bx #25
951-2457   H-Files 21 mm 6/bx #30
951-2459   H-Files 21 mm 6/bx #35
951-2461   H-Files 21 mm 6/bx #40
951-2487   H-Files 21 mm 6/bx #15-40
951-2579   H-Files 31 mm 6/bx #15-40
951-2583   H-Files 31 mm 6/bx #45-80

Rotary File System
902-0400   Pow-R Engine Files .02 21 mm #15 6/pkg
902-4002   Pow-R Engine Files .02 21 mm #20 6/pkg
902-4004   Pow-R Engine Files .02 21 mm #25 6/pkg
902-4006   Pow-R Engine Files .02 21 mm #30 6/pkg
902-4008   Pow-R Engine Files .02 21 mm #35 6/pkg
902-4010   Pow-R Engine Files .02 21 mm #40 6/pkg
902-0424   Pow-R Engine Files .02 21 mm #15-40 6/pkg
902-4026   Pow-R Engine Files .02 21 mm #45-80 6/pkg
902-4030   Pow-R Engine Files .02 25 mm #15 6/pkg
902-4032   Pow-R Engine Files .02 25 mm #20 6/pkg
902-4034   Pow-R Engine Files .02 25 mm #25 6/pkg
902-4036   Pow-R Engine Files .02 25 mm #30 6/pkg
902-4038   Pow-R Engine Files .02 25 mm #35 6/pkg
902-4040   Pow-R Engine Files .02 25 mm #40 6/pkg
902-4054   Pow-R Engine Files .02 25 mm #15-40 6/pkg
902-4056   Pow-R Engine Files .02 25 mm #45-80 6/pkg
902-4060   Pow-R Engine Files .04 21 mm #15 6/pkg
902-4062   Pow-R Engine Files .04 21 mm #20 6/pkg
902-4064   Pow-R Engine Files .04 21 mm #25 6/pkg
902-4066   Pow-R Engine Files .04 21 mm #30 6/pkg
902-4068   Pow-R Engine Files .04 21 mm #35 6/pkg
902-4070   Pow-R Engine Files .04 21 mm #40 6/pkg
902-4080   Pow-R Engine Files .04 21 mm #15-40 6/pkg
902-4082   Pow-R Engine Files .04 21 mm #45-80 6/pkg
902-0490   Pow-R Engine Files .04 25 mm #15 6/pkg
902-0492   Pow-R Engine Files .04 25 mm #20 6/pkg
902-0494   Pow-R Engine Files .04 25 mm #25 6/pkg
902-0496   Pow-R Engine Files .04 25 mm #30 6/pkg
902-0498   Pow-R Engine Files .04 25 mm #35 6/pkg
902-4100   Pow-R Engine Files .04 25 mm #40 6/pkg
902-4110   Pow-R Engine Files .04 25 mm #15-40 6/pkg
902-4112   Pow-R Engine Files .04 25 mm #45-80 6/pkg

Endo Stops
951-9792   Silicone Endo Stops Round 100/bx Asst
951-9790   Silicone Endo Stops Tear Shape 100/bx Asst
813-3700   Sure-Stop Endo Stop Dispenser 200/bx Red
997-0282   Sure-Stop Endo Stop Dispenser 200/bx Yellow
997-1866   Sure-Stop Endo Stop Dispenser 200/bx Blue

Pluggers and Spreaders
951-8910   Dr. Luks Plugger SE #1
951-8912   Dr. Luks Plugger SE #2
951-8914   Dr. Luks Plugger SE #3
951-8916   Dr. Luks Plugger SE #4
271-9095   Holmstrom Plugger/Spreader Set of 5

951-8225   Self-Locking Pliers
854-6930   Pathfinders 21 mm
954-6935   Pathfinders 25 mm

Heat Obturation Systems

954-3150	Touch 'n Heat #5004
954-3156	Heat Carrier Standard Anterior #500-001
954-3158	Heat Carrier Standard Posterior #500-002
954-3156	Heat Carrier Narrow Anterior #500-003
954-3154	Heat Carrier Narrow Posterior #500-004
813-5200	Densfil Thermal Endo Obturators
699-5722	SuccessFil Oven
844-1876	SuccessFil Gutta Percha Syringe
844-1878	SuccessFil Titanium Cores 6/pkg #20
844-1880	SuccessFil Titanium Cores 6/pkg #25
844-1890	SuccessFil Titanium Cores 6/pkg #30
844-1892	SuccessFil Titanium Cores 6/pkg #35
844-1894	SuccessFil Titanium Cores 6/pkg #40
844-1896	SuccessFil Titanium Cores 6/pkg #45
844-1898	SuccessFil Titanium Cores 6/pkg #50
844-1900	SuccessFil Titanium Cores 6/pkg #20-40
844-1902	SuccessFil Titanium Cores 6/pkg #45-80

Paper Points and Gutta Percha Points

951-7614	Absorbent Points Assortment #15-40 200/bx
951-7640	Absorbent Points Assortment #45-80 200/bx
271-7240	Absorbent Paper Points 60 mm #15-25 60/bx
271-7241	Absorbent Paper Points 60 mm #30-40 60/bx
271-7242	Absorbent Paper Points 60 mm #45-55 60/bx
271-7243	Absorbent Paper Points 60 mm #60-80 60/bx
951-1802	Endo-Aide Organizer w/400 Absorbent Points
951-1803	Endo-Aide Organizer w/400 Absorbent Points and Gutta Percha Points 15-40
951-1800	Endo-Aide Organizer w/240 Gutta Percha Points #15-80
271-7215	Gutta Percha Points 60 mm #15-25 60/bx
271-7216	Gutta Percha Points 60 mm #30-40 60/bx
271-7217	Gutta Percha Points 60 mm #45-55 60/bx
271-7218	Gutta Percha Points 60 mm #60-80 60/bx
951-4350	Gutta Percha Points Standard 25 mm #15-40 Asst 120/bx
951-4352	Gutta Percha Points Standard 25 mm #45-80 Asst 120/bx
951-4330	Gutta Percha Points Standard 25 mm #15 100/bx
951-4331	Gutta Percha Points Standard 25 mm #20 100/bx
951-4332	Gutta Percha Points Standard 25 mm #25 100/bx
951-4333	Gutta Percha Points Standard 25 mm #30 100/bx
951-4334	Gutta Percha Points Standard 25 mm #35 100/bx
951-4335	Gutta Percha Points Standard 25 mm #40 100/bx
951-4336	Gutta Percha Points Standard 25 mm #45 100/bx
951-4337	Gutta Percha Points Standard 25 mm #50 100/bx
951-4338	Gutta Percha Points Standard 25 mm #55 100/bx
951-4339	Gutta Percha Points Standard 25 mm #60 100/bx
951-4340	Gutta Percha Points Standard 25 mm #70 100/bx
951-4341	Gutta Percha Points Standard 25 mm #80 100/bx

Endodontic Medicaments and Restoratives

952-0052	Sodium Hypochlorite pt
950-2423	Calcium Hydroxide Powder lb
834-0850	Hypo Cal (Calcium Hydroxide Paste)
813-1200	Dycal Ivory Complete
952-3250	Zinc Oxide Powder lb
951-2081	Eugenol 4 oz

Curing Lights and Accessories

955-7400	Model 100 Curing Light Gun

951-9152   Protective Glasses Ladies
950-9614   Protective Glasses Mens
950-9617   Protective Glasses Clip-On
950-9616   Protective Glasses Flip-Up
950-9029   Protective Visible Light-Cure Shield

Restoratives

Glass Ionomers
878-1180   Ketac Bond Intro Package
878-1192   Ketac Bond Powder 10 gm Yellow
878-1192   Kctac Bond Powdcr 10 gm Gray
878-1185   Ketac Bond Liquid Only 12 ml
953-7802   Fuji II LC Improved Resin Reinforced Glass Ionomer Material
867-7200   Vitrebond Light Cure Glass Ionomer Intro Kit
867-7210   Vitrebond Light Cure Powder Only 9 gm
867-7205   Vitrebond Light Cure Liquid 5.5 ml

Self-Cured Acrylic Resin
859-1000   Jet Repair Acrylic Professional Pkg. 4 oz Powder 120 cc Liquid Pink
859-1001   Jet Repair Acrylic Professional Pkg. 4 oz Powder 120 cc Liquid Pink Fibered
859-1005   Jet Repair Acrylic Professional Pkg. 4 oz Powder 120 cc Liquid Clear
859-1020   Jet Repair Acrylic Pound Package 16 oz Powder 240 cc Liquid Pink
859-1040   Jet Repair Acrylic Pound Package 16 oz Powder 240 cc Liquid Pink Fibered
859-1025   Jet Repair Acrylic Pound Package 16 oz Powder 240 cc Liquid Clear
933-3030   Jet Repair Acrylic Powder 4 oz Pink
933-3032   Jet Repair Acrylic Powder 4 oz Pink Fibered
933-3034   Jet Repair Acrylic Powder 4 oz Clear
859-1055   Jet Repair Powder 1 lb Pink
859-1045   Jet Repair Powder 1 lb Pink Fibered
859-0106   Jet Repair Powder 1 lb Clear
878-0534   Protemp Garant Starter Pack A3

Impression Materials—Rubber-Based
867-1000   Express Hydrophilic Introductory Kit
867-1005   Express Light Body Fast Set Refills
867-1007   Express Light Body Regular Set Refills
867-2532   Express Regular Body Refill
867-2522   Putty Kit Firm Set

CISLAK MANUFACTURING INC.

Periodontal Instruments

P1	#4 Mouth Mirror	Slimline Handle
P1-XL	Featherweight XL Handle	
	(#3 Size & #5 Size Mirror Available Upon Request)	
P2	3,6,9,12,15,18 mm Probe/23 Explorer	Standard Handle
P2-XL		Featherweight XL Handle
P2F	3,6,9,12 mm Small Probe/23 Explorer	Standard Handle
P2F-XL		Featherweight XL Handle
POW/23	QOW Probe/Explorer	Standard Handle
POW/23-XL		Featherweight XL Handle
EN1	DE Explorer/Endo Explorer TU17/23	Standard Handle
EN1-XL		Featherweight XL Handle
UNC15/23	(All Marking 1–15 mm)/23 Probe Explorer	Standard Handle
UNC15/23-XL		Featherweight XL Handle
EXP11/12	ODU 11/12 DE Probe	Standard Handle
EXP11/12-XL		Featherweight XL Handle
P3	U15/J30 Towner/Jacquette Scaler	Standard Handle
P3-XL		Featherweight XL Handle
P4	J31/J32 Jacquette Scaler	Standard Handle
P4-XL		Featherweight XL Handle
P5	McCall 13S/14S Scaler	Standard Handle
P5-XL		Featherweight XL Handle
P6	McCall 13/14 Curette	Standard Handle
P6-XL		Featherweight XL Handle
P7	J34/J35 Jacquette Scaler	Standard Handle
P7-XL		Featherweight XL Handle
P8	Barnhart 5/6 Curette	Standard Handle
P8-XL		Featherweight XL Handle
P9	Mc Call 17/18	Standard
P9 XL		Featherweight XL Handle
P10	Columbia 13/14 Curette	Standard Handle
P10-XL		Featherweight XL Handle
P11	H6/H7 Offset Sickle Scaler	Standard Handle
P11-XL		Featherweight XL Handle
P12	204S Interproximal Scaler	Standard Handle
P12-XL		Featherweight XL Handle
P12SD	204SD Interproximal Scaler	Standard Handle
P12SD-XL		Featherweight XL Handle
P13	U15/J33 Towner Jacquette Scaler	Standard Handle
P13-XL		Featherweight XL Handle
P14	H5/J33 Sickle.Jacquette Scaler	Standard Handle
P14-XL		Featherweight XL Handle
P15	H51H48 Sickle Hoe	Standard Handle
P15 XL		Featherweight XL Handle
P19	Gracey-Small 1S/2S Feline Curette	Standard Handle
P19-XL		Featherweight XL Handle
P20	Gracey 11/12 Standard Gracey	Standard Handle
P20-XL		Featherweight XL Handle
P21	Gracey 13/14 Standard Gracey	Standard Handle
P21-XL		Featherweight XL Handle
P22	Gracey 3/4 Standard Gracey	Standard Handle
P22-XL		Featherweight XL Handle
P23	Gracey 7/8 Standard Gracey	Standard Handle
P23-XL		Featherweight XL Handle

P24	Gracey-Small 5S/6S Feline Curette	Standard Handle
P24-XL		Featherweight XL Handle
P25	Gracey-Small 7S/8S Feline Curette	Standard Handle
P25-XL		Featherweight XL Handle
P26	Gracey-Small 11S/12S Feline Curette	Standard Handle
P26-XL		Featherweight XL Handle
P27	Gracey-Small 13S/14S Feline Curette	Standard Handle
P27-XL		Featherweight XL Handle
P28	Gracey-Small 11S/14S Feline Curette	Standard Handle
P28-XL		Featherweight XL Handle
P29	Gracey-Small 12S/13S	Standard Handle
P29-XL		Featherweight XL Handle
P35	Heavy Tartar Hoe	Standard Handle
P35-XL		Featherweight XL Handle
P36	Small Version of Barn 5/6	Standard Handle
P36-XL		Featherweight XL Handle
P37	Small Version of Col 4R/4L	Standard Handle
P37-XL		Featherweight XL Handle
P38	Small Version of McCall 13/14	Standard Handle
P38-XL		Featherweight XL Handle
P46	Gracey-Long 1/2 Deep Curette	Standard Handle
P46-XL		Featherweight XL Handle
P47	Gracey-Long 3/4 Deep Curette	Standard Handle
P47-XL		Featherweight XL Handle
P48	Gracey-Long 5/6 Deep Curette	Standard Handle
P48-XL		Featherweight XL Handle
P49	Gracey-Long 7/8 Deep Curette	Standard Handle
P49-XL		Featherweight XL Handle
P50	Gracey-Long 9/10 Deep Curette	Standard Handle
P50-XL		Featherweight XL Handle
P51	Gracey-Long 11/12 Deep Curette	Standard Handle
P51-XL		Featherweight XL Handle
P52	Gracey-Long 13/14 Deep Curette	Standard Handle
P52-XL		Featherweight XL Handle
M0/00	Feline Anterior Scaler	Standard Handle
M0/00-XL		Featherweight XL Handle
H3/7	Hirschfeld 3/7 Root Planing File	Standard Handle
H5/11	Hirschfeld 5/11 Root Planing File	Standard Handle
H 9/10	Hirschfeld 9/10 Root Planing File	Standard Handle

Oral/Perio Surgery Instruments

Bone Chisels

C4	#4 Chandler Large Straight Bone Chisel
C5	#5 Chandler Large Angled Left Bone Chisel
C6	#6 Chandler Large Angled Right Bone Chisel
C13	#13 Chandler Small Bone Gouge
C15	#15 Chandler Large Bone Gouge
G1	#1 Gardner Small Straight Bone Chisel
G2	#2 Gardner Medium Straight Bone Chisel
M18	#18 McFarland Tooth Splitting Chisel
W1	#1 Wakefield Bi-Bevel Bone Chisel
W2	#2 Wakefield Bi-Bevel Bone Chisel

Bone Files

BF1	Single-Cut Bone File (Miller 21)
BF2	Single-Cut Curved Bone File (Wahl 2)
BF3	Cross-Cut Bone File (#1X)
BF4	Cross-Cut Bone File (#2X)

BF5   Cross-Cut Bone File (#3X)

Elevators

EX3   Large Straight Surgical Elevator (34S)
EX4   Small Straight Surgical Elevator (301)
EX5   Feline Straight Surgical Elevator (301S)
EX5E   Eisner Back-Bent Toy Breed Elevator
EX5EH   Eisner Back-Bent Toy Breed Elevator with Holmstrom Notch
EX5H   Feline Straight Surgical Elevator with Holmstrom Notch
EX12   Small Curved Surgical Elevator (46)
EX14   Straight Pointed Surgical Elevator (HO-1)
EX15   Chisel Edged Inside Curved Elevator (Feline Specific)
EX15H   Chisel Edged Inside Curved Elevator with Holmstrom Notch
EX16   Chisel Edged Outside Curved Elevator (Feline Specific)
EX16H   Chisel Edged Outside Curved Elevator with Holmstrom Notch
EX17   Left Flag Elevator (#44 Cryer)
EX18   Right Flag Elevator (#45 Cryer)
100C   Slim/Backbent Feline Elevator
100CH   Slim/Backbent Feline Elevator with Holmstrom Notch
301MX   Small Spade Shaped Elevator
301W   Small Straight Chisel Edged Elevator
301WS   Small Backbent Surgical Elevator
304   Large Pointed Surgical Elevator
Cameron   Large Scoop Shaped Elevator
1.3 S   Straight Root Elevator
1.3 IC   Inside Curved Root Elevator
1.3 OC   Outside Curved Root Elevator

Elevators (Luxating Type)

Lux2S   2 mm Straight Luxating Type Elevator
Lux2C   2 mm Curved Luxating Type Elevator
Lux3S   3 mm Straight Luxating Type Elevator
Lux3C   3 mm Curved Luxating Type Elevator
Lux4.5S   4.5 mm Straight Luxating Type Elevator
Lux4.5CC   4.5 mm Curved Luxating Type Elevator
Lux5S   5 mm Straight Luxating Type Elevator
Lux5C   5 mm Curved Luxating Type Elevator

Elevators (Winged)

EX-W1   Winged Elevator Extra-Small
EX-W2   Winged Elevator Small
EX-W3   Winged Elevator Medium
EX-W4   Winged Elevator Large

Forceps

EX23   Large Extraction Forcep (#32A Parmly)   (Economy Grade)
EX23-1171   Large Extraction Forcep (#32A Parmly)   (German Grade)
EX24   Upper Universal Extraction Forcep (#150 Cryer)   (Economy Grade)
EX24-1192   Upper Universal Extraction Forcep (#150 Cryer)   (German Grade)
EX25   Lower Universal Extraction Forcep (#151 Cryer)   (Economy Grade)
EX25-1198   Lower Universal Extraction Forcep (#151 Cryer)   (German Grade)
EX26   Lower Small Breed Extraction Forcep (#151SK)   (Economy Grade)
EX26-1203   Lower Small Breed Extraction Forcep (#151SK)   (German Grade)
EX27   Small Breed Universal Forcep   (Economy Grade)
EX27-1143   Small Breed Universal Forcep   (German Grade)
EX28   Tartar Breaking Forcep   (Economy Grade)
EX28-1416   Tartar Breaking Forcep   (German Grade)
2162   #300 Root Forcep   (German Grade)
2163   #301 Root Forcep   (German Grade)

2187	#351S Root Forcep Profile Handle	(German Grade)
2188	#333S Root Forcep Profile Handle	(German Grade)
2204	#246 Root Forcep Profile Handle	(German Grade)
2205	#251 Root Forcep Profile Handle	(German Grade)
4658	Root Forcep #4658	(German Grade)
5217	Peets Forcep #5217	(German Grade)

Needle Holders

EX47	Crile-Wood Stainless Needle Holder	(Economy Grade)
EX47-4051	Crile-Wood Stainless Needle Holder	(German Grade)
EX49	Derf Stainless Needle Holder	(Economy Grade)
EX49-4052	Derf Stainless Needle Holder	(German Grade)
4057	Olsen-Hegar Needle Holder 14 cm Stainless	(German Grade)
4065	Derf Carbide Needle Holder	(German Grade)
4068	Crile-Wood Carbide Needle Holder 16cm	(German Grade)
4070	Olsen-Hegar Carbide Needle Holder 14cm	(German Grade)
4699	Olsen-Hegar Carbide Needle Holder	(German Grade)
4954	Olsen-Hegar Needle Holder Micro Stainless	(German Grade)

Perio Chisels

Och1	Ochsenbein SE Perio Chisel #1
Och2	Ochsenbein SE Perio Chisel #2
Och3	Ochsenbein DE Perio Chisel #3
Och4	Ochsenbein DE Perio Chisel #4

| Fed1 | Fedi #1 DE Small Perio Chisel |
| Fed2 | Fedi #2 DE Small Perio Chisel |

Perio Knives/Furcation Files

O12	Orban 1/2 Gingivectomy Knife
K1516	Kirkland 15/16 Gingivectomy Knife
S1S2S	Sugarman 1S/2S Furcation File
S3S4S	Sugarman 3S/4S Furcation File

Periosteals

EX1	#9 Molt Periosteal
EX6	SE Periosteal (#5 Molt)
SP-7	Special Single-End Periosteal
EX7	DE Feline Periosteal
EX8	DE Feline Periosteal
EX9	DE Extra Small Feline Periosteal
Freer	Freer Nasal Periosteal
Freer15	Freer Periosteal/Slight Curved Retracting End
MF15	Mini Version of Freer 15
Freer16	Freer Periosteal/Strong Curved Retracting End
MF16	Mini Version of Freer 16
PR-3	Retractor /Periosteal Combination
Shan-RT4	Mini PR-3 Periosteal

Retractors

S23	#23 Seldin Retractor
R6	U of MN Retractor
R9	Small Feline Tissue Retractor

Rongeurs

EX31	Mini-Friedman Rongeur	(Economy Grade)
EX31-4111	Friedman Rongeur	(German Grade)
4112	Micro-Friedman Rongeur	(German Grade)

Root Elevators/Root Picks

WA1	Straight Feline Root Tip Pick
WA2	Left Feline Root Tip Pick
WA3	Right Feline Root Tip Pick
WA23	Double-End Left & Right Feline Root Tip Pick

RT1	Straight Larger Root Tip Pick
RT2	Left Larger Root Tip Pick
RT3	Right Larger Root Tip Pick
RT4	Double-End Left & Right Larger Root Pick

WJS	Rounded Tip Straight Root Elevator

Scissors

EX45	Goldman-Fox Curved Scissor	(Economy Grade)
EX45-4017	Goldman-Fox Curved Scissor	(German Grade)
4015	LaGrange Double-Curved Scissor #4015	(German Grade)
4034	Precision Scissor Serrated #4034	(German Grade)

Surgical Curettes

EX2	#10 Miller Surgical Curette
EX2F	Feline Miller Surgical Curette
EX20	SE Surgical Curette Small (#2 Molt)
EX21	SE Surgical Curette Large (#4 Molt)
EX20/21	DE Surgical Curette (#2/4 Molt)

Restorative and Endodontic Instruments

Composite #1–#21 Various Patterns of Titanium-Coated Instruments for Non-Stick Composite Work

EN2	Double-End Endodontic Explorer (DG16)	Standard Handle
EN2-XL		Featherweight XL Handle

EN8	Small Endo Excavator (#31L)
EN9	Larger Endo Excavator

Holm20	#20 Holmstrom Plugger/Spreader
Holm35	#35 Holmstrom Plugger/Spreader
Holm50	#50 Holmstrom Plugger/Spreader
Holm65	#65 Holmstrom Plugger/Spreader
Holm90	#90 Holmstrom Plugger/Spreader

RES14	Double-End Burnisher (#2)
RES15	Double-End Ball Burnisher (#27/29)
RES20	Double-End Plugger (H1 Plugger)
RES24	Single-End Cement Spatula

RES30	Wedelstadt Chisel 1/2
RES31	Wedelstadt Chisel 3/4
RES32	Wedelstadt Chisel 5/6

Special Kit Numbers for Cislak Kits

P-100	Basic Prophy Set-Up
P-101	Advanced Prophy Set-Up
P-102	Feline Scaler/Curette Kit

EX-100	Basic Extraction Set-Up
EX-101	Feline Elevator Kit
EX-102	Advanced Feline Elevator Kit

H-100   Holmstrom Elevator Kit
H-101   Holmstrom Plugger/Spreader Kit

SKIT   Cislak Two-Stone Sharpening Kit

HENRY SCHEIN DENTAL SUPPLIES

Item	Description
100-8267	Master Push-Button Handpiece
101-8028	Master Push-Button Handpiece Less Swivel
101-3251	Master Swivel Coupling 4 Hole
100-7566	Master Replacement Cartridge
100-2289	Master Replacement End Cap
100-6493	Master Standard Handpiece 2 Hole
100-2231	Master Standard Handpiece 4 Hole
100-8734	Bur Changer
100-2670	Replacement Cartridge
100-4112	Replacement End Cap
772-4896	Quick-Air L with Power Lever
772-7989	Replacement Cartridge
100-0700	Master Miniature Handpiece 2 Hole
100-7111	Master Miniature Handpiece 4 Hole
100-8511	Replacement Cartridge
100-7843	Bur Changer

Fiber-Optic Handpieces

100-1922	Masterlight Fiber-Optic Handpiece, power pac tubing, AC wall adaptor and bulb w/coiled tubing
100-3969	Masterlight Fiber-Optic Handpiece, power pac tubing, AC wall adaptor and bulb w/straight tubing
100-9970	Masterlight Fiber-Optic Handpiece
100-6978	Masterlight Replacement Tubing—coiled
100-7481	Masterlight Replacement Tubing—straight
100-4365	Masterlight Replacement Lamp
808-8586	StarFlex Swl Fiber-Optic Handpiece
808-9065	FiberOptic Swivel Assembly
808-9245	Fiber-Optic Swivel Assembly with Lamp
808-7430	StarFlex K Handpiece with Auto Chuck 4 Hole
808-0928	Steel Bearing Auto Chuck Turbine
808-8888	Swivel & Turbine End Cap Tightening Wrench
772-4775	Midwest XGT Fiber-Optic Handpiece Less Coupler
772-2891	5-hole Coupler
772-0421	6-pin Coupler

Maintenance

100-2037	Lubricant Oil
102-8721	Spray & Clean

Low-Speed Handpieces and Accessories

100-3206	Master Torque Handpiece 2 Hole
100-0701	Master Torque Handpiece 4 Hole
100-2234	Straight Nose Cone
100-7121	Angle Nose Cone w/Latch Angle
100-2702	Latch Type Angle
100-8613	Friction Grip Angle
100-7458	Prophy Angle Snap-on
100-3776	Prophy Angle Screw-on
100-8727	Lynx Low-Speed Prophy Handpiece 4000 RPM
100-5233	Lynx Basic Low-Speed Air Motor Only
101-9965	Lynx Prophy Nose Cone Only
100-9814	Lynx Standard Nose Cone Only

Contra Angles

100-0026	10:1 reduction gear
100-8643	Contra angle #200 latch style
100-3003	Contra angle #200 latch style deluxe sectional

Prophy Cups

100-5078	White, webbed—pure rubber snap-on
100-6188	White, webbed—pure rubber screw type
100-1800	Gray, ribbed, soft screw type
100-6461	Gray, webbed, soft snap-on

Prophy Angles

100-2652	Seal-Tite prophy angle snap-on
100-8453	Seal-Tite prophy angle screw type
136-2503	Disposable prophy angles firm cup
136-2867	Disposable prophy anglcs soft cup
817-8867	The twist disposable prophy angles (oscillating)
928-2280	Prophy-matic (autoclavable, oscillating prophy angle)

Dental Burs

100-7205	Carbide FG 1/4 Plain Round
100-3995	Carbide FG 1/2 Plain Round
100-4907	Carbide FG 1 Plain Round
100-0288	Carbide FG 2 Plain Round
100-4535	Carbide FG 4 Plain Round
100-3220	Carbide FG 6 Plain Round
100-6131	Carbide FG 8 Plain Round
100-6373	Carbide RA 1/2 Plain Round
100-6319	Carbide RA 1 Plain Round
100-6411	Carbide RA 2 Plain Round
100-1847	Carbide RA 4 Plain Round
100-8765	Carbide RA 6 Plain Round
100-1401	Carbide RA 8 Plain Round
100-5860	Carbide HP 1/2 Plain Round
100-7176	Carbide HP 1 Plain Round
100-2095	Carbide HP 2 Plain Round
100-0899	Carbide HP 4 Plain Round
100-9086	Carbide HP 6 Plain Round
100-6137	Carbide HP 8 Plain Round
100-0703	Carbide FG 33 1/2 Inverted Cone
100-8454	Carbide FG 34 Inverted Cone
100-2484	Carbide FG 35 Inverted Cone
100-9299	Carbide FG 37 Inverted Cone
100-6637	Carbide RA 33 1/4 Inverted Cone
100-7735	Carbide RA 34 Inverted Cone
100-2431	Carbide RA 35 Inverted Cone
100-2407	Carbide RA 37 Inverted Cone
100-8612	Carbide HP 35 Inverted Cone
999-9782	Carbide HP 36 Inverted Cone
999-7718	Carbide HP 37 Inverted Cone
100-9613	Carbide FG 699 Crosscut Taper Fissure
100-4546	Carbide FG 701 Crosscut Taper Fissure
100-7228	Carbide FG 701L Crosscut Taper Fissure
100-9464	Carbide FG 702 Crosscut Taper Fissure
100-3108	Carbide FG 703 Crosscut Taper Fissure
100-0405	Carbide RA 701 Crosscut Taper Fissure
100-9229	Carbide HP 701 Crosscut Taper Fissure
100-9941	Carbide HP 702 Crosscut Taper Fissure
100-6111	Carbide HP 703 Crosscut Taper Fissure
195-1823	Finishing Burs White pointed Cone FG
195-5811	Finishing Burs White Frame
195-7905	Finishing Burs Dura-green FG
195-7328	Finishing Burs Dura-green CA

100-3307	Carbide FG 557 Crosscut Fissure
100-3104	Carbide FG 558 Crosscut Fissure
100-3795	Carbide RA 557 Crosscut Fissure
100-4895	Carbide HP 558 Crosscut Fissure
378-7246	SC5 Diamond Burs Premier Two-Striper FG Crown Cut
378-7797	SC8 Diamond Burs Premier Two-Striper FG Crown Cut
378-7938	SC10 Diamond Burs Premier Two-Striper FG Crown Cut
378-8202	ST6 Diamond Burs Premier Two-Striper FG Crown Cut
378-8463	ST8 Diamond Burs Premier Two-Striper FG Crown Cut
378-8770	ST8 Diamond Burs Premier Two-Striper FG Crown Cut
100-7117	Diamond Disc #914 Single Sided HP
100-2689	Diamond Disc #915 Double Sided HP
387-5547	Diaflex Diamond Disc 347/190 3/4" HP
387-7683	Diaflex Diamond Disc 345/190 3/4" HP

Radiography

263-4478	Dental vet-70 X ray system top mount wall unit
263-0438	Dental vet-70 X ray system mobile stand
100-0798	GX-770 X ray unit Gendex without installation

Radiographic Film

D-Speed Film

100-5871	DX-57 #2 Double Film paper pack 150/bx
100-9761	DX-57 #2 Double Film Flexisoft vinyl pack 150/bx
100-7066	DX-58 #2 1 Film per pack 150/pack
100-1243	DX-58 #2 Double Film paper pack 150/bx

Kodak Ultraspeed Film

111-3261	DF-42 #3 1 Film per packet paper pack 100/bx
111-1262	DF-50 #4 1 Film per packet paper pack 25/box
111-8995	DF-53 #0 1 Film per packet polysoft 100/box
111-2822	DF-54 #0 1 Film per packet polysoft 100/box
111-4039	DF-57 #2 Films per packet paper pack 150/bx
111-4404	DF-57 #2 Films per packet polysoft 150/box
111-2876	DF-58 #2 Films per packet polysoft 150/box
111-2082	DF-38 #1 (Anterior bite wing 1 Film per packet paper pack 50/bx)
	Kodak Ektaspeed Film
111-0811	EP-21p #2 1 Film per packet polysoft 150/box

Film Hangers

100-7570	1 clip—long
100-4133	2 clip—long
100-3176	4 clip—long
100-0125	6 clip
100-0398	8 clip
100-1268	10 clip—short
100-4042	10 clip—long
100-0921	Single clip 12/box

Chairside Darkrooms

173-1381	Insta-veloper
189-4677	Chairside Darkroom—Rinn
189-7385	Chairside Mini-Darkroom—Rinn

Processing Solutions

101-7275	Peril-mix Developer & Fixer (Automatic developer)
189-4910	RRP Rapid Process Developer & Fixer—Rinn (Manual)
111-3842	GBX—Kodak Developer & Fixer (Manual)

173-0233   Insta-Neg/Insta-Fix Gallon Combo
173-1606   Insta-Neg Develop Gallon
173-2932   Insta-Neg Fixer Gallon

Intraoral Processors
698-5024   Peri-Pro with daylight loader
698-4713   Peri-Pro without daylight loader
698-3114   Perio pro Film Carrier Pedo Film #0
698-1649   Perio pro Film Carrier Adult Film #1
698-4320   Perio pro Film Carrier Bite Wing Film #3
698-6037   Perio pro Film Carrier Occlusal Film #4

Mouth Props
568-8953   The Wedge Veterinary Mouth Prop small (cats and dogs under 20 lb)
568-6710   The Wedge Veterinary Mouth Prop large (dogs over 20 lb)

Patient Monitoring Devices
425-3944   Cardell Veterinary Blood Pressure Monitor—Sharn
301-8670   Palco Multi-Parameter Monitor 500V
656-3525   Palco Multi-Parameter Monitor 500VP w/Printer
301-5511   Palco Veterinary Oximeter 340V
301-1347   Palco Veterinary ECG 100V
568-5604   EC-60 ECG/Respiratory monitor—Silogic
762-7919   Arc 2000 Veterinary Monitor—Silogic
120-8855   Burdick EK-10 ECG
310-4019   Audio Patient Monitor—Bickford
568-7368   Doppler Ultrasonic Blood Pressure Monitor—Jorvet

Periodontal Instruments

Explorers, Probes, and Explorer/Probes
101-2098   Probe 11/23 Explorer
101-3149   Probe 12/23 Explorer
600-6803   Expro 23/UNC15
100-4335   Goldman-Fox Probe/17 Explorer
100-0805   Probex 1/23
100-4807   Explorer/Probe ST-4
100-9279   Explorer DG-16
600-7964   Color Coded Probe CP8-3-6-8 mm
600-3452   Color Coded Probe CP3-6-8-11 mm
600-5389   Color Coded Probe CP12-3-6-9-12 mm
115-8371   Explorer DE #12/12

Scalers
100-6703   Scaler DE #12
100-9848   Scaler Jacquette #2/3
100-6930   Scaler ST-2
100-4186   Scaler Sickle 23 8/E SE
600-2147   Scaler 240SD DE

After Five Curettes—Hu-Friedy
600-9397   Gracey DE 1/2 AF
600-3140   Gracey DE 5/6 AF
600-0925   Gracey DE 7/8 AF
600-1311   Gracey DE 11/12 AF
600-1527   Gracey DE 13/14 AF
600-4808   Gracey DE 15/16 AF

Mini Five Curettes—Hu-Friedy
600-6312   #1/2
600-5551   #7/8
600-7227   #11/12
600-7297   #13/14

Henry Schein Curettes
100-2126   Gracey DE #13/14
100-1982   Gracey DE #11/12
100-5418   Gracey DE #7/8
100-4313   Columbia DE #13/14
100-6523   McCalls DE #13/14

Sharpening
365-2875   Buffalo Arkansas Sharpening Stone
600-6804   Conical Sharpening Stone #299
600-2191   India Wedge #6 Medium
600-8408   India Wedge #4 Fine
600-1691   India Wedge #309
600-6671   Sharpening Manual Hu-Friedy
600-5390   Sharpen-Ez Oil
600-6480   Acrylic Test Stick 6/Pkg
518-5675   RX System II Perio Set—RX Honing
378-2355   Disc Sharpener—Premier
107-7210   Prophy & Synthetic Stone
563-0374   Neivert Whitter

Mechanized Instruments for Calculus Removal and Dental Care
362-1875   Ultima 500
362-3530   Ultima 500 II S
362-4967   Ultima 500 II SF
362-3829   Ultima 2000
192-9296   Vetroson Millennium 25/30 Ultrasonic Scaler
192-7097   Vetroson Portable Water Tank
192-4521   Vetroson "SS" Insert #3 25K
192-6417   Vetroson "SS" Insert #3 30K
192-5716   Vetroson "SS" Insert #10 25K
192-7126   Vetroson "SS" Insert #10 30K
192-3284   Vetroson "SS" Insert Universal perio 30K
888-3408   Biosonic US 100 Ultrasonic Scaler
888-6576   Biosonic Insert #10 25K
888-1642   Biosonic Insert #10 30K
888-5589   Biosonic Insert Slim 25K
888-1219   Biosonic Insert Slim 30K
192-8895   Vetroson Millennium Motor Pack
192-5824   Vetroson Powder/Polisher/Stain Eraser
192-7532   Vetroson Polishing Powder
167-0335   Bobcat Ultrasonic Scaler
100-8209   Prophy Mate Polisher
100-6454   Plastic Disposable Prophy Angles 100/Pkg
167-3341   Cavitron SPS Ultrasonic Scaler
167-6580   Cavitron Jet w/SPS Scaler & Air Polisher
167-2563   Cavitron Prophy Jet Air Polishing System
167-0358   Air Polishing Insert Nozzle for Cavitron Jet each
167-5452   Air Polishing Insert Nozzle for Cavitron Jet 3/Pk
167-8887   Air Polishing Nozzle for Prophy Jet 30 each
167-2299   Air Polishing Nozzle for Prophy Jet 30 3/Pk
167-7553   Prophy Jet Cleaning Powder
389-5671   Henry Schein Polisher
389-5330   Henry Schein Micro Motor Polisher 30,000 RPM

389-2397   Henry Schein Ultrasonic Scaler & Polisher
389-4705   Henry Schein Ultrasonic Scaler

Cavitron Ultrasonic Inserts
167-6513   P10
167-7752   EWPP
167-1805   P3
167-0340   25K TFI-1
167-1083   25K TFI-3
167-3452   25K TFI-7
167-1005   25K TFI-9
167-3203   25K TFI-10
167-5512   25K TFI-1000
167-2142   25K TFI-EWPP
167-3162   30K TFI-3
167-4351   30K TFI-9
167-4055   30K TFI-10
167-0062   30K TFI-EWPP
167-6675   30K TFI-1000
167-5906   Slimline Assorted 3 Pak 30K
167-7498   Slimline Assorted 3 Pak 25K
167-6905   Slimline 30K SLI-10S Straight
167-6907   Slimline 30K SLI-10R Right
167-6906   Slimline 30K SLI 10L Left
167-7753   Slimline 25K SLI-10S Straight
167-0574   Slimline 25K SLI-10R Right
167-0322   Slimline 25K SLI-10L Left

Anesthetics
465-1150   Lidocaine HCL 2% w/Epinephrine 1:100,000 50/Box
465-1050   Lidocaine HCL 2% w/Epinephrine 1:50,000 50/Box
856-0233   Carbocaine HCL 3% Plain 50/can
856-7407   Marcaine HCL 0.5% w/Epinephrine 1:200,000 50/can
100-0731   Benzo-Jel Topical Anesthetic Gel 1 oz Banana
101-7804   Benzo-Jel Topical Anesthetic Gel 1 oz Cherry
101-0436   Benzo-Jel Topical Anesthetic Gel 1 oz Mint
101-9442   Benzo-Jel Topical Anesthetic Gel 1 oz Bubble Gum
101-3099   Benzo-Jel Topical Anesthetic Gel 1 oz Piña Colada
101-1993   Benzo-Jel Topical Anesthetic Gel 1 oz Strawberry
100-4612   Aspirating Syringe Astra Type
101-8629   Aspirating Syringe Replacement Tip
194-1613   Monoject #400 needles 27g x 3/4" 100/Box
194-0506   Monoject #400 needles 27g x 1 1/4"
194-5141   Monoject #400 needles 30g x 3/4"
194-1753   Monoject #400 needles 30g x 1/2"

Periodontal Care
198-6048   Freer Elevator
600-6125   #2 Molt
600-9526   #4 Molt
100-4888   #9 Molt
600-1398   Ochsenbein Chisel SE #1
600-4456   Ochsenbein Chisel SE #2
600-4205   Ochsenbein Chisel SE #3
600-3405   Ochsenbein Chisel SE #4
100-8976   SS Surgical Blades #10 100/Bx
100-5794   SS Surgical Blades #11 100/Bx
100-0247   SS Surgical Blades #12 100/Bx
100-0249   SS Surgical Blades #15 100/Bx

953-6343	SS Surgical Blades #12B 100/Bx
953-7101	SS Surgical blades #15C 100/Bx
100-7520	Surgical Handle #3
100-3973	Surgical handle #4
100-2492	Needle Holder Crile Wood 6"
600-5636	Needle Holder Crile Wood 6" Grooved
100-1125	Needle Holder Olsen Hegar 5 1/2"
100-2146	Needle Holder Castroviejo 5 1/2"
102-7557	Needle Holder Castroviejo 7" Locking
658-0753	Set-Up Trays w/Microban 13 1/2" x 9 5/8" x 7/8" Flat Blue
658-0941	Set-Up Trays w/Microban 13 1/2" x 9 5/8" x 7/8" Flat Yellow
658-0399	Set-Up Trays w/Microban 13 1/2" x 9 5/8" x 7/8" Flat Green
658-9643	Set-Up Trays w/Microban 13 1/2" x 9 5/8" x 7/8" Flat White
658-0645	Set-Up Trays w/Microban 13 1/2" x 9 5/8" x 7/8" Flat Mauve
658-2663	Set-Up Trays w/Microban 13 1/2" x 9 5/8" x 7/8" Flat Blue
658-3013	Set-Up Trays w/Microban 13 1/2" x 9 5/8" x 7/8" Flat Yellow
658-3182	Set-Up Trays w/Microban 13 1/2" x 9 5/8" x 7/8" Flat Green
658-3469	Set-Up Trays w/Microban 13 1/2" x 9 5/8" x 7/8" Flat White
658-3482	Set-Up Trays w/Microban 13 1/2" x 9 5/8" x 7/8" Flat Mauve
658-4975	Adjustable Tray Rack
658-5844	Clear Tray Cover
658-5353	Procedure Tubs w/Microban 10 1/4" x 9 1/4" x 2 1/2" Blue
658-5401	Procedure Tubs w/Microban 10 1/4" x 9 1/4" x 2 1/2" Yellow
658-5429	Procedure Tubs w/Microban 10 1/4" x 9 1/4" x 2 1/2" Green
658-4824	Procedure Tubs w/Microban 10 1/4" x 9 1/4" x 2 1/2" White
658-5713	Procedure Tubs w/Microban 10 1/4" x 9 1/4" x 2 1/2" Mauve

Dental Antibiotics

178-8113	Antirobe Aquadrops 12/Box
178-6592	Antirobe Capsules 25 mg 600/Bt
178-7271	Antirobe Capsules 75 mg 200/Bt
178-7600	Antirobe Capsules 150 mg 100/Bt
178-4957	Doxirobe Gel Syringe Kit 3/Bx

Teeth Cleaning Products

100-7869	Zircon-F Prophy Paste 10 oz jar
100-9102	Uni-Pro Prophy Paste 200/Bx Coarse Mint
101-5159	Uni-Pro Prophy Paste 200/Bx Coarse Mint
101-0203	Uni-Pro Prophy Paste 200/Box Coarse Cherry
100-9016	Uni-Pro Prophy Paste 200/Box Medium Orange
101-5462	Uni-Pro Prophy Paste 200/Box Medium Mint
101-9609	Uni-Pro Prophy Paste 200/Box Medium Cherry
100-8742	Uni-Pro Prophy Paste 200/Box Fine Cherry
555-3052	Nupro Prophy Paste 200/Box Coarse Orange
555-1186	Nupro Prophy Paste 200/Box Coarse Mint
555-1026	Nupro Prophy Paste 200/Box Coarse Fruit
555-6355	Nupro Prophy Paste 200/Box Coarse Cherry
555-4705	Nupro Prophy Paste 200/Box Coarse Grape
555-0828	Nupro Prophy Paste 200/Box Medium Orange
555-1604	Nupro Prophy Paste 200/Box Medium Mint
555-2639	Nupro Prophy Paste 200/Box Medium Cherry
555-2742	Nupro Prophy Paste 200/Box Medium Grape
555-1056	Nupro Prophy Paste 200/Box Fine Orange
555-1961	Nupro Prophy Paste 200/Box Fine Mint
555-1056	Nupro Prophy Paste 200/Box Fine Fruit
555-0424	Nupro Prophy Paste 200/Box Fine Cherry
555-9392	Nupro Prophy Paste 200/Box Fine Grape
555-5996	Nupro Prophy Paste 120 oz jar Coarse Orange
555-2793	Nupro Prophy Paste 120 oz jar Coarse Mint

555-9729   Nupro Prophy Paste 120 oz jar Coarse Fruit
555-3270   Nupro Prophy Paste 120 oz jar Coarse Cherry
555-9891   Nupro Prophy Paste 120 oz jar Coarse Grape
555-3201   Nupro Prophy Paste 12 oz jar Medium Mint
555-1732   Nupro Prophy Paste 12 oz jar Medium Fruit
555-3402   Nupro Prophy Paste 12 oz jar Medium Grape
312-6573   Topex Prophy Paste 200/Bx Coarse Cherry
312-8753   Topex Prophy Paste 200/Box Coarse Mint
312-9056   Topex Prophy Paste 200/Box Coarse Piña Colada
312-2675   Topex Prophy paste 200/Box Coarse Chocolate Mint
312-5152   Topex Prophy Paste 200/Box Medium Chocolate Mint
312-9158   Topex Prophy Paste 200/Box Medium Cherry
312-9429   Topex Prophy Paste 200/Box Medium Mint
312-9643   Topex Prophy Paste 200/Box Medium Piña Colada
312-5533   Topex Prophy Paste 200/Box Fine Bubble Gum
312-0230   Topex Prophy Paste 200/Box Fine Mint

Disclosing Solutions
100-2491   Reveal Disclosing Solution 2 oz
100-7940   Reveal Disclosing Solution 8 oz
889-8871   Young 2-Tone Disclosing Solution 2 oz
889-7033   Young 2-Tone Disclosing Tablets 250/Pkg

Topical Fluorides
100-3322   Thixo-Gel 32 oz Orange
100-0590   Thixo-gel 32 oz Strawberry
101-9350   Acclean 1.23% APF Fluoride Foam 4.4 oz Strawberry
101-1102   Acclean 1.23% APF Fluoride Foam 4.4 oz Bubble Gum
101-4580   Acclean 1.23% APF Fluoride Foam 4.4 oz Mint
101-4927   Acclean 1.23% APF Fluoride Foam 4.4 oz Grape
247-6783   Perfect Choice Neutral Gel 2% 1 oz Peppermint
247-4186   Perfect Choice Neutral Gel 2% 1 oz Vanilla Orange
247-7414   Perfect Choice Neutral Gel 2% 1 oz Wild Berry
247-4272   Perfect Choice Perio Rinse 10 oz
100-8570   Fluoride Phosphated Topical Gel 1.23% Bubble Gum
100-0797   Fluoride Phosphated Topical Gel 1.23% Pint Cherry
100-2105   Fluoride Phosphated Topical Solution Pint Cherry
309-0143   FluaFom 1.23% APF 5.5 oz
100-2322   Home Care Gel .4% Stannous Fluoride 4.3 oz 12/Bx Mint
100-3853   Home Care Gel .4% Stannous Fluoride 4.3 oz 12/Bx Bubble Gum
100-4162   Home Care Gel .4% Stannous Fluoride 4.3 oz 12/Bx Berry
100-0906   Home Care Gel .4% Stannous Fluoride 4.3 oz 12/Bx Grape
100-0438   Home Care Gel .4% Stannous Fluoride 4.3 oz 12/Bx Cinnamon
103-5565   Pet-Gel .4% Stannous Fluoride

Home Care Rinses
309-8903   CET Oral Hygiene Rinse
309-3732   CET Oral Lavage Kit
121-9219   Maxi-Guard Oral Cleansing Spray 4 oz
995-4123   Novaldent 4 oz 12/Box
995-4925   Novaldent 8 oz each

Home Care Gels
309=5373   CET Oral Hygiene Gel
121-5581   MAXI/GUARD Oral Gel 4 oz each

Toothbrushes
309-7925   CET Finger Toothbrush 12/Box
309-6372   CET Cat Toothbrush 12/Box

309-0398 CET Dual Ended Toothbrush 12/Box
309-2697 Dentivet Finger Brush 12/Box
100-1946 Junior Toothbrushes 72/Box

Dentrifices

309-6777 CET Chews Small/Medium 5 oz 12/Box
309-2458 CET Chews Small/Medium 16 oz 4/Box
309-5126 CET Chews Large 5 oz 12/Box
309-5655 CET Chews Large 16 oz 4/Box
309-4444 CET Chews X-Lg 8 oz each
309-9478 CET Starter Kit 12/Box
309-9207 CET Dentifrices for Pets 70 gm Malt 12/Box
309-8309 CET Dentrifices for Pets 2.5 oz Mint 6/Box
309-3310 CET Dentrifices for Pets 70 gm Poultry 12/Box
309-6372 CET Dental Kits for Cats 21/box

Endodontics

100-5170 Gates Glidden Drills RA 6/Vial #1
100-6481 Gates Glidden Drills RA 6/Vial #2
100-0661 Gates Glidden Drills RA 6/Vial #3
100-2107 Gates Glidden Drills RA 6/Vial #4
100-6716 Gates Glidden Drills RA 6/Vial #5
100-1410 Gates Glidden Drills RA 6/Vial #6
100-9919 Gates Glidden Drills RA 6/Vial Assorted 1–6
100-6351 Barbed Broaches Veterinary 47 mm Assorted 12/Pkg
100-4473 Barbed Broaches 22 mm 10/Box XXXF-Purple 0
100-4259 Barbed Broaches 22 mm 10/Box XXXF-White 1
100-3577 Barbed Broaches 22 mm 10/Box XXF-Yellow 2
100-1403 Barbed Broaches 22 mm 10/Box XF-Red 3
100-4472 Barbed Broaches 22 mm 10/Box Fine-Blue 4
100-4256 Barbed Broaches 22 mm 10/Box Medium-Green 5
100-3568 Barbed Broaches 22 mm 10/Box Coarse-Black 6
100-3883 Endoflex H-Files 2/mm 6/Bx #15
100-4074 Endoflex H-Files 2/mm 6/Bx #20
100-0765 Endoflex H-Files 2/mm 6/Bx #25
100-4196 Endoflex H-Files 2/mm 6/Bx #30
100-4368 Endoflex H-Files 2/mm 6/Bx #35
100-4055 Endoflex H-Files 2/mm 6/Bx #40
100-4722 Endoflex H-Files 2/mm 6/Bx #15-40
100-4137 Endoflex H-Files 2/mm 6/Bx #45-80
100-5139 Endoflex H-Files 25 mm 6/Box #15
100-5318 Endoflex H-Files 25 mm 6/Box #20
100-5362 Endoflex H-Files 25 mm 6/Box #25
100-5429 Endoflex H-Files 25 mm 6/Box #30
100-4085 Endoflex H-Files 25 mm 6/Box #35
100-5678 Endoflex H-Files 25 mm 6/Box #40
100-0069 Endoflex H-Files 25 mm 6/Box #15-40
100-4596 Endoflex H-Files 25 mm 6/Box #45-80
100-8146 Veterinary Hedstrom Files 40 mm 6/Box #15-40
100-9141 Veterinary Hedstrom Files 40 mm 6/Box #45-80
100-9291 Veterinary Hedstrom Files 40 mm 6/Box #90-140
100-7643 Veterinary Hedstrom Files 60 mm 6/box #15-40
100-8303 Veterinary Hedstrom Files 60 mm 6/box #45-80
100-8583 Veterinary Hedstrom Files 60 mm 6/box #90-140
100-3132 Veterinary Hedstrom Files 60 mm 6/box #15 only
100-6848 Veterinary Hedstrom Files 60 mm 6/box #20 only

Rotary File System

317-8662 Pow-R Engine Files .02 21 mm 6/Pkg #15

317-9086   Pow-R Engine Files .02 21 mm 6/Pkg #20
317-2315   Pow-R Engine Files .02 21 mm 6/Pkg #25
317-5152   Pow-R Engine Files .02 21 mm 6/Pkg #30
317-3492   Pow-R Engine Files .02 21 mm 6/Pkg #35
317-1394   Pow-R Engine Files .02 21 mm 6/Pkg #40
317-4231   Pow-R Engine Files .02 21 mm 6/Pkg #15-50
317-6147   Pow-R Engine Files .02 21 mm 6/Pkg #45-80
317-6364   Pow-R Engine Files .02 25 mm 6/Pkg #15
317-4658   Pow-R Engine Files .02 25 mm 6/Pkg #20
317-2427   Pow-R Engine Files .02 25 mm 6/Pkg #25
317-8582   Pow-R Engine Files .02 25 mm 6/Pkg #30
317-9542   Pow-R Engine Files .02 25 mm 6/Pkg #35
317-6877   Pow-R Engine Files .02 25 mm 6/Pkg #40
317-0281   Pow-R Engine Files .02 25 mm 6/Pkg #15-50
317-4157   Pow-R Engine Files .02 25 mm 6/Pkg #45-80
317-6364   Pow-R Engine Files .04 21 mm 6/Pkg #15
317-9086   Pow-R Engine Files .04 21 mm 6/Pkg #20
317-2315   Pow-R Engine Files .04 21 mm 6/Pkg #25
317-5152   Pow-R Engine Files .04 21 mm 6/Pkg #30
317-3492   Pow-R Engine Files .04 21 mm 6/Pkg #35
317-1394   Pow-R Engine Files .04 21 mm 6/Pkg #40
317-4231   Pow-R Engine Files .04 21 mm 6/Pkg #15-50
317-6147   Pow-R Engine Files .04 21 mm 6/Pkg #45-80
317-8662   Pow-R Engine Files .04 25 mm 6/Pkg #15
317-4658   Pow-R Engine Files .04 25 mm 6/Pkg #20
317-2427   Pow-R Engine Files .04 25 mm 6/Pkg #25
317-8582   Pow-R Engine Files .04 25 mm 6/Pkg #30
317-9542   Pow-R Engine Files .04 25 mm 6/Pkg #35
317-6877   Pow-R Engine Files .04 25 mm 6/Pkg #40
317-0281   Pow-R Engine Files .04 25 mm 6/Pkg #15-50
317-4157   Pow-R Engine Files .04 25 mm 6/Pkg #45-80

Endo Stops

100-5271   Silicone Endo Stops Round 100/Box Asst
100-0560   Silicone Endo Stops Tear Shaped 100/Box Asst
222-1540   Sure-Stop Endo Stop Dispenser 200/Box Red
222-3050   Sure-Stop Endo Stop Dispenser 200/Box Yellow
222-3548   Sure-Stop Endo Stop Dispenser 200/Box Blue
222-5685   Sure Stop Endo Stop Dispenser 200/box Black

Pluggers and Spreaders

100-8337   Dr. S. Luks Plugger SE #1
100-6578   Dr. S. Luks Plugger SE #2
100-0971   Dr. S. Luks Plugger SE #3
100-3095   Dr. S. Luks Plugger SE #3
102-7918   Holmstrom Pluggers/Spreaders 28 mm #20
102-3240   Holmstrom Pluggers/Spreaders 28 mm #35
102-5334   Holmstrom Pluggers/Spreaders 45 mm #50
102-8126   Holmstrom Pluggers/Spreaders 45 mm #65
102-4718   Holmstrom Pluggers/Spreaders 45 mm #90
100-9062   Pluggers/Spreaders Dr. Green #608 DE
100-0936   Spreaders SE #3
100-2806   Spreaders SE #D-11
100-3172   Spreaders SE #D-11 T
100-0264   Self-Locking Pliers
123-3063   Path Finders 21 mm
123-3344   Path Finders 25 mm

Heat Obturation Systems

114-5154	Touch 'n Heat #5004
114-8682	Heat Carrier Standard Anterior
114-9696	Heat Carrier Standard Posterior
114-1884	Heat Carrier Narrow Anterior
114-9964	Heat Carrier Narrow Posterior
114-1552	Touch 'n Heat Spoon Tip
114-0883	Hot Pulp Test Tip
114-0516	Plugger Tips Thick
114-0226	Plugger Tips Thin
222-7739	Densfil Thermal Dental Obturator System
222-7351	DensHeat Oven
547-6344	SuccessFil Gutta Percha Syringe
547-7689	SuccessFil Titanium Cores 6/Pkg #20
547-8273	SuccessFil Titanium Cores 6/Pkg #25
547-8355	SuccessFil Titanium Cores 6/Pkg #30
547-8566	SuccessFil Titanium Cores 6/Pkg #35
547-8642	SuccessFil Titanium Cores 6/Pkg #40
547-8830	SuccessFil Titanium Cores 6/Pkg #45
547-8888	SuccessFil Titanium Cores 6/Pkg #50
547-9838	SuccessFil Titanium Cores 6/Pkg #45-80
107-3379	Soft-Core Endodontic Obturator & Heating Device
107-0754	Soft-Core Endodontic Obturators 6/Pkg #20
107-2172	Soft-Core Endodontic Obturators 6/Pkg #25
107-5096	Soft-Core Endodontic Obturators 6/Pkg #30
107-4281	Soft-Core Endodontic Obturators 6/Pkg #35
107-1920	Soft-Core Endodontic Obturators 6/Pkg #40
107-8031	Soft-Core Endodontic Obturators 6/Pkg #45
107-6370	Soft-Core Endodontic Obturators 6/Pkg #50
107-4840	Soft-Core Endodontic Obturators 6/Pkg #55
107-9380	Soft-Core Endodontic Obturators 6/Pkg #60
107-1474	Soft-Core Endodontic Obturators 6/Pkg #70
107-7062	Soft-Core Endodontic Obturators 6/Pkg #80
107-8152	Soft-Core Endodontic Obturators 6/Pkg #90
107-7365	Soft-Core Endodontic Obturators 6/Pkg #100

Paper Points & Gutta Percha Points

100-0672	Absorbent Points Asst #15-40 200/Box
100-2142	Absorbent Points Asst #45-80 200/Box
100-1776	Absorbent Points Asst #90-140 200/Box
100-2683	Paper Points Veterinary Length 55 mm Extra Fine 100/box
100-8242	Paper Points Veterinary Length 55 mm Medium 100/box
100-9339	Paper Points Veterinary Length 55 mm Coarse 100/box
100-6590	Endo-Aide "P" Asst 315-80 400/box
100-8226	Gutta Percha Points Veterinary Length 45 mm Medium 50/box
100-6273	Gutta Percha Points Standard Length 25 mm #15-40 150/box
100-9997	Gutta Percha Points Standard Length 25 mm #45-80 150/box
100-1871	Gutta Percha Points Standard Length 25 mm #90-140 150/box
100-8393	Endo Aide "G" Asst #15-80 240/box
317-9617	Gutta Percha Points Standard 25 mm 50/vial #15
317-0632	Gutta Percha Points Standard 25 mm 50/vial #20
317-0995	Gutta Percha Points Standard 25 mm 50/vial #25
317-1814	Gutta Percha Points Standard 25 mm 50/vial #30
317-2446	Gutta Percha Points Standard 25 mm 50/vial #35
317-4460	Gutta Percha Points Standard 25 mm 50/vial #40
317-4996	Gutta Percha Points Standard 25 mm 50/vial #45
317-5353	Gutta Percha Points Standard 25 mm 50/vial #50
317-5672	Gutta Percha Points Standard 25 mm 50/vial #55
317-6918	Gutta Percha Points Standard 25 mm 50/vial #60

317-7077   Gutta Percha Points Standard 25 mm 50/vial #70
317-7393   Gutta Percha Points Standard 25 mm 50/vial #80
317-8266   Gutta Percha Points Standard 25 mm 50/vial #15-40
317-2055   Gutta Percha Points Standard 25 mm 50/vial #45-80

Endodontic Medicaments and Restoratives
100-7562   Sodium Hypochlorite 16 oz
100-0036   Calcium Hydroxide Powder lb
295-1036   Hypo Cal
222-5882   Dycal Ivory Complete Pkg
222-2269   Dycal Ivory Standard pkg
100-4540   Zinc Oxide Powder lb
100-3688   Eugenol 1 oz
100-1757   Eugenol 4 oz

Curing Lights and Accessories
100-5151   Economy Curing Light
398-8212   Hilux 250 Curing Light
222-9223   QHL 75 Curing Light
100-3244   Protective Glasses Ladies
100-4634   Protective Glasses Mens
100-5661   Protective Glasses Clip-On
134-4539   Veratti Bonding Eyewear
549-0514   Protective Light Shield

Restoratives

Glass Ionomers
378-2618   Ketac Bond Powder 10 gm Yellow
378-5748   Ketac Bond Liquid Only 12 ml
333-7932   Fugi II LC Improved Package
777-2647   Vitrebond Light Cure Glass Ionomer Intro Kit
777-3504   Vitrebond Light cure Glass Ionomer Powder Only
777-3947   Vitrebond Light Cure Glass Ionomer Liquid Only

Self Curved Acrylic Resin
125-1546   Jet Repair Acrylic Professional Pkg Pink 120 cc 4 oz Powder
125-4928   Jet Repair Acrylic Professional Pkg Pink Fibered 120 cc 4 oz Powder
125-5710   Jet Repair Acrylic Professional Pkg Clear 120 cc 4 oz Powder
125-8203   Jet Repair Acrylic Pound Pkg Pink 16 oz powder 240 cc
125-6151   Jet Repair Acrylic Pound Pkg Pink Fibered 16 oz powder 240 cc
125-9608   Jet Repair Acrylic Pound Pkg Clear 16 oz powder 240 cc
125-5942   Jet Repair Powder Only 4 oz Pink
125-6560   Jet Repair Powder Only 4 oz Pink Fibered
125-7242   Jet Repair Powder Only 4 oz Clear
125-0542   Jet Repair Powder Only lb Pink
125-3337   Jet Repair Powder Only lb Fibered
125-4048   Jet Repair Powder Only lb Clear
125-6401   Jet Repair Liquid Only 120 ml
125-0406   Jet Repair Liquid Only 240 ml
125-5142   Jet Repair Liquid Only Qt
101-2894   Maxi-Temp Intro Package Universal, refills (101-0275)

Impression Materials
777-8798   Express Hydrophilic Intro Kit
777-9468   Express Light Body, Fast Set Refills
777-0125   Express Light Body, Regular Set Refills
777-8201   Express Regular Body Refills
101-5208   VP Mix Putty 4 Pack

Orthodontic Care

547-4425	Flexibole Small
547-4106	Flexibole Medium
547-3089	Flexibole Large
547-9846	Flexibole X-large
547-9611	Flexibole Jumbo
365-7743	Buffalo Spatulas 4" Flexible
365-3203	Buffalo Spatulas 3-1/4" Stiff
365-0211	Buffalo Spatulas 4" Stiff
365-2142	Buffalo Spatulas 4-1/4" Extra Stiff
365-6828	Buffalo Spatulas 3-1/2" Flexible
100-5292	Alginate Regular
100-5455	Alginate Fast Set
222-2723	Jeltrate Regular
222-3864	Jeltrate Fast Set
569-6330	Green Stone 25 lb
665-0993	Green Stone 50 lb
569-3164	Dentstone White
365-3554	Vibrator #1A Buffalo Dental
100-4157	Vibrator 110 Volt
100-8844	Vibrator 220 Volt
365-6944	Model Trimmer
106-9748	Massel Chair Blue 15'
106-9990	Massel Chair Pink 15'
106-0335	Massel Chair Red 15'
106-6684	Lingual Buttons Flat
106-7408	Lingual Buttons Curved
106-3732	Ortho Bracket Adhesive Kit
106-6184	Bracket Forcep Anterior
106-6564	Bracket Forcep Posterior
100-8740	Bending Pliers, Clasp Adjusting
100-7712	Bending Pliers, Wire Bending
106-0439	Arch Wire .014
106-6348	Bird Beak Pliers
918-1230	Ortho Pliers #026 Digital End Cutter
918-9926	Ortho Pliers #020 Pin and Ligature Cutter
600-4325	Coon Pliers
106-0001	How Pliers

Oral Surgery

600-0069	Elevator #81
100-7934	Elevator #301 Apical
100-5293	Elevator #302 Apical
100-6873	Elevator #303 Apical
600-1429	Heidbrind #1
189-4332	Cryer #44
189-1740	Cryer #45
600-6511	Crane #8
888-3220	Luxator Kit

Lasers

192-6545	Vetroson Diode Laser Twilite Model

RECOMMENDED SUPPLIERS OF DENTAL EQUIPMENT, MATERIALS, AND SERVICES

Supplier	Supplies	Phone Number	E-mail/Web Address	Contact
Addison Biologic Laboratories Inc.	Oral hygiene products	800-331-2530	www.addisonlabs.com	J. Bruce Addison Chuck McCutcheon
AFP Imaging	Dental radiographic units, automatic processors	800-592-6666 800-346-3636, ext. 7018	www.afpimaging.com sybrondental.com	Alan Haber
Analytic Technology	Endodontic materials and equipment	800-428-2808		
Brassler USA Inc.	Hand, endodontic instruments, burs	800-841-4522	www.brasslerusa.com	John McCoy
Burns Veterinary Supply	Complete line of dental equipment and materials	800-258-5157 ext. 7273	www.burnsvet.com	Adrienne Silkowitz
CBi (Charles Brungart, Inc.)	Ultrasonic scalers, NitAir high-speed delivery system	800-654-5705		Charles Brungart
Centrix Inc.	Centrix syringes and tips	800-235-5862	www.centrixdental.com	Kerin Finch
Chapel Associates Architects, Inc.	Architect for dental operatory	800-229-5903	dchapel@ chapelarchitects.htm	Dan Chapel
Cislak Manufacturing, Inc.	Dental hand instruments	800-239-2904	ken@zolldental.com	Ken Zoll
CK Dental Specialties, Inc.	Dental instruments	800-675-2537	ckeyler@aol.com	Chuck Keyler
CliniPix	Dental cameras	866-254-6749	www.clinipix-on-line.com	Fred Freidman
Coltene Whaledent Inc.	General dental supplies for endodontics	201-512-8000, 800-221-3046 ext. 8131	www.coltenewhaledent.com	
Darby Dental	Complete line of dental instruments, materials, equipment	800-448-7323	www.darbyspencermead.com	Lynn Golden, ext. 6204
DentaLabels	Stick-on veterinary dental charts	800-662-7920	Dentalabels@aol.com	Nancy Ehrlich
Dentalaire	High/low-speed delivery systems, hand instruments	800-844-7377	dentalaire@aol.com	Nicole Parks
Dentsply International	High/low-speed handpieces, instruments	800-877-0020	www.dentsply.com	
Dr. Shipp's Laboratories	Veterinary dental equipment and materials	800-442-0107	www.drshipp.com	Jay Haenert

Supplier	Supplies	Phone Number	E-mail/Web Address	Contact
Ellman International	Electrosurgical equipment	800-835-5355	www.ellman.com	Richard Noss, ext. 60
Film carrier Film Tran	Bisco International, Inc.	708-544-6308 800-247-3368	www.bisco.com	
Fujifilm	Digital cameras	800-659-3854	www.fujifilm.com	Bruce Mitchell
Gates Hafen Cochrane	Architect dental suites	800-332-4413	ghc@ghcarch.com www.ghcarch.com	Mark Hafen Larry Knecht
Gralen Company	Kong veterinary products	800-523-7979	Jan@gralencompany.com	Jennifer Maraga
Greenies S&M NuTec	Dental chews	816-221-8538	www.greenies.com	Arch McGulian
Hampton Research and Engineering	Dental units	800-800-6369	www.hamptondental.com	Dr. Harris
HESKA	Anesthesia monitoring equipment	800-GO-HESKA	www.heska.com	Dr. Paul Cleland
Hills Pet Nutrition, Inc.	Tartar control diet for dogs and cats	800-354-4557	www.hillspet.com	
Honing Machine Corporation	Motorized instrument sharpening	800-346-6464	rxhoning@michiana.org	R. J. Watson
Hu-Friedy Company	Hand instruments	800-729-3743	www.hufriedy.com	Linda Parson
iM3 Inc.	Dental delivery systems, disposable oscillating prophy angle, iM3 Model 42-12 ultrasonic scaler	800-664-6348 360-254-2981	www.iM3vet.com Imthree@pacifier.com	Vern Dollar
J. Morita	Panavia, photo core build-up material, dental bonding systems	949-581-9600	www.Jmoritausa.com	Kristen Towers
Kodak	Dental radiograph film, digital camera, local anesthesia		www.kodak.com/go/dental	Ruth Arbuckle
Kong Company	Dental chew devices	303-216-2626	Kong@kongcompany.com	Joe Markham
Lake Superior X-Ray Inc.	Desktop dental view box	800-777-4518	www.lsxray.com	Terry Hart
3M ESPE	Full line of dental materials	800-634-2249	www.3mespe.com www.dental@mmm.com	Kathy Cohort
MAXI/GUARD	Dental gel to help prevent plaque and gingivitis	800-331-2530	alabrat@coin.com www.addisonlabs.com	Chuck Mc Cutcheon

Supplier	Supplies	Phone Number	E-mail/Web Address	Contact
MedRx Inc.	Veterinary imaging system	888-392-1234	www.medrx-usa.com	Byron Uppercue
Microscopy	Portable darkroom	800-235-1863	www.microcopydental.com	
Nutramax Laboratories, Inc.	Consil synthetic bone graft particulate	410-776-4000	www.nutramaxlabs.com	Sean Brennan
Nylabone Products	Dental chew toys	251-633-9633	www.tfh.com	Dr. Andrew Duke
Orascoptic	Dental magnification loupes and lights	800-369-3698	www.orascoptic.com	Claude Allen
Ortho Arch	Light cured resin orthodontic buttons	800-423-3527	www.orthoarch.com	
Parkell Products Inc.	Ultrasonic scalers, endodontic equipment	800-243-7446	www.parkell.com	
Pentron Clinical Technologies Inc.	Flowable composite, restoratives, impression material	800-551-0283	www.pentron.com	
Petosan Kanalveien 51c N-5068 Bergen Norway	Twin head dental brush	+47 55 29 66 21	www.petosan.com	Ole Barman
Precision Ceramics Dental Laboratory	Crowns and orthodontic appliances	800-223-6322	www.precisionceramics.com	Mark Jackson or Jason Stone
Ribbond Inc.	Dental splinting material	800-624-4554	www.ribbond.com	
Satelec Inc.	Piezoelectric scaler, perio, and ultrasonic endodontic attachments	800-289-6367	www.acteongroup.com	Wyatt Wilson, ext. 25
Henry Schein	Dental equipment and materials	800-872-4346	dennis.mcguire@henryschein.com	Dennis McGuire
Schroer Manufacturing Company (Shor-Line)	Dental cabinetry, scalers, polishers, thermal heating pad	800-444-1579 ext. 2309	www.shor-line.com	Larry Haake
Stellar Pets Inc.	Havaball	800-786-9981 303-673-0709	www.stellarpets.com	
Suburban Surgical Co, Inc	Stainless steel veterinary equipment and laminated cabinetry	800-323-7366 ext. 3496	suburbansurgical.com www.suburbansurgical.com	Scott Robins/ Jeff Kahn
Summit Hill Laboratories	Dental scalers, high-speed delivery systems, electrosurgical and lasers	800-922-0722	vmstntnfls@aol.com	Charles Rahner, Jr.

Supplier	Supplies	Phone Number	E-mail/Web Address	Contact
SybronEndo	Kerr and analytic endodontic products	800-346-3636 ext. 144	www.k3endolcom sybrondental.com lipscombl@sybrondental.com	Lance Lipscomb
Thermafil	Heated gutta percha materials and equipment	800-662-1202	www.tulsadental.com	Marc Contreras, ext. 1395
Warren Freedenfeld and Associates	Dental suite architect	617-338-0050	warren@freedenfeld.com	Warren Freedenfeld, AIA
Wayne Usiak P.C. BDA Architecture	Dental operatory architect	800-247-5387	wayneusiak@bdaarc.com /bdaarch.com	
VetSpecs	Anesthesia monitoring equipment	888-657-9967	www.vetspecs.com	Casey Bishop
Virbac	Home care products	800-338-3659	www.virbaccorp.com	Greg Underwood

Index